The Neuropsychologist's Roadmap

The Neuropsychologist's Roadmap | *A Training and Career Guide*

Edited by
Cady Block

Foreword by Antonio E. Puente

 AMERICAN PSYCHOLOGICAL ASSOCIATION

Published by
American Psychological Association
750 First Street, NE
Washington, DC 20002
https://www.apa.org

Order Department
https://www.apa.org/pubs/books
order@apa.org

In the U.K., Europe, Africa, and the Middle East, copies may be ordered from Eurospan
https://www.eurospanbookstore.com/apa
info@eurospangroup.com

Typeset in Charter and Interstate by Circle Graphics, Inc., Reisterstown, MD

Printer: Sheridan Books, Chelsea, MI
Cover Designer: Blake Logan, New York, NY

Library of Congress Cataloging-in-Publication Data

Names: Block, Cady, editor.
Title: The neuropsychologist's roadmap : a training and career guide / edited by Cady Block.
Description: Washington, DC : American Psychological Association, [2021] | Includes bibliographical references and index.
Identifiers: LCCN 2021005944 (print) | LCCN 2021005945 (ebook) | ISBN 9781433832987 (paperback) | ISBN 9781433833243 (ebook)
Subjects: LCSH: Neuropsychiatry—Vocational guidance. | BISAC: PSYCHOLOGY / Neuropsychology | PSYCHOLOGY / Education & Training
Classification: LCC RC341 .N87 2021 (print) | LCC RC341 (ebook) | DDC 616.80023—dc23
LC record available at https://lccn.loc.gov/2021005944
LC ebook record available at https://lccn.loc.gov/2021005945

https://doi.org/10.1037/0000250-000

Printed in the United States of America

10 9 8 7 6 5 4 3 2 1

A journey of a thousand miles begins with a single step.

−Lao Tzu, *Tao Te Ching*

Don't panic.

−Douglas Adams, *The Hitchhiker's Guide to the Galaxy*

Contents

Contributors

Joseph Ackerson, PhD, Ackerson and Associates, Birmingham, AL, United States

Claire Alexander, BS, Department of Psychology, Ohio University, Athens, OH, United States

Patrick Armistead-Jehle, PhD, ABPP, Munson Army Health Center, Fort Leavenworth, KS, United States

Beth C. Arredondo, PhD, ABPP, Department of Neurology, Ochsner Health Center, Covington, LA, United States

Michelle Babicz, MA, Department of Psychology, University of Houston, Houston, TX, United States

Stephanie D. Bajo, PsyD, Department of Psychiatry and Neurobehavioral Sciences, University of Virginia, Charlottesville, VA, United States

Mark Barisa, PhD, ABPP, Performance Neuropsychology, Frisco, TX, United States

Heather G. Belanger, PhD, ABPP, United States Special Operations Command (USSOCOM), St. Michael's Inc., Department of Psychology; and Department of Psychiatry and Behavioral Neurosciences, University of South Florida, Tampa, FL, United States

Cady Block, PhD, Department of Neurology, Emory University School of Medicine, Atlanta, GA, United States

Douglas Bodin, PhD, ABPP, Department of Pediatric Psychology & Neuropsychology, Nationwide Children's Hospital; Department of

Pediatrics, The Ohio State University Wexner Medical Center, Columbus, OH, United States

Brittany Cerbone, PhD, Barrow Neurological Institute, Phoenix, AZ, United States

Derin Cobia, PhD, Department of Psychology and Neuroscience Center, Brigham Young University, Provo, UT, United States

Robert Collins, PhD, ABPP, Neurocognitive Specialty Group, Houston, TX, United States

C. Munro Cullum, PhD, ABPP, Psychology Department, University of Texas Southwestern Medical Center, Dallas, TX, United States

Lucas D. Driskell, PsyD, Department of Neurology, Yale University, New Haven, CT, United States

Matthew J. Euler, PhD, Department of Psychology, University of Utah, Salt Lake City, UT, United States

Joanne R. Festa, PhD, Icahn School of Medicine at Mount Sinai, New York, NY, United States

Laura Flashman, PhD, ABPP, Department of Neurology, Wake Forest Baptist Health, Winston-Salem, NC, United States

Daryl Fujii, PhD, ABPP, Veterans Affairs Pacific Island Health Care Services, Department of Psychiatry, University of Hawaii, Honolulu, HI, United States

Christopher Grote, PhD, ABPP, Department of Psychiatry and Behavioral Sciences, Rush University Medical Center, Chicago, IL, United States

Leslie Guidotti Breting, PhD, ABPP, Department of Psychiatry & Behavioral Sciences, Northshore University Health System, Evanston, IL, United States

Amy Heffelfinger, PhD, ABPP, Department of Neurology, Medical College of Wisconsin, Milwaukee, WI, United States

Robin Hilsabeck, PhD, ABPP, Department of Neurology, The University of Texas at Austin Dell Medical School, Austin, TX, United States

Julie Janecek, PhD, Department of Neurology, Division of Neuropsychology, Medical College of Wisconsin, Milwaukee, WI, United States

Emily Kellogg, PhD, Behavioral Health Program, Michael E. DeBakey VA Medical Center, Houston, TX, United States

Laura Kenealy, PhD, ABPP, Division of Pediatric Neuropsychology, Children's National Health System, Rockville, MD, United States

Stephanie Kielb, PhD, Department of Psychiatry and Behavioral Health, Section of Neurobehavioral Health, The Ohio State University Wexner Medical Center, Columbus, OH, United States

Cynthia S. Kubu, PhD, ABPP-CN, Department of Neurology, Cleveland Clinic, Cleveland, OH, United States

Laura Lacritz, PhD, ABPP, Department of Psychiatry, University of Texas Southwestern Medical Center, Dallas, TX, United States

Adeline León, PhD, Department of Psychiatry and Behavioral Sciences, Rush University Medical Center, Chicago, IL, United States

Shawn McClintock, PhD, Department of Psychiatry, University of Texas Southwestern Medical Center, Dallas, TX, United States

Christopher Nguyen, PhD, Department of Psychiatry and Behavioral Health, Section of Neurobehavioral Health, The Ohio State University Wexner Medical Center, Columbus, OH, United States

Christina A. Palmese, PhD, ABPP, Icahn School of Medicine at Mount Sinai, New York, NY, United States

Michael Parsons, PhD, ABPP-CN, Department of Psychiatry, Massachusetts General Hospital, Boston, MA, United States

Edward Peck III, PhD, ABPP, Neuropsychological Services of Virginia, Richmond, VA, United States

Antonio E. Puente, PhD, Department of Psychology, University of North Carolina, Wilmington, NC, United States

Dalin Pulsipher, PhD, ABPP, Department of Neurology, University of Rochester Medical Center, Rochester, NY, United States

Lucien Roberts III, MHA, FACMPE, Neuropsychological Services of Virginia, Richmond, VA, United States

Brad Roper, PhD, ABPP, Department of Veterans Affairs Medical Center, Memphis, TN, United States

Octavio Santos, PhD, Department of Psychology, The Ottawa Hospital, Ottawa, ON, Canada

Mike R. Schoenberg, PhD, ABPP, Department of Neurology, University of South Florida, Tampa, FL, United States

Jason R. Soble, PhD, ABPP, Department of Psychiatry, University of Illinois College of Medicine, Chicago, IL, United States

Scott Sperling, PsyD, Center for Neurological Restoration, Department of Neurology, Cleveland Clinic, Cleveland, OH, United States

Yana Suchy, PhD, ABPP, Department of Psychology, University of Utah, Salt Lake City, UT, United States

Julie Suhr, PhD, Department of Psychology, Ohio University, Athens, OH, United States

Daniel Tranel, PhD, Department of Psychological and Brain Sciences, The University of Iowa, Iowa City, IA, United States

Dede Ukueberuwa, PhD, Department of Rehabilitation Medicine and Human Performance, Icahn School of Medicine at Mount Sinai, New York, NY, United States

Douglas M. Whiteside, PhD, ABPP, Department of Rehabilitation Medicine, University of Minnesota, Minneapolis, MN, United States

Steven Paul Woods, PsyD, Department of Psychology, University of Houston, Houston, TX, United States

Foreword

What It Means to Be a Neuropsychologist in an Evolving Field

In graduate school, when I first started dating my girlfriend—who subsequently became my wife—she asked me what my career was going to be. I responded with "clinical neuropsychology," to which she replied, "What is that, and how do you become a neuropsychologist?" My response was "Don't know, but I will get back to you." This book is the answer to all of her questions.

I was among the first wave of early scientists and professionals that came after the real pioneers, scientists like Roger Sperry with his studies on split-brain patients; clinicians such as Ralph Reitan, who developed the first widely used battery in neuropsychology; and others such as Manfred Meier, who established the foundations for modern-day neuropsychological practice and training. All of us went into a professional world that did not yet exist but that held promise and great opportunity for discovery and service. Like the formation of the American Psychological Association (APA) in 1892, neuropsychology emerged in the 1970s and 1980s from a diverse combination of disciplines and from a wide variety of individuals, who forged a vision from which all reading this book are descendants and to whom we are all greatly indebted.

As I have written before, in terms of the development of the profession of neuropsychology (as early as 1988), we have emerged from the related specialties of clinical psychology, psychometrics, physiological psychology, and neuroscience with clear influence from related fields such as neurology, psychiatry, and law; even the sports industry has brought a new perspective to psychology. Similarly, I have recently begun to argue that the emergence of clinical neuropsychology as the largest and most vibrant of all professional specialties within the APA should be reframed not as emergence of a specialty per se, but as a return to the roots of psychology (Puente, 2019).

In searching for psychology's historical roots, we look to the three geographical origins from which psychology owes it greatest influence: Germany, Russia, and the United States. This should be focused on the work of forbearers in each of these geographic locations—Wilhem Wundt, Ivan Pavlov, and William James. The founders of psychology were physicians steeped in understanding of the physiological—specifically the brain—and considered the brain the basis of behavior and mind. Wundt's *Principles of Physiological Psychology* (1874), Pavlov's *Conditioned Reflexes* (1968), and James's *Textbook of Psychology* (1892) were essentially the earliest neuropsychology textbooks. All were largely, if not completely, devoted to the explanation of how the brain formulates behavior and thinking. For example, Wundt focused almost exclusively on how the brain contributes to behavior. The subtitle of Pavlov's book is an investigation of the physiological activity of cerebral cortex. In Chapter 3 of James's book, he focused on functioning of the cerebral hemispheres. In many ways, the emergence of neuropsychology as the largest, most robust, and possibly most important specialty in psychology represents the return to psychology's roots of over 125 years ago.

However, those roots were clearly academic, research-focused, and had little to do with the practice of neuropsychology. It has taken over a century for the promise of that seminal work to emerge as a professional reality (Barth et al., 2003). The origin of the significant gains of psychology in the professional realm can be traceable to World War II and the Veterans Administration. Despite the large percentage of veterans returning with brain injuries, as evidenced by the work of individuals such as Kurt Goldstein at St. Elizabeth's Hospital in Washington, DC (1942), it was not until the founding of the Division of Clinical Neuropsychology (Society for Clinical Neuropsychology, Division 40) of the APA and the National Academy of Neuropsychology in the 1980s that neuropsychology became formally organized as a professional pursuit. Solidifying these efforts were the development of neuropsychology's professional boards, American Board of Clinical Neuropsychology and the American Board of Professional Neuropsychology (now American Board of Neuropsychology), also during the 1980s. The Houston Conference, as outlined in other chapters in this book, was the first time that education and training guidelines were developed (despite the fact that many early neuropsychologists, including myself, and some members of the Houston conference would not have met the Houston guidelines).

It is not until this book that the complete path of education and training in clinical neuropsychology is finally found in one location. Though it has taken several decades for clinical neuropsychology to clearly outline what is to be a neuropsychologist, how one is educated and trained as well as licensed and credentialed, a clear roadmap is finally available for implementation, recognition, and evolution. This text provides a foundational, theoretical, and practical description of the path(s) necessary to achieve an understanding of what it is to be a neuropsychologist and how one achieves such a title and certification. Additionally, as reimbursement patterns shift, a change is occurring from merely getting paid for doing an activity to an emphasis on obtaining results. In other words, neuropsychologists will be getting paid not just for doing but for performing measurable and empirically supported activities. In achieving that, the focus on competency as fundamental to performance is outlined. Along these lines, the focus on objective, patient-centered, and performance-based outcome is emphasized as the state of the specialty. Similarly, clinical neuropsychology has clearly developed into psychology's specialty most readily accepted by other health professionals, insurance carriers, and society in general. Its growth, its impact, and its easy extension from traditional medicine to encapsulate psychological principles have been some of the reasons for this significant success. Likewise, the emphasis on the uniformity of education and training as well as certification has been critical to this success as well.

However, success is by no means cause for celebration, arrogance, complacency, or comfort with the status quo. Many questions have yet to be answered, and new horizons are evolving in ways that had not previously been envisioned. One emerging example is that of teletesting. With the advent of COVID-19 came an immediate need for shifting from just in-person, face-to-face testing. With that came abrupt shifts in practice patterns and questions of scientific support for such practices. As you use this book, here are some questions to consider:

- Is the present education and training model developed more to provide support for those involved in education and training than for future students, health care delivery systems, or societal needs and questions (e.g., Coetzer, 2017)? Should our focus be on understanding the marketplace and societal needs, and then develop training that reflects that instead of programs that reflect the needs of the faculty and their research programs?

- Is the emphasis on uniformity, professionalism, and certification (which has resulted in initial significant growth and acceptance both within psychology and health care) likely to affect the infusion of new ideas (e.g., artificial intelligence), personnel (e.g., underrepresented groups or other countries), or venues (e.g., business and economics) that will assure the continued growth and acceptance that occurred in the first half-century of neuropsychology (e.g., Costa, 1988)? Could it be that an unintended consequence of increased professionalism is that novel ideas and alternative training pathways become extinguished in favor of professional uniformity?

- Are evidence-based and immediate performance metrics enough to capture a holistic perspective and specific patient circumstance, or does the present empirical approach ignore a Luria–Vygotsky paradigm and bypass critical sociohistorical-cultural contexts (Ardila et al., 1994)? Should qualitative perspectives and understanding difficult-to-measure concepts be integrated in our strict empirical psychometric traditions?

- There is strong internal validity for our instruments and practices, but do they hold ecological utility and construct validity, especially with evolving demographics in North American and Europe and the need for a truly universal (not just a Western-focused) neuropsychology (e.g., Furtado et al., 2019)? Should the development of our specialty also take into consideration those we are seeking to understand and serve? If so, should these questions not mirror shifting demographics nationally and a broader international perspective?

Reliance on uniformity, professionalism, and certification is important to ensure that our specialty should not allow itself to settle into complacency. Instead, the status quo and our present success should be a call to action. Be understanding and mindful of the present; encourage, digest, and practice what has been described so well in this book. After all, the success of psychology's first and most important specialty hinges on providing pathways for the future. May its past and present success become a challenge to all involved with neuropsychology—pioneers and students alike—to question and improve the specialty.

—*Antonio E. Puente*

REFERENCES

Ardila, A., Rosselli, M., & Puente, A. E. (1994). *Neuropsychological evaluation of the Spanish speaker*. Plenum Press.

Barth, J. T., Pliskin, N., Axelrod, B., Faust, D., Fisher, J., Harley, J. P., Heilbronner, R., Larrabee, G., Puente, A., Ricker, J., & Silver, C. (2003). Introduction to the NAN 2001 definition of a clinical neuropsychologist NAN policy and planning committee. *Archives of Clinical Neuropsychology, 18*(5), 551–555. https://doi.org/10.1093/arclin/18.5.551

Coetzer, R. (2017). *The notebook of a new clinical neuropsychologist: Stories from another world.* Routledge.

Costa, L. (1988). Clinical neuropsychology: Prospects and problems. *Clinical Neuropsychologist, 2*, 3–11. https://doi.org/10.1080/13854048808520079

Furtado, M., Ríos-Vázquez, I., Sanderson Brown, S., & Belén, K. (2019). The false hope of becoming a neuropsychologist: A call for action! *Archives of Clinical Neuropsychology, 34*(7), 1299. https://doi.org/10.1093/arclin/acz029.66

Goldstein, K. (1942). *After effects of brain injuries in war.* Grune & Straton.

James, W. (1892). *Textbook of psychology.* Macmillan.

Pavlov, I. P. (1968). *Conditioned reflexes: An investigation of the physiological activity of cerebral cortex.* Dover.

Puente, A. E. (2019, August 8–11). *Neuropsychology: The origins and the future of psychology* [Paper presentation]. American Psychological Association 127th Annual Convention, Chicago, IL, United States.

Wundt, W. M. (1874). *Principles of physiological psychology.* Wilhelm Engelmann.

Acknowledgments

Over the years, I've had the pleasure of working with many fine people whom I would like to acknowledge. First, I would like to specifically thank my many personal mentors: Brad Roper, Leanne Cianfrini, Tom Novack, Katherine Fabrizio, Joseph Ackerson, Russell Adams, Jim Scott, Corwin Boake, Robert Bornstein, David Loring, and Dan Drane. You have all been critical guideposts in my own journey into neuropsychology.

I also want to recognize many of my peers and colleagues. First and foremost, Katie Osborn, who was an immeasurable inspiration for this text. In addition to the individuals named above, I would like to also recognize (in alphabetical order) Alexander Tan, Amanda Gooding, Anny Reyes, Ben Hill, Callie Beck Dunn, Christopher Nguyen, Dalin Pulsipher, Derek Phillips, Derin Cobia, Doug Bodin, Doug Johnson-Greene, Emily Duggan, Jennifer Koop, Joshua Fox-Fuller, Julia Maietta, Juliette Galindo, Kelly Coulehan, Lucas Driskell, Maia Feigon, Missy Lancaster, Neil Pliskin, Octavio Santos, Ozioma Okonkwo, Preeti Sunderaraman, Scott Sperling, Seth Margolis, Shawn McClintock, Tanya Diver, Victor Del Bene, William McBride, and all the other amazing people that serve our profession (and whom I have had the distinct honor of serving with). There is unfortunately not enough space to name others in this book, but you know who you are and that you are appreciated.

I would also like to thank some of those closest to me. Ed, you have been my rock throughout this book and I never could have done this without your love and support. I also thank my family, who have been my personal cheerleaders all along the way—but in particular, for these past few years, which have been challenging both professionally and personally. Last but certainly not least, I dedicate this text to my father—who I know would have been incredibly proud of all that I've been able to accomplish. This is for you, Dad.

The
Neuropsychologist's
Roadmap

INTRODUCTION

On Becoming a Neuropsychologist

CADY BLOCK

We each have our own journey to becoming a neuropsychologist. For some of us, the road is clear and straight. For others, the road is winding and with many detours. Though my own journey in many ways fell squarely under the latter, I still recall it fondly. It actually began in experimental psychology, specifically in the realm of human factors research. Then, I discovered that one could blend the empirical study of the human brain with clinical practice—and I was *hooked*. But at that time I had no clue about the Houston Conference Guidelines or various neuropsychological organizations. I also didn't know much about what it took to be a competitive applicant for graduate school or what it took to be a successful and productive student. I felt a little lost and not quite sure what to do next. It was around this time that I encountered the first of several pivotal individuals in my professional journey.

Dr. Scott Sautter was a local neuropsychologist in my hometown, and he was kind enough to provide me with the mentorship and support needed to get started. When I didn't make it into graduate school the first time I applied out of my undergraduate program, he wouldn't let me feel deterred; instead, he offered me a job as a psychometrist. I accepted it gladly. That

https://doi.org/10.1037/0000250-001
The Neuropsychologist's Roadmap: A Training and Career Guide, C. Block (Editor)

summer, I attended my very first American Psychological Association (APA) convention in San Francisco with the brilliant and talented Melissa Pence (another mentor of mine). One of the talks I attended was a panel discussion that outlined all of the various steps involved to becoming a neuropsychologist. I'll never forget watching the first speaker at the podium, then-chair of the Association of Neuropsychology Students in Training (ANST), Zoe Proctor-Weber. She was poised, articulate, confident. She spoke with such passion for service in the profession. I nudged the friend next to me, and said, "One day, I want to be like her." Little did I know the true prescience of those words.

Several years later (and with some more experience under my belt), I was a graduate student in the medical–clinical psychology doctoral program at the University of Alabama–Birmingham (UAB). It was then that I met another pivotal individual in my professional journey, a fellow graduate student and good friend of mine, Jacquelynn Copeland. For all of the work that I do in neuropsychology governance, I credit her for opening that door. I have a favorite memory of her coming to class one day, excitedly holding in hand the application paperwork to start our own ANST chapter at UAB. I readily agreed. I was always astounded by her boundless energy as we worked to grow our chapter.

Were it not for Jacquie, I might never have met Erica Kalkut. She was the new chair of ANST and had placed a call for applications for the national officer committee. I initially dismissed the email, assuming that the opportunity would go to better and more capable individuals. But then I found myself reading the email again and again. For several days my internal dialogue wavered back and forth. I think I was trying to convince myself that I was qualified enough to submit an application. In a moment of pluck, my finger struck the "send" button. Not only was I accepted onto the committee, when Erica's term was over she offered the chair position to me. I knew I had big shoes to fill. This initial involvement within ANST has since catapulted me to other opportunities within the Society for Clinical Neuropsychology (SCN), National Academy of Neuropsychology (NAN), American Academy of Clinical Neuropsychology (AACN), International Neuropsychological Society (INS), and Clinical Neuropsychology Synarchy (CNS). Through my educational and professional experiences, I've learned much about the journey to becoming a neuropsychologist. I also discovered a passion for helping others navigate their own path. In a way, this is where the story of *The Neuropsychologist's Roadmap* begins. Its pages are filled with the wisdom of mentors, colleagues, and friends. I hope that you find it an invaluable guide to your own journey. I do caution you, dear reader: Even though this text is neatly organized into a series of discrete steps, in real life things may look a little messier. At times, you may even wonder if you took a wrong turn somewhere. This is okay. We all ultimately have our own journey to make, and collectively they enrich our field. For what is a roadmap but a collection of different paths?

● ● ● ● ● ●

In the decade since graduate school, I have been fortunate to serve the profession in various capacities including roles across organizations like the Society for Clinical Neuropsychology, International Neuropsychological Society, National Academy of Neuropsychology, and the American Academy of Clinical Neuropsychology. One particularly critical exposure during my work within these organizations was the concept of professional competencies. Since 2002, there has been a competency movement within clinical psychology—and neuropsychology has recently begun to adopt and refine this approach (thanks to excellent neuropsychologists like Brad Roper, Celiane Rey-Casserly, and Russell Bauer). But what are competencies, exactly? Broadly speaking, *foundational competencies* refer to the knowledge, attitudes, and values required of all entry-level neuropsychologists. In contrast, *functional competencies* refer to the activities of actual practice of entry-level neuropsychologists. More clearly stated, these competencies represent developmentally acquired knowledge and applied skills—gained over the course of education and training—that you (the trainee) should seek to achieve by the time you begin your first professional job.

The idea of the *Roadmap* began years ago, as a solely stage-specific text that would cover the developmental steps required for entry into graduate school, internship, postdoctoral fellowship, and first job. However, being exposed to neuropsychology competencies helped to foster a different sort of conceptualization for this text. It seemed important that student and trainee (and prospective student/trainee) readers not only get a sense of the overall journey from graduate school to first job, but also a more detailed understanding of the diversity of knowledge and skills that should be acquired and mastered along the way.

Consequently, the *Roadmap* began to take a very different shape compared with its original form. The organization of this text diverged into two separate but interrelated sections. The first represents an overview of the timeline for neuropsychology training and career entry. Chapters 1 through 3 offer detailed, practical advice on applying to graduate school, internship, and fellowship. The authors of these chapters represent not only some of the best supervisors and training directors in the country, but also trainees themselves, who provide valuable insight and information based on their own experience. Chapter 4 helps to bridge the gap between fellowship and board certification on a topic that I find is covered less frequently in advice provided by mentors: professional licensure and credentialing. This chapter was primarily authored by a neuropsychologist with personal experience serving on a state psychology board, who provides accurate and helpful advice in this area.

No text on the neuropsychology training and education journey would be completed without some inclusion of board certification. Chapter 5 serves as an excellent review of the process of applying for board certification, as well as going through the examination steps involved in this process. This chapter is authored by several neuropsychologists, among them a former member of the board of directors of one board-certifying body within neuropsychology, the American Board of Clinical Neuropsychology (ABCN). Other board-certifying bodies include the American Board of Professional Neuropsychology (ABN) and the American Board of Pediatric Neuropsychology (ABPdN). The issue of board certification can be a contentious one, and the fact that this text was only able to review one such option was an editorial decision based on limitations of space and not any intent to exclude other potential boards; indeed, I know and hold in high regard a number of excellent neuropsychologists who are boarded through ABN and ABPdN. I highly encourage student and trainee readers to do their own research, reviewing and considering all potential options to arrive at the best fit for themselves.

For students and trainees, Chapters 6 and 7 represent the end goal: getting that first job. But where does one end up: A clinical position? A research position? One that is a blend of the two? Not all clinical neuropsychologists are, in fact, clinical; rather, a number of neuropsychologists serve as research faculty in graduate institutions or academic medical centers, or as advisors to private industry or governmental entities such as the U.S. National Institutes of Health (NIH) and the National Aeronautics and Space Administration (NASA). Rather than restricting this topic to one chapter, it felt necessary to allow sufficient space to cover the breadth and depth of career options across governmental, private practice, and academic medical clinical positions, as well as between academic medical and academic psychology department research positions. The authors of these respective chapters are well-regarded neuropsychologists with extensive experience serving in clinical and/or research sectors.

The second section of the *Roadmap* opens up with a chapter that sets the tone for the rest of the text. Brad Roper, one of the original drivers of the competency movement in neuropsychology, leads the way on this chapter, reviewing the history behind neuropsychology competencies with which all students and trainees should be familiar, as well as important definitions and associated initiatives. This chapter is a critical one, as it provides important context for the chapters that follow.

Each of the *Roadmap*'s subsequent chapters breaks down a specific competency domain, providing strategies, steps, and/or tips for readers to follow. Chapters 9 through 11 review clinical competencies related to teaching and supervision, evidence-based practice, assessment, and intervention. Chapters 12 and 13 review basic knowledge and skills critical to research, such as cultivating a research idea and funding your research, as well as how to write up and present your research. To close out the text, Chapters 14 through 20 cover a range of topics important to one's professional identity. This includes ethical and legal standards, cultural competency, working within integrated care teams, cultivating self-care and work-life integration, seeking mentorship, leadership development, and professional advocacy. These chapters are all authored by well-regarded leaders in our field, who populate the *Roadmap*'s pages with their own personal wisdom, advice, and -isms.

The field of neuropsychology is ever-evolving. The *Roadmap* represents a cross section of the field, reviewing training steps, issues, and competencies pertinent at this point in time. However, these are likely to change as the field continues to grow. It is also by no means wholly comprehensive, as the development of a neuropsychologist doesn't simply cease upon entry into the first job; rather, there is continued learning, advancement, and refinement through the early career and midcareer periods—and even well into the later part of one's career. Plus, as neuropsychology continues to expand globally, this text may grow to encompass an even greater diversity of neuropsychological clinical and scientific education, training, and practices. But these are issues for another time, another future edition of this book. For now, I truly hope that you enjoy your journey through this *Roadmap*.

PART **I** TIMELINE FOR TRAINING AND CAREER ENTRY IN NEUROPSYCHOLOGY

1 APPLYING AND GETTING INTO GRADUATE SCHOOL

JULIE SUHR, STEVEN PAUL WOODS, CLAIRE ALEXANDER, AND MICHELLE BABICZ

Neuropsychology is one of many specialty areas in health service psychology and is formally recognized by the American Psychological Association (APA) and the Canadian Psychological Association (Smith, 2018). Training in neuropsychology is a long road that culminates in a postdoctoral fellowship, though specialization often begins in a doctoral program in clinical psychology (see Hannay et al., 1998). The goal of this chapter is to offer advice to students applying to doctoral clinical psychology programs with training in neuropsychology. In writing this chapter, we introspected on our own personal experiences, informally surveyed other neuropsychology faculty and trainees across the United States, read the limited empirical literature, and gathered information from other sources of support for prospective students. We organized the tidbits of wisdom we collected into a baker's dozen of tips.

Our thanks to faculty who provided us with their comments and ideas, including (in alphabetical order): Daniel N. Allen, University of Nevada, Las Vegas; Tania Giovannetti, Temple University; Paul J. Massman, University of Houston; Monica Rivera Mindt, Fordham University; Antonio E. Puente, University of North Carolina Wilmington; Becky Ready, University of Massachusetts Amherst; Lynn A. Schaefer, Nassau University Medical Center; Paula Shear, University of Cincinnati; Yana Suchy, University of Utah; Elizabeth W. Twamley, University of California, San Diego.

https://doi.org/10.1037/0000250-002
The Neuropsychologist's Roadmap: A Training and Career Guide, C. Block (Editor)

TIPS FOR GETTING INTO GRADUATE SCHOOL

Table 1.1 provides a brief summary of our tips for quick reference. The tips are also elaborated further in a helpful timeline in Table 1.2.

Tip 1: Steps in this process will take longer than you think. In our decades of advising and mentoring students, we have found that the most common hurdle to getting into graduate school in clinical psychology is waiting too long to begin key tasks. Although there is no formulaic pathway guaranteeing successful admittance to a doctoral program, Table 1.2 outlines a timeline to guide your planning, starting in the first year of undergraduate schooling. There are several "typical" pathways towards successful admission, including applying: (a) during your senior year, (b) after working for one to two years in a clinical- and/or research-related job, and (c) after completing a terminal master's program. While each pathway is different, all require intentional long-term planning. The tasks in Table 1.2 are relevant to all applicants, but the timeframe may vary depending on the particular pathway.

Tip 2: Assess your readiness for graduate training. There are many elements to readiness for graduate training to consider, including level of interpersonal maturity, academic preparation, financial resources, and social and professional supports (e.g., mentors). Each of these elements change over the course of any student's pathway; being aware of them as early as possible allows you to think proactively about ways to increase your readiness by the time you sit down to prepare your graduate school applications.

TABLE 1.1. Tips for Getting Into Graduate School

Tip	Suggestion
1	Steps in this process will take longer than you think.
2	Assess your readiness for graduate training.
3	Determine the type of program that's right for you.
4	Do your homework when determining where to apply.
5	Do your very best on the Graduate Record Examination (GRE).
6	Craft an effective personal statement.
7	Polish your curriculum vitae (CV).
8	Secure glowing letters of recommendation.
9	Submit your applications early and stay focused.
10	Knock their socks off at the interview.
11	Seal the deal.
12	Stay realistic about your prospects.
13	Make alternative timelines and plans.

TABLE 1.2. Suggested Timeline to Guide Students in the Graduate Application Process

Time	Task
Sophomore year *Summer to fall*	✓ Plan your undergraduate courses in accordance with graduate school program prerequisites.
	✓ Seek work in neuropsychology-related research laboratories (e.g., psychological laboratories that do applied work with neuropsychological populations).
	✓ Draft an initial CV to update as you gain relevant experiences, and have your mentors look it over.
	✓ Take advantage of graduate school preparation resources and workshops through your university or conferences.
Junior year *Summer to fall*	✓ Continue to gain relevant research experience.
	✓ Coauthor presentations and publications.
	✓ Gain relevant clinical experience (e.g., hotline counselor, psychometrist).
	✓ Actively self-reflect and seek feedback on your readiness and competitiveness for graduate school.
	✓ Make self-corrections to your preparation and training.
Junior year *Spring*	✓ Start to identify graduate programs of interest and ensure that neuropsychology faculty are accepting applications.
	✓ Prepare for and take the general and psychology GRE (so that you have time to take it again if necessary).
	✓ Continue to gain research/clinical experience.
	✓ Gain presentation/authorship experience.
	✓ Build relationships with academic clinical psychologists who may write letters of reference.
	✓ Speak with a professor in your major about opportunities to complete a senior thesis research project.
Junior year *Summer*	✓ Solidify your list of potential graduate programs.
	✓ Begin organizing and collecting necessary materials for the application to each graduate program.
Senior year *Fall*	✓ Prepare for and take the general and psychology GRE.
	✓ Complete one or more practice interviews with letter writers or through your university's career center.
Senior year *Winter to spring*	✓ Continue to gain research and clinical experiences.

Note. CV = curriculum vitae; GRE = Graduate Record Examination.

With regard to interpersonal maturity, students should consider the length of training. Doctoral training can take 4 to 7 years, including internship; an additional 2 years of postdoctoral fellowship in neuropsychology is required (Hannay et al., 1998; Smith, 2018). Upon starting their first job, newly minted neuropsychologists have invested about 23 years in school/training. Students intrinsically motivated and comfortable working towards long-term goals are suited for this challenge. Those who have difficulty with delayed gratification should evaluate whether this career path is right for them.

Students also should consider their personal readiness for the challenging graduate student lifestyle, which requires a great deal of self-regulation. Graduate students face many different, challenging, and sometimes ambiguous requirements. Graduate school courses are more intense, challenging, discussion-based, and driven by larger critical writing and research components than undergraduate courses. There is also required practical training, such as conducting clinical interviews, administering neuropsychological and other psychological tests, and learning effective therapy methods and skills. Sometimes students who have always been strong in instructor-led coursework where learning is evaluated by tests and essays/papers find "hands on" practical training experiences that require integration and demonstration of applied skills to be difficult; others find they have strengths in the practical training elements but struggle with the increasingly challenging didactic components. Students are also expected to become involved in research (at minimum, completing thesis and dissertation projects) and to maintain work responsibilities required of their stipend. It is difficult to manage all of these responsibilities, particularly when some come with clear expectations and deadlines (e.g., a test in a course in 3 days) and others have ambiguous demands and deadlines (e.g., writing a thesis proposal sometime in the future). Graduate school is not a 9-to-5 job, and this commitment can be difficult, especially when students compare themselves to peers who "clock-out" at the end of the day.

Perseverance and determination are necessary qualities to self-assess before beginning graduate study. Graduate school introduces a new evaluative culture, which can be a challenge. Chapter author Julie Suhr often reminds first-year graduate students that because they were likely above average students in the undergraduate setting, it can be disconcerting to just be "average" among a population full of high-achieving graduate students. Further, accredited doctoral programs use competency-based evaluation to determine whether students are showing appropriate development of profession-wide competencies. Evaluative feedback may not be a grade, but instead a note of "meeting expectations," a term that may not be satisfying for students used to "A" grades. A research manuscript draft that may have gotten an A in an undergraduate course may be returned multiple times with extensive edits on its way to a thesis committee or a peer-reviewed journal, which can be disheartening. Being evaluated as "below expectations" can strike fear into the hearts of students who have yet to encounter things at which they aren't naturally "good."

Students should also consider their own psychological needs. An important competency in clinical practice is the ability to "engage in self-reflection regarding one's personal and professional functioning" and "engage in activities to maintain and improve performance, well-being, and professional effectiveness" (APA Commission on Accreditation [APA CoA], 2015, p. 18; see also Rey-Casserly et al., 2012). The stress of graduate school can also exacerbate psychological concerns. When students try to "push through" their psychological or personal difficulties, it can negatively affect progress in the program, and, more important, the clinical care they offer to patients. Before entering graduate school, it is a good idea to consider and address your own psychological and personal needs (see Chapter 16, this volume).

With regard to overall personal readiness to apply, some students feel ready for graduate school fresh out of college; others feel that a gap year or two before going to graduate school is in their best interests. Speaking to the point above regarding the importance of developing a network of professional support, it is recommended that you have a frank conversation with a trusted mentor about your readiness, in addition to engaging in honest self-reflection about your personal and professional preparedness. If you decide to wait, make those gap years count with relevant experiences that increase your readiness to succeed. You can take additional postbaccalaureate courses, volunteer to work in a research laboratory, or secure a paid research position. You can gain general experience working in a lab, publishing and presenting research projects, and/or attending scientific meetings. Prioritize postbaccalaureate experiences that will make you competitive for the type of program to which you are applying.

With regard to educational readiness, getting relevant research experience is crucial. This means more than just working in a lab; you should work to develop and then assess your skills in writing, statistics, and oral presentation, as these are key to graduate school success. The most competitive applicants developed skills that result in lead-authored national presentations and subsequent publication (see Chapter 12). A recent survey of faculty in doctoral programs of clinical psychology emphasized research experience as well as coauthorships on publications and presentations as things they expect in ideal graduate school candidates (Karazsia & Smith, 2016).

Course-wise, graduate programs value a solid background in psychology, including experimental design/research methods, statistics, assessment, diversity, psychopathology, and behavioral neuroscience (though you should confirm program-specific requirements on the graduate program's website; Karazsia et al., 2013).

For perspective on grades, you can examine program websites. Programs may report minimum grade point averages (GPAs) and some provide median and mean GPAs for current students under the heading Student Admissions, Outcomes, and Other Data. As for other relevant skills, ask for honest feedback from lab supervisors, course instructors, and work supervisors about your level of readiness for graduate-level responsibilities and take advantage of opportunities and resources to develop your own skills.

Nearly half of all neuropsychology trainees report that finances were the most limiting factor in their training (Whiteside et al., 2016). While many graduate programs pay their graduate students a stipend and provide tuition waivers, many don't, and the degree to which the stipend covers living expenses can vary dramatically depending on where the program is located. Fortunately, accredited graduate programs are required to provide this information, including student fees, within one click on their website (under the domain of Student Admissions, Outcomes, and Other Data). In examining their financial readiness, students can research cost of living in that area to determine whether the stipend offers a livable wage. Students should also assess the "hidden" costs that can accrue based on the program or city (e.g., textbooks and supplies, cost of rent, public or personal transportation, health insurance) and what additional financial supports may be available (e.g., loans).

Tip 3: Determine the type of program that's right for you. When considering doctoral programs, the first step is to determine whether to pursue a doctor of philosophy (PhD) or doctor of psychology (PsyD) degree. Most neuropsychology training programs reside within clinical psychology programs and are either PhD or PsyD in nature. PsyD programs tend to train clinicians, while PhD programs train students to be both researchers and practitioners (Karazsia & Smith, 2016). A "fit factor" for the prospective student is to consider how much of their graduate school time and future career will focus on research and scholarship (PhD) versus clinical work (PsyD). Another important distinction is the tuition waiver and stipend that many PhD programs offer, compared to the out-of-pocket cost of most PsyD programs. PhD programs tend to place more emphasis on undergraduate experience in scientific methodology, research experience, fit with potential research mentors, and GRE scores, relative to PsyD programs. However, all programs value interpersonal skills, fit with mentors in the program, and applied experiences, in addition to relevant coursework (Karazsia & Smith, 2016).

The next step is to consider what kind of training orientation best matches your career goals. Even though it is no longer required by APA accreditation standards, some programs still identify their training as scientist–practitioner, clinical scientist, or practitioner–scholar orientation. In a scientist–practitioner orientation, there is relatively equal balance between scientific training and clinical training. Clinical scientist programs place more emphasis on scientific/research training and tend to offer the PhD. Practitioner–scholar programs place a stronger emphasis on clinical training, training students to be consumers of research rather than active contributors to research and tend to offer the PsyD. Your interest in a future career that emphasizes research or clinical work should influence your decision to apply to programs with a clear training emphasis in one area versus the other.

Another important consideration when thinking about the differences in degree types or training orientations is the length of time you will be in the program (e.g., often longer for programs with a research orientation), which will ostensibly affect the overall cost of your education (e.g., higher loan burden) and lead to longer delay to your first professional salary. Another is the competitiveness of the program (i.e., scientist–practitioner and clinical scientist programs tend to accept far fewer students and thus are more competitive to get into). Yet another is the success of program graduates. Data from the Association of Psychology Postdoctoral and Internship Centers (APPIC, 2018) show that the rate of obtaining accredited psychology internships, required to become a licensed psychologist in many states, is much lower for students in PsyD programs than PhD programs. Data from the Association of State and Provincial Psychology Boards (2017) show that the pass rate for the national licensing exam is much higher for PhD than PsyD graduate students. There is heterogeneity across programs that offer the PhD and PsyD degrees, so it's important to do your homework on the specific programs to which you're applying.

As noted above, some students apply to master's degree programs and/or to jobs in a clinical research area, either as a first step towards obtaining a doctoral degree, or as backup if they are not successful in doctoral applications (see Tips 12 and 13). When graduate students were informally polled about why they chose to complete a master's degree program, common answers included: to demonstrate academic competence in graduate level courses that their undergraduate GPA may not reflect, to gain research and clinical experience, and to solidify their interest in the field. Graduate students employed in clinical research positions reported gaining more clinical and research experience, solidifying their interest in the field, and saving money for graduate school as the main factors in their decision.

Another way to get a better sense of whether you enjoy research and/or clinical interactions (while also building your curriculum vitae [CV]) is to find a research assistantship in a clinical research lab. The best places to seek clinical research jobs are in the labs or clinics of neuropsychologists in research universities or academic medical centers. You can search their human resource websites for relevant positions (e.g., research assistant, research coordinator, psychometrist), often under departments of psychology, psychiatry, and neurology. These roles are ideal for gaining clinical experience with patients, as well as being surrounded by professionals in your future field. Another option is to use the Council of University Directors of Clinical Psychology (CUDCP) website to search for research assistant positions (https://clinicalpsychgradschool.org/positions/).

Your professional network of professors and mentors is also a great resource to ask about any labs or centers that they recommend or know are hiring. When interviewing for these positions, it is helpful to ask (a) whether others in that position have gone on to a graduate program, and (b) whether there are opportunities to be involved in research and publications. You will be an employee first and an aspiring graduate student second, meaning that research and publication opportunities will likely need to be completed on your own time in addition to your work responsibilities.

While neuropsychology requires the doctoral degree, earning a master's degree first might also make you more competitive for doctoral programs. The key word here is "might," as it depends upon the quality of the master's program. Master's programs are currently not accredited by the APA, although there are plans to accredit health service psychology master's programs in the near future (APA CoA, 2020). So for now you must do your own homework to determine whether a master's program will help you be more competitive for admittance to a doctoral program. First, check to see if the program offers you the opportunity to gain research experience with neuropsychologists (or at least topics relevant to neuropsychology), which will be more likely for master of science programs than for master of arts programs. Second, you can check to see if the program offers you direct clinical assessment and intervention experience with neuropsychological populations. Finally, you can use website information or send emails to the directors of the master's training programs to determine where graduates of the program usually end up. Oftentimes the primary goal of master's programs is to allow graduates to be certified or licensed as mental health practitioners (not psychologists) in a specific state, which may not increase the likelihood that you will successfully gain admittance to a doctoral program after their completion. It is important to keep in mind that completing a master's degree will not necessarily speed up your completion of a doctoral degree. Some doctoral programs may allow you to transfer credits from some of your master's work, and some may count your master's thesis project as meeting their thesis requirements; however, in other doctoral programs you may be "starting over."

Tip 4: Do your homework when determining where to apply. The first step in deciding where to apply to graduate school is to determine where there are accredited programs that provide training in neuropsychology. We strongly recommend that you only seek to attend accredited doctoral programs, because this will provide some assurances on the quality of your training and minimize any barriers to obtaining a license down the road. Accredited programs are required to provide this information clearly on their websites, but there are other ways to quickly obtain lists of accredited programs in the United States and Canada. A source of information unique to neuropsychology is the Society of Clinical Neuropsychology Training Directory (http://training.scn40.org), which lists self-identified neuropsychology training programs. They request that self-identified programs follow the guiding principles of the Houston Conference Guidelines (Hannay et al., 1998) and the *Taxonomy for Education and Training in Clinical Neuropsychology* (Sperling et al., 2017), which are the most widely-accepted standards for training neuropsychologists. By using this site, potential graduate students can determine whether programs self-identify as offering exposure, experience, emphasis, or a major area of study in neuropsychology. Not all programs that train in neuropsychology are identified on this resource. Another source of information is the APA Graduate Study in Psychology search tool (http://www.apa.org/pubs/databases/gradstudy), which is available online for a small fee. Another great resource, which is free, is the Getting Into Clinical Psych Grad School website sponsored by the CUDCP (http://clinicalpsychgradschool.org). This site includes a list of all accredited programs in clinical psychology, including neuropsychology.

Other programs can be identified by using your professional network. Ask your mentor or other professors at your undergraduate institution about good programs in neuropsychology. Talk with neuropsychologists in the field and ask them where they trained. Talk with conference attendees who are presenting research that you are particularly interested in and find out where they are on faculty or in training. If you already have a well-defined research interest, do a literature search to identify the major researchers in that area, determine where they are located and if they are associated with a doctoral training program. Regardless of how you identify potential programs, visit the programs' websites to determine whether they provide training to be successful in obtaining an internship and postdoctoral fellowship in neuropsychology, even if the program did not identify itself as offering neuropsychology as a major area of study. You can examine whether the course offerings, practical experiences, and research opportunities provide appropriate foundational training consistent with Houston Conference Guidelines, as well as with your own interests. For example, are there opportunities to work with a specific population of interest (such as geriatrics, pediatrics, or Spanish-speaking individuals)? Another thing to look for is where their students go on internship, and whether those internships are in settings (e.g., veterans affairs, academic medical centers, community mental health, integrated primary care) of interest to you.

Since the proof is in the pudding, as Dr. Yana Suchy, professor in the Department of Psychology at the University of Utah, advises, pay close attention to internship placements of recent graduates from that program, and whether graduates from that program went on to obtain postdoctoral fellowships in neuropsychology and eventually became board certified. You want to ascertain that the program is capable of launching you successfully on your desired career path. Chapter author Steven Paul Woods offers the most pragmatic way to examine this factor: ask yourself where you want to be in 10 years and examine whether that program has recently produced graduates who are already there. As Dr. Suchy also notes, a potential advisor's publication record within the field of neuropsychology and their general involvement with the profession (e.g., governance of major neuropsychological organizations) is also a good indicator. It is also worth considering the number of faculty and clinical supervisors available to train in the area of neuropsychology. With only one or two faculty and supervisors, your training may be more limited (or even in jeopardy if there are sudden faculty issues like illness, change in institution, retirement, death, etc.) than if an institution has a well-established program with many faculty and supervisors available for training.

The next step for the applicant is identifying potential mentors, who are specific professors within a program who would be a good research fit for you (and thus you a good fit for their program). Research fit has been described as key to a student's competitiveness and successful application in both formal (Karazsia & Smith, 2016; Karazsia et al., 2013) and informal surveys of neuropsychology program faculty and students. Keep in mind that if you are set on studying a very specific population and/or a very specific area of research, you will likely not find a "perfect" fit with very many potential mentors. While it is important to consider fit, you should also consider ways in which a program and a potential mentor's research "flexibly fit" your general research and training goals. Mentor fit at this stage is primarily based on fit with the area of research; other mentor fit factors (e.g., personality, mentoring style) cannot be determined until interviews, at which time you'll often have an opportunity for extended interactions with the mentor and lab members.

Once you have narrowed your search to mentors with similar research interests, it is important to learn whether these mentors are taking students in the year you are applying. Faculty don't always accept a student every year. Some programs offer this information on their websites, while others don't. Dr. Suhr recommends that students email potential mentors to express their interest and ask the mentor whether they are taking students, either the summer before or early fall of the application year. See Table 1.3 for advice for sending emails to potential faculty mentors. Keep in mind that you may not hear back from potential mentors you email. In this case, as Dr. Suhr tells her students, a clear negative ("I am not taking students this year") is very useful, as you will not waste time and financial resources on applying to that program. A clear positive ("I am taking students this year") is also useful, as they may now be more likely to watch for your application, and you know that it might be worth your time and money to apply there. A lack of response may mean many things, including that the mentor is someone who just doesn't typically answer these emails or that your email went to the spam filter at the university and the faculty member didn't read it. If you continue to be strongly interested in a mentor from whom you have not received an email response, you could follow-up with a phone call.

TABLE 1.3. Tips for Emailing Potential Mentors

Do	Do not
✓ Use a professional email address, preferably one attached to your school (.edu) or one that uses your actual name (Firstname.Lastname@gmail.com).	✗ Ask questions that are easily answered on the websites of the program and/or lab.
✓ Include a relevant subject line, such as "potential graduate applicant seeking information."	✗ Include links or attachments to your initial email, which may trigger spam filters or burden mentors.
✓ Include in your email a brief summary of your reasons for interest in the mentor's laboratory and a summary of your relevant experiences to date.	✗ Definitely do not send an email addressed to the wrong person or mentioning the wrong program! Always check for spelling, grammar, and content errors.

Dr. Paula Shear, chair of the Department of Psychology at the University of Cincinnati, notes that most programs are not able to accommodate on-site informational visits or lengthy email conversations prior to formal application reviews and official offers for interviews. However, a quick chat over email or telephone can help mentors match a name to an enthusiastic applicant.

The next step in determining where you might apply is to identify and weigh your personal fit factors. Some were described above; however, there are others to consider, including geographical location. If you are strongly tied for personal reasons to a particular geographic area, it may be difficult to be far away from that area for the many years of graduate school. Certain geographical regions are also more expensive to live in, which might be a consideration in the context of your own personal financial situation, as well as the program itself and their financial support. Personal fit factors to evaluate during interview season might include the learning environment (e.g., diversity, emphasis on competitiveness vs. cooperative team science), mentoring style (e.g., supportive, individualized, philosophy on communicating successes and areas in need of improvement), and the psychological health and well-being of the laboratory, program, and department (e.g., do current graduate students seem glad to be there?).

Tip 5: Do your very best on the GRE. The Graduate Record Examination (GRE) is used by many programs as a predictor of success in graduate school. There is a GRE General Test and then there are subject specific tests, including Psychology. The General Test includes a Verbal Reasoning section, a Quantitative Reasoning section, and an Analytical Writing section. The GRE website (https://www.ets.org/gre) gives detailed descriptions of these sections, as well as sample items. Accredited programs include the GRE percentile scores for their admitted students in the past 7 years on their websites, so you can determine if your score is competitive at the schools you are interested in. In addition, be aware of the ScoreSelect option, which allows you to send only select administrations of the GRE to the schools you are applying to, and details of sending prior scores to programs (available under Scores at https://www.ets.org/gre).

The Psychology GRE subject test is currently not used by a lot of doctoral programs as part of their admissions requirements, but it likely will be in the future because of the new Standards of Accreditation for Health Service Psychology (APA, 2019). These standards went into effect January 1, 2017, and allow programs to potentially use GRE Psychology test subtest scores to help streamline training by waiving some program requirements. The GRE Psychology test can also be a useful tool to demonstrate competence when coming from an educational background that isn't necessarily traditional for graduate study in clinical neuropsychology (e.g., biological science major, human neuroscience major).

In terms of preparing to do your best on the GRE, there are several companies that offer courses and workbooks to help students study for the exam (including Manhattan Prep, Kaplan, Princeton Review, and Educational Testing Service [ETS]). They differ in price, and many of Dr. Suhr's prior undergraduate students felt that doing the workbooks was more valuable than paying for expensive courses. The ETS website (https://www.ets.org/gre) allows users to take two online practice tests for free, which are similar to the look, feel, and difficulty of the official test. It also offers a free test preview tool and a sample test for the Psychology subject test. Several students found that familiarization with the question types and length of the test were the most valuable preparation. In addition, improving (or refreshing) your vocabulary can help you gain several points on the verbal section; there are many free smartphone applications to aid this goal, including several GRE vocabulary flashcards apps.

Generally, how you performed on other standardized tests (e.g., the SAT) are predictive of your GRE scores, so you can judge your readiness for the GRE somewhat on your prior performance on those exams. Taking appropriate level math in college can be helpful for the quantitative section, which includes basic arithmetic, algebra, and geometry questions. For the Psychology test, studying a good introduction to psychology textbook is a great way to review. Dr. Suhr found that being a peer tutor for psychology courses is another great way to prepare for the Psychology test. One factor to consider is that you may benefit from taking the GRE during your undergraduate studies or soon after so that the material is "fresh" in your mind.

Tip 6: Craft an effective personal statement. An effective personal statement tells a compelling, coherent, and professional story about your preparedness and goals as a future neuropsychologist. The personal statement should complement, not recite, your CV by clearly and concisely communicating to your prospective program and mentors that you have: (a) the interpersonal characteristics (e.g., curiosity, ambition, drive), background knowledge, academic skills, and clinical experiences to thrive in graduate school; (b) clear short-term training goals in neuropsychology that fit with the program's offerings and your prospective mentor's research; and (c) a long-term career plan that aligns with the program. Table 1.4 lists a few common mistakes to avoid in your personal statement.

The best personal statement (in our opinion) seamlessly integrates your background, interests, and goals with that of the laboratory to which you

TABLE 1.4. Tips for Personal Statements

Do	Do not
✓ Contextualize your CV with your training goals and fit with the program.	✗ Simply restate details/experiences from your curriculum vitae.
✓ Communicate your unique background and passions about neuropsychology.	✗ Provide too much personal information about you or your family.
✓ Directly address obvious weaknesses or oddities in your application materials (e.g., low scores, long gaps in training).	✗ Sell your qualifications short by being overly critical of your background, experiences, and standardized test scores.
✓ Carefully proofread your final document for each school to which you apply for typographical, grammatical, and content errors.	✗ Mention the wrong person or the wrong program!

Note. CV = curriculum vitae.

are applying. This is no easy task, as perfect research matches are rare, and when they do occur, they can raise questions about the added value of the training site, the risks of being pigeonholed, and so forth. It is very common (and also valuable) in neuropsychology for trainees to have had different populations and constructs be the focus of their research as they move from undergraduate placements to postbaccalaureate jobs to their graduate mentor's lab. Your charge as an applicant is threefold: (a) do your homework on the overarching aims and current projects of the laboratories to which you're applying, (b) discover specific areas in which your background and skills could be leveraged to advance your own emergent line of clinical research in a way that gets your potential mentor excited about how your work will complement and extend that of the laboratory, and (c) articulate that in a paragraph that is uniquely tailored to each program. The rationale shouldn't be a simple, direct comparison, or an overly generalized statement. The modal, safe (but not at all exciting) personal statement says straightforwardly: "I'm particularly interested in Dr. Jones's research on memory and traumatic brain injury, so we're a good fit, right?" A far more compelling rationale might look something like this: "Dr. Jones's program of research on episodic memory in the long-term daily functioning outcomes of traumatic brain injury in adults may be a fruitful setting in which to examine the role of individual differences in underlying attentional processes, which I have previously studied in the context of Alzheimer's disease in Dr. Smith's laboratory. In particular, I would hypothesize that. . . ." This more thoughtful, integrative approach increases your chances of getting the prospective mentor excited about the clinical science you could accomplish together. However, this is also a very difficult approach that will invariably need multiple revisions and edits from your mentors. Dr. Rebecca Ready, professor and director of Clinical Training at the University of Massachusetts at Amherst, recommends that you start early and seek feedback often. Having two or three individuals review the materials is a good idea. Solicit examples from graduate students to help get you started.

Tip 7: Polish your CV. Your CV is the primary vehicle for communicating your background, qualifications, and accomplishments to prospective programs and future employers. There are many different templates for formatting a CV, so seek out examples from graduate students in your laboratory and trusted online sources. Keep in mind that a busy reader should be able to easily glean a few key elements from your CV, which include educational background, research experience, clinical experience, publications and presentations, and relevant coursework, certifications, and organizational memberships. There are a few common CV mistakes that you'd be well advised to avoid if you can, including (a) cosmetic flaws, like cluttered formatting, nonstandard fonts, and typographical errors; (b) passive rather than active words; (c) "padding," for example, by double listing presentations and abstracts or including dubious qualifications; and (d) inclusion of hobbies and unrelated work, which may lead reviewers to question your professionalism.

Tip 8: Secure glowing letters of recommendation. Despite the fact that letters of recommendations are variable in their quality, accuracy, and transparency (e.g., Johnson et al., 2008), they are nevertheless rated as highly important among evaluators of neuropsychology graduate applicants (Karazsia et al., 2013). Programs typically request three letters of recommendation from professionals who can knowledgeably comment on your strengths and training needs in academics, research skills, and clinical acumen, as well as your interpersonal readiness for graduate-level studies. It's our experience that the most influential letters of recommendation come from academic neuropsychologists with whom we have had some level of collaboration and/or who are well-known for high-quality research and training. It is quite unusual to have all of your letters written by academic neuropsychologists and, of course, not all of your recommenders can comment on all aspects of your qualifications. We advise soliciting letters from three professionals who, together, give the clearest possible picture of your academic, research, clinical, and interpersonal dimensions. Letters from other types of professionals (e.g., attorneys, nondoctoral clinicians), undergraduate course instructors who have only seen your performance in one class, or relatives or family friends are not viewed favorably.

When contacting potential letter writers, be sure to determine if they would be willing to write you a *strong* recommendation letter. Provide your letter writers with (a) advance notice a few months prior to the first due date; (b) updated copies of your application materials, including your CV, relevant grade and test data (i.e., GPA, GRE scores), and personal statement; (c) specific achievements, accomplishments, or anecdotes you believe are worth including in the letter—these should be personalized to the letter writer, as a previous professor may speak better to your educational aptitude, while your current supervisor may speak better to your clinical skills; (d) a list of programs and mentors to which you are applying; and (e) information about how and when the letters should be sent. Send a follow-up reminder a few weeks prior to the submission deadline along with updates on how you progress through the application process. Once the recommendation is sent, be sure to send a prompt thank-you note.

Tip 9: Submit your applications early and stay focused. We recommend creating a spreadsheet to track each program's application details (due dates, required materials, application processes, fees, recommendation letters, potential mentors), and progress toward completing them. Dr. Suhr encourages applicants to read submission instructions carefully because programs vary in what types of materials are required, how they are formatted, and to where they are submitted. Application submission deadlines are typically firm (usually in late fall), and, as Dr. Woods tells his students, there is almost never a penalty for submitting applications a little early, but the consequences of being late can be devastating. Once you have submitted your applications, there is a waiting period of a few months prior to interviews. After you submit your materials, email prospective mentors to update them on official submission of your application, and that you're excited about the possibility of learning more about the lab and the program.

Tip 10: Knock their socks off at the interview. If you've gotten one or more interview offers: Congratulations! This means that your qualifications on paper place you in about the top 10% of a very large and competitive pool of applicants. Now it is time to prepare yourself for the interview process, because the more daunting news is that your peer group at this stage is also much stronger and more competitive. Historically, interviews are 1- to 2-day events that are held on-site at the university campus and involve informational sessions (e.g., overviews of the program's coursework, clinical training, and research), interviews with faculty and students, and social events (e.g., group dinners, happy hours). Graduate school interviews are less about your basic qualifications and more about your professional fit. In this way, you are also evaluating the laboratories that you'll be visiting for fit to your training and professional goals.

Interview scheduling can be challenging, and you will likely have over-lapping interview dates. Some programs offer a single date, others offer multiple dates, and others will go the extra mile to organize alternate dates. Many programs post their interview dates in advance, so if you know on which date your top choice has interviews, you can try to schedule alternate dates for other programs. Be respectful, flexible, and enthusiastic in navigating scheduling conflicts. Let prospective programs know that you are highly interested in visiting their program but are unfortunately committed to another interview on that specific day, and thus hope that there is an opportunity for either a formal or informal alternate interview day.

Build on the research on potential mentors and the individual programs you did in preparing your application materials, and revisit and elaborate on that groundwork to develop targeted, thoughtful questions for your interviews. For example, you might read a recent research paper from the lab that inspires questions about how you might fit into (or extend) their ongoing work. It is critical for you to also know the fundamental details of your own research (e.g., an "elevator speech" that articulates the over-arching aims, hypotheses, independent and dependent variables, basic statistics, implications, and limitations). You'll want to ask questions that are generic enough to compare across programs, but specific enough to get a sense of each program's unique qualities. We recommend broad, standard questions that you can ask of people on whom you haven't done your home-work, which can also help you get multiple perspectives on training and program issues. It is always a good idea to have practice interviews with mentors, peers, and other students, especially if you have the opportunity to practice with people you don't know well. Practicing in a formal environ-ment will help you overcome nerves on your real interviews.

At this point, you're ready for your interviews! Standard professional etiquette for white-collar jobs applies, which means arriving early and dressing professionally. We recommend that you turn off and stow away your personal electronic devices for the entire day. It's helpful to bring several copies of your updated CV, which helps unfamiliar interviewers (e.g., non-neuropsychology faculty). We also recommend bringing along a notepad to hold your list of questions and jot down observations about the program, which will help down the road when you're sending thank-you letters and ranking programs. As you may be interviewing at several programs, referring back to these notes will also be helpful in your decision-making process. Interview formats and styles vary widely across programs, labs, and mentors. Some programs host an "open house," which typically involves an informational session and small group discussions, while other programs prefer a multiday interview process that includes informational sessions, individual faculty and student interviews, and social events.

Interview styles vary quite a bit within and across programs. Dr. Woods prefers a mixed-methods approach, using standardized questions across all applicants during the first phase of the interview that transitions into a more free-flowing casual interaction. Dr. Daniel Allen of University of Nevada Las Vegas notes that interviews are an opportunity to share your personality in a professional, appropriate manner to determine "fit" with your prospective lab. Keep in mind that you are likely being "interviewed" during the most casual of encounters (e.g., social events) during the interview process, so be on your best behavior. Send a thank-you note to coordinating staff, students, and faculty to express your appreciation for the time invested and (if relevant) your continued strong interest in attending that program.

Tip 11: Seal the deal. For each program to which you've applied, there are one of three primary postinterview outcomes that are possible: (a) an offer of admission, (b) a spot on the waitlist, or (c) a denial of admission. Of course, there is variability in each of these outcomes, which are not mutually exclusive; for example, you could receive an offer of delayed admissions into a program. Unlike an internship or postdoctoral fellowship, there is no algorithmic match procedure for graduate admissions. Instead, you are your own booking agent for the next few months. Programs usually try to make offers to their top candidates as soon as possible after interviews have been completed, but a variety of issues could delay those decisions for weeks. So you may begin to field offers of admission, waitlist notifications, and/or rejections as early as January or as late as April.

The order of notification and the accompanying content of the news rarely aligns with your program rankings. It is not typical for an applicant's first notification to be an unqualified offer of admissions from their top-ranked program after all other interviews have been completed. Instead, you are more likely to experience something like this: Your fourth-ranked program makes you an offer while you're at the airport traveling to interviews for your third-ranked program, while your second-ranked program waitlisted you several days ago, and you haven't heard a peep from your first-ranked program, even though you interviewed with them a week ago and things seemed to have gone well. How do you handle this chaos? Fortunately, most programs adhere to the Council of Graduate Schools (2019) uniform decision day, which allows applicants to make a final decision no later than mid-April (usually April 15). Thus, you can "hold" the offer from your fourth-ranked program until you know your final standing with your higher ranked programs, which enables you to make an informed decision.

Programs understand that they may not be your top choice (and vice versa), so it is reasonable to thank them for the kind offer, express your enthusiasm for the training program and opportunities, and let them know that you have not yet completed the interview or decision process, but will keep them informed and notify them as soon as you can. Then do just that.

The CUDCP guidelines are fairly self-explanatory, but a few practical bits of advice are worth mentioning here. First, read the CUDCP guidelines so that you know your rights and those of the programs (https://cudcp. wildapricot.org). Second, don't release an offer from a lower ranked program that made your final acceptable list unless you have a better offer in hand from a higher ranked program. No matter how high you are on the waitlist of the higher-ranked program, that is not a guarantee of admissions. Third, don't hold on to an offer from a program if you do have an offer from one that ranks more highly on your list. Remember that other students are on the waitlist for that program and, like you, are eager to hear some good news. Fourth, if you haven't heard any news for a while, feel free to politely check in with a potential mentor or program on the status of your application. Fifth, if you begin to feel undue pressure from a potential mentor or program to make a decision before you are ready and entitled to do so, revisit the CUDCP guidelines to make sure you are within your rights, consult with a trusted mentor on the best course of action, and think carefully about whether that pressure may be a red flag for experiencing problems with the program if you decide to attend there.

Tip 12: Stay realistic about your prospects. As you go through the months involved in Tips 10 and 11, you should watch for signs that you may not meet your goal of admission to a doctoral program in that year. Signs might include the following: (a) not getting any interviews before the beginning of February (especially if online sources, such as https://thegradcafe.com, indicate that the schools you applied to have already invited students, or their posted interview dates are coming too fast for you to have arranged travel there); (b) not getting more than one or two interviews (which leaves you with limited options, given the low base rate of admittance); (c) not hearing back from a program, or a mentor of a program, after your interview (unless the site has a policy against such contact); and (d) not hearing back by any dates the program stated as typical for notifications (again, online sources, such as https://www.studentdoctor.net, will inform you of dates that offers are being made by programs you are interested in). If you experience these signs, a follow-up call or email to the programs you applied to might help you determine whether you need a backup plan for the upcoming year. Watch for these signs along the way to ensure that the opportunity to apply to other programs is still possible. If you wait until mid-to-late spring (see Tip 13) to begin thinking about a backup plan, you will likely be too late to meet application deadlines for alternative programs.

Tip 13: Make alternative timelines and plans. If you have not been notified about in-person interviews by mid-to-late spring, then it is unlikely that you will be admitted into a program for the coming fall. Do not despair: talented applicants who will one day become leaders in neuropsychology are sometimes derailed at various points along their journey, including doctoral admissions. Getting admitted to graduate school is an exceptionally competitive process that involves perseverance, hard work, and a little luck. Now is the time to dive head-first into Plan B for next year. Begin by querying your current mentors and the advisors of labs to which you applied, thank them for the opportunity to be considered, and ask them for a quick, but frank commentary on the strengths and weaknesses of your application. Reaffirm your interests in neuropsychology and their lab and let them know that you're eager to improve your skills and portfolio so that you can improve your chances next year. Then go do those things.

REFERENCES

American Psychological Association. (2019). *Standards of accreditation for health service psychology and accreditation operating procedures*. https://www.apa.org/ed/accreditation/about/policies/standards-of-accreditation.pdf

APA Commission on Accreditation (APA CoA). (2015). *Implementing regulations: Section C: IRs related to the standards of accreditation*. American Psychological Association. http://www.apa.org/ed/accreditation/section-c-soa.pdf

APA Commission on Accreditation (APA CoA). (2020). *Master's level accreditation: A status update from the Master's Accreditation Work Group*. CoA Update. [Blog post]. American Psychological Association. https://www.apa.org/ed/accreditation/newsletter/2020/03/masters-accreditation

Association of Psychology Postdoctoral and Internship Centers. (2018). *APPIC match statistics*. https://www.appic.org/Internships/Match/Match-Statistics

Association of State and Provincial Psychology Boards. (2017). *Psychology licensing exam scores by doctoral program*. https://cdn.ymaws.com/www.asppb.net/resource/resmgr/eppp_/2017_Doctoral_Report.pdf

Council of Graduate Schools. (2019). *April 15 Resolution: Resolution regarding graduate scholars, fellows, trainees, and assistants*. https://cgsnet.org/april-15-resolution

Hannay, H. J., Bieliauskas, L. A., Crosson, B. A., Harmneke, T. A., Hamsher, K. deS., & Koffler, S. P. (1998). Proceedings of the Houston conference on specialty education and training in clinical neuropsychology. *Archives of Clinical Neuropsychology, 13*(2), 157–250. https://doi.org/10.1093/arclin/13.2.160

Johnson, W. B., Forrest, L., Rodolfa, E., Elman, N. S., Robiner, W. N., & Schaffer, J. B. (2008). Addressing professional competence problems in trainees: Some ethical considerations. *Professional Psychology, Research and Practice, 39*(6), 589–599. https://doi.org/10.1037/a0014264

Karazsia, B. T., & Smith, L. (2016). Preparing for graduate-level training in professional psychology: Comparisons across Clinical PhD, Counseling PhD, and Clinical PsyD programs. *Teaching of Psychology, 43*(4), 305–313. https://doi.org/10.1177/0098628316662760

Karazsia, B. T., Stavnezer, A. J., & Reeves, J. W. (2013). Graduate admissions in clinical neuropsychology: The importance of undergraduate training. *Archives of Clinical Neuropsychology, 28*(7), 711–720. https://doi.org/10.1093/arclin/act056

Rey-Casserly, C., Roper, B. L., & Bauer, R. M. (2012). Application of a competency model to clinical neuropsychology. *Professional Psychology: Research and Practice, 43*(5), 422–431. https://doi.org/10.1037/a0028721

Smith, G. (2018). Education and training in clinical neuropsychology: Recent developments and documents from the clinical neuropsychology synarchy. *Archives of Clinical Neuropsychology, 34*(3), 418–431. https://doi.org/10.1093/arclin/acy075

Sperling, S. A., Cimino, C. R., Stricker, N. H., Heffelfinger, A. K., Gess, J. L., Osborn, K. E., & Roper, B. L. (2017). *Taxonomy for Education and Training in Clinical Neuropsychology*: Past, present, and future. *The Clinical Neuropsychologist, 31*(5), 817–828. https://doi.org/10.1080/13854046.2017.1314017

Whiteside, D. M., Guidotti Breting, L. M., Butts, A. M., Hahn-Ketter, A. E., Osborn, K., Towns, S. J., Barisa, M., Santos, O. A., & Smith, D. (2016). 2015 American Academy of Clinical Neuropsychology (AACN) student affairs committee survey of neuropsychology trainees. *The Clinical Neuropsychologist, 30*(5), 664–694. https://doi.org/10.1080/13854046.2016.1196731

2

PREPARING FOR AND OBTAINING A PREDOCTORAL INTERNSHIP IN NEUROPSYCHOLOGY

EMILY KELLOGG, BRITTANY CERBONE, LAURA KENEALY, AND ROBERT COLLINS

The predoctoral internship is a requirement for graduation from a doctoral program in professional psychology and necessary for licensure. Most psychologists-in-training complete the internship as a year-long, full-time placement in the last year of graduate school. Internship helps to solidify much of the experiences gained over the years through graduate course work, various externships, and knowledge passed down from supervisors and mentors. However, internship is not only a time to hone clinical skills in your selected area of clinical focus; it is also your last chance to have broad clinical training before further specializing during your postdoctoral residency. Internship is a very important year of both personal and professional growth, and no doubt you are hoping to find one that's a great fit for you. In this chapter, we introduce you to the purpose behind a neuropsychology internship and discuss how to identify internship sites that work for you. We cover the application process and interviews, and provide tips for how to manage the stress and anxiety of the internship match.

https://doi.org/10.1037/0000250-003
The Neuropsychologist's Roadmap: A Training and Career Guide, C. Block (Editor)

ROLE OF THE PREDOCTORAL INTERNSHIP ON THE PATH TO NEUROPSYCHOLOGY SPECIALIZATION

Reviewing the history behind the neuropsychologist training requirements is beyond the scope of this chapter, as we are focusing on the internship application process. Readers are encouraged to review the history, as it may give additional perspective and insight into the rational for training programs (e.g., Bieliauskas & Matthews, 1987).

Germane to the neuropsychology internship, a report from the International Neuropsychological Society and the American Psychological Association's (APA's) Society for Clinical Neuropsychology/Division 40 suggested that adequate training in neuropsychology would require at least 50% immersion in neuropsychology at the predoctoral internship level (INS/Division 40 Task Force, 1987). While some internship programs still adhere to a 50% neuropsychology experience (e.g., Association for Internship Training in Clinical Neuropsychology member programs), this should not be considered a universal requirement. An applicant's selection of the appropriate program should occur within the context of the guidelines developed at the Houston Conference on Specialty Education and Training in Clinical Neuropsychology (Hannay et al., 1998), which suggest that a clinical neuropsychologist should not only have training in both general psychology principals and clinical care, but should also have advanced training in brain–behavior relationships (e.g., functional neuroanatomy, neurological disorders) and the foundations of the practice of clinical neuropsychology (e.g., research in neuropsychology, professional issues and ethics of neuropsychology). In selecting an appropriate internship program, applicants need to consider the neuropsychological knowledge and skills they acquired at the doctoral level in order to (a) assess their own individual readiness for advancement to internship training, and (b) identify areas of growth that may be filled while on internship.

Fortunately, there is a good chance that your graduate program has properly prepared you for pursuing advanced training in neuropsychology. In a survey by the American Academy of Clinical Neuropsychology, 77% of respondents on internship and 91% in postdoctoral training positions reported that their graduate school programs followed the Houston Conference Guidelines (Whiteside et al., 2016). Certainly, individuals pursuing a career in neuropsychology should familiarize themselves with the Houston Conference Guidelines, which remain a cornerstone document for board certification, as well as the more recently developed neuropsychology taxonomy, which provides a common language all programs should use to describe their training experiences, including the percentage of time spent supervised in clinical neuropsychology and the number of didactics (Sperling et al., 2017). Thus, programs that offer neuropsychology internships with at least 50% of training activities in the discipline could describe their program as a "Major Area of Study," while programs offering less intensive neuropsychology experiences would use different descriptors (e.g., Emphasis, Experience, Exposure). A full review of these training-related documents is beyond the scope of this chapter, but it is important for applicants at this level to have a familiarity with these resources.

STEPS TOWARD SECURING A PREDOCTORAL INTERNSHIP IN NEUROPSYCHOLOGY

Now that you are familiar with some of the background behind the neuropsychology internship and have some guidance regarding what to pay attention to when looking at program brochures, the following six steps are meant to provide a guideline for you to follow throughout the application process (see Table 2.1). Within each section, we have provided advice and helpful resources to help increase your knowledge about the process so that you can focus on presenting your best self in your application materials and in person.

Step 1: Assess Your Readiness for Internship Training

One of the main goals for doctoral programs in psychology is to help their students achieve the knowledge and skills needed to prepare them for a doctoral internship program. Therefore, almost everything you do as a graduate student will be a step toward readiness for internship. In order to have a better sense of where you stand on your readiness and competitiveness for internship programs, we recommend that you regularly reflect on your progress towards this goal and discuss your timeline with your advisor. Table 2.2 and Exhibit 2.1 provide helpful guides that graduate students can use to get a better understanding of the application timeline and assessing their readiness in several domains essential for a competitive application and successful internship year.

Tip 1: Complete academic coursework. One of the first considerations regarding readiness for internship is whether you will have completed all academic coursework requirements (aside from your dissertation) by the time your internship year begins. In addition to general foundation courses, internship programs with neuropsychological training will highly value, and sometimes require, that prospective students will have taken courses in

TABLE 2.1. Steps and Tips for Getting a Predoctoral Internship in Neuropsychology

Step	Suggestion
1	Assess your readiness for internship training.
	Tip 1: Complete academic coursework.
	Tip 2: Complete comprehensive or qualifying exams.
	Tip 3: Obtain and track graduate training hours.
	Tip 4: Seek diverse practicum experiences and fill gaps in training.
	Tip 5: Ensure dissertation progress.
	Tip 6: Maintain research productivity.
2	Assess potential internship programs.
	Tip 1: Review the program's public materials.
	Tip 2: Review the program's specific materials.
3	Decide where to apply.
	Tip 1: Consider accreditation status.
	Tip 2: Consider personal factors.
4	Submit your application.
	Tip 1: Be familiar with all application components.
	Tip 2: Complete your cover letter.
	Tip 3: Polish your curriculum vitae.
	Tip 4: Write your essays.
	Tip 5: Seek letters of recommendation.
5	Attend the interview(s).
	Tip 1: Be familiar with the various interview formats.
	Tip 2: Prepare yourself for a range of interview questions.
6	Rank internship programs and wait for Match Day.
	Tip 1: Consider how you want to rank internship programs.
	Tip 2: Endure the waiting game.
	Tip 3: Look for your results on Match Day.
	Tip 4: Be familiar with what to do if you do not match.

neuropsychology. Sample coursework topics could include brain–behavior relationships, structural and functional neuroanatomy, neuropsychological populations, neuropsychological models and theory, principles of neuro-psychological testing and interpretation, and multicultural considerations and professional issues in neuropsychology.

Tip 2: Complete comprehensive or qualifying exams. Comprehensive or qualifying examinations are an integral part of a doctoral student's training that help demonstrate acquired competencies and skills within their specialty field. Most doctoral programs will require that you complete these exams prior to applying for internship, and therefore it is important to develop a time-line of when you anticipate the completion of your program's examination

TABLE 2.2. Suggested Timeline to Guide Students in the Internship Application Process

Time	Task
January–July	✓ Assess anticipated readiness to apply for internship for the following fall semester, including completion of courses, clinical hours, comprehensive exams, and dissertation proposal.
	✓ At the beginning of July, join the APPIC Match-News Email List.
Early August	✓ Create an account on the APPIC Application for Psychology Internships (AAPI) website and familiarize yourself with the Applicant Portal.
	✓ Create an account on the National Matching Service website to obtain your match number, and add it to your APPIC application.
	✓ Determine your training goals and needs.
	✓ Begin researching APPIC internship sites on various online outlets, including APPIC, SCN/Division 40, and AITCN.
	✓ Reach out to those within your professional network (e.g., faculty advisor, alumnae within your program, practicum supervisors) to obtain a preliminary list of reputable training sites.
	✓ Create a checklist with anticipated completion dates of required steps for the application process.
Late August–early September	✓ Create a spreadsheet of site information, including match number, submission deadline, required materials, rotations, etc.
	✓ Reduce list of sites to approximately 15–20.
	✓ Identify and contact your references regarding letters of recommendation.
	✓ Request transcripts from graduate programs.
	✓ Draft general essays (aim for one essay written per week).
Middle–late September	✓ Edit and finalize curriculum vitae.
	✓ Finalize essays.
	✓ Finalize your site list.
	✓ Request a letter from your director of clinical training.
	✓ Draft your first cover letter.
Early–middle October	✓ If not already done, propose dissertation before application deadlines.
	✓ Begin filling out APPIC application.
	✓ Create individual cover letters for each site.

(continues)

TABLE 2.2. Suggested Timeline to Guide Students in the Internship Application Process (*Continued*)

Time	Task
	✓ Tally up and finalize your intervention, assessment, and supervision hours, as well as number of reports written.
	✓ Identify an integrated assessment and/or treatment summary report for submission.
	✓ Check in with letter writers about their progress and anticipated submission date.
Late October	✓ Review your application checklist.
	✓ Proof-check application materials.
	✓ Add final list of sites to your APPIC application.
	✓ Upload all applicable materials to the APPIC website.
	✓ Send any final reminder emails regarding reference letters.
	✓ Review and finalize APPIC application.
	✓ Submit and relax!
November 1	✓ Deadline for all predoctoral internship applications.
Middle of January	✓ Begin submitting your rank order to APPIC.
Early–middle February	✓ Beginning of February, finalize your Phase I rank order.
	✓ Phase I Match Day takes place in the middle of February.
Late February	✓ If you did not match in Phase I, during this time you can submit your application to programs who are participating in Phase II of the Match.
March	✓ Finalize your Phase II rank order.
	✓ Phase II Match Day is towards the end of March.

Note. APPIC = Association of Psychology Postdoctoral and Internship Centers; SCN = Society for Clinical Neuropsychology; AITCN = Association for Internship Training in Clinical Neuropsychology.

EXHIBIT 2.1. Self-Checklist for Internship Readiness

Task

☐ Complete academic coursework.
☐ Complete comprehensive/qualifying exams.
☐ Successfully propose dissertation project.
☐ Set a realistic timeline of dissertation completion.
☐ Obtain and track intervention hours.
☐ Obtain and track assessment hours.
☐ Obtain and track supervision hours.
☐ Complete a sufficient number of integrated reports.
☐ Seek diverse practicum experiences and fill gaps in training.
☐ Maintain research productivity.

process. Make sure to allow sufficient time in case of possible unexpected obstacles (e.g., having to retake your exam to receive a passing grade) since this could delay the process and impede your ability to apply for internship.

Tip 3: Obtain and track graduate training hours. A hot topic for psychology doctoral students relates to the acquisition of training hours (e.g., hours spent engaged in assessments, interventions, in supervision, etc.,) and especially the minimum number of hours needed to be competitive for internship. You will document these hours when you complete the standard application for psychology internships, called the AAPI (APPIC Application for Psychology Internships; APPIC stands for Association of Psychology Post-doctoral and Internship Centers). Start tracking your hours in the first year of graduate school. Being proactive in recording all of your clinical, support, and supervision hours will save you time (and headaches) down the road. Many students use online tracking websites, such as Time2Track or PsyKey, or an AAPI-compatible Excel spreadsheet. While there is a cost to subscribe, there are benefits of using an online service to track your hours, including user-friendly ways of entering and calculating hours, easy access to your information from any computer, protection against loss of information (e.g., crashing, accidental deletion, overwriting), access to APPIC applicant statistics, AAPI-compatible format and view options, and direct transfer of your hours onto the AAPI web portal (for Time2Track). If you decide to choose the more economical option of an Excel spreadsheet, be sure your spreadsheet includes all the information that the AAPI web portal requests at the time of the application (e.g., client age, race/ethnicity, gender, sexual orientation). This information can be found on the AAPI Online Applicant Help Center web page.

Unfortunately, because of variability across individuals and graduate programs, no solid consensus exists on how many hours should be completed. Nonetheless, there are several ways to obtain a general "ballpark" estimate of training hours. Time2Track provides estimates of matched APPIC applicants who are members of their website, and reports total intervention and assessment hours ranging from a low average of 500 to high average of 1,375. It is important to keep in mind that these numbers include students from different degree programs (e.g., PhD and PsyD; clinical or counseling psychology), areas of focus (e.g., adult, child, neuropsychology, forensics), and years in the program. According to a 2012 internship survey completed by supervising neuropsychologists (Ritchie et al., 2012), competitive applicants had a median of 400 neuropsychological assessment hours ($M = 575$, $SD = 506$). Another way of determining a minimum threshold for acceptable number of training hours is by researching prospective internship sites and identifying whether they have minimum hours specified. This information is available on the APPIC website or on individual programs' webpages. Lastly, some graduate programs will provide students with a range of hours based on the experience of alumni within their program.

In general, for neuropsychology students, the assessment to intervention ratio should be more balanced (e.g., 400 hours of assessment and 400 hours of intervention), compared with those without a neuropsychology training focus and who may have more intervention hours. In addition, it is important to track the number of integrated reports you have completed while on externships or in other supervised experiences, as this is frequently reviewed and considered by internship sites with neuropsychological training. According to APPIC (2021), an integrated report is defined as "a report that includes a review of history, results of an interview, and at least two psychological tests from one or more of the following categories: personality measures, intellectual tests, cognitive tests, and neuropsychological tests."

Tip 4: Seek diverse practicum experiences and fill gaps in training. According to a 2012 survey of internship programs, clinical experience in neuropsychological assessment, particularly within university-affiliated or VA medical center settings, is considered to be the most important criterion for neuropsychology supervisor rankings of intern applicants (Ritchie et al., 2012). It is also expected that students are supervised by neuropsychologists within these training settings. A majority of survey respondents indicated that it is essential or very important for applicants to have prior experiences with flexible battery and process approaches compared with a fixed battery approach, as well as objective personality assessment experience (e.g., Minnesota Multiphasic Personality Inventory–2). Preferences for experience with certain patient populations varied, with general neuropsychology populations (e.g., traumatic brain injury, neurodegenerative diseases) being most essential, followed by referrals from neurology and psychiatry departments. Consider these factors when making decisions about practicum experiences during graduate training.

While it is important to consider the quantity and quality of your neuropsychological practicum experiences, it is also very important for clinical psychologists to receive training in psychotherapy and intervention services. Internship sites will seek well-rounded trainees who have sufficient competencies in and desire to learn clinical interventions; the Houston Conference Guidelines consider the provision of treatment and interventions to be a core clinical skill for neuropsychologists. In addition, the "match" between the applicant's clinical experience and the internship opportunities matter in terms of age of patients, treatment modality, and therapeutic orientation. For example, if you are interested in pediatric neuropsychology and hope for an internship at a children's hospital, you will be most competitive if you have experience providing treatment to relevant populations (e.g., behavioral medicine intervention experience with children; cognitive behavior therapy with kids and adolescents).

Tip 5: Ensure dissertation progress. An applicant is more competitive if they have successfully proposed their dissertation prior to internship application deadlines. According to the 2016 APPIC Applicant Survey, those who proposed their dissertation prior to applying for internship had a 91% match rate, compared with a 79% match rate among those who had not yet completed the dissertation proposal (Keilin, 2017). In 2018, 90% of applicants reported having proposed their dissertation prior to application deadlines (Keilin, 2018). Overall, nine out of 10 neuropsychology internship supervisors consider dissertation proposal approval prior to internship to be essential or very important, and a third consider it very important for students to have completed their dissertation prior to beginning internship (Ritchie et al., 2012). Since the completion of your dissertation is a necessary component to graduate from your doctoral program, internship sites will want to ensure that you have a reasonable timeline to complete your dissertation prior to the culmination of your internship training year. Therefore, it is essential to consider a realistic timeline for anticipated dates of proposal, data collection, data analysis, and defense, prior to applying for internship.

Tip 6: Maintain research productivity. Neuropsychology internship programs rank research productivity to be the fifth most important consideration for an applicant's competitiveness (Ritchie et al., 2012). In this survey, applicants were expected to have a median of one publication ($M = 1.66$, $SD = 1.08$) and three professional presentations ($M = 3.86$, $SD = 2.39$). In addition, approximately 50% of neuropsychology supervisors considered peer-reviewed publication and presentations at national conferences to be essential or very important for applicants. More competitive sites and those where research is highly valued in general (e.g., academic medical centers) may particularly look for research productivity as evidence that someone is a "star" applicant. Furthermore, it is also important to consider your future goals and research interests when identifying training sites, as sites that emphasize research productivity are probably the best fit for trainees whose long-term goals include a significant research component. Reflection on these goals will help determine which sites best fit your needs and professional aspirations.

Step 2: Assess Potential Internship Programs

In conjunction with determining individual readiness for internship, there are many factors a doctoral student should consider when applying to programs. Some of these factors can be discerned from public materials that all accredited programs are required to list, whereas other factors will require additional investigation for an applicant and should, at least in part, be guided by a self-assessment of readiness discussed previously. For example, do you lack exposure to populations with acute neurologic injury, presurgical populations requiring specialized assessment techniques (e.g., intracarotid evaluations for epilepsy), severe mental illness, and so on? Ultimately an applicant will need to consider these factors as they relate to their training development and competency.

Tip 1: Review the program's public materials. All training programs accredited by the American Psychological Association Commission on Accreditation (APA CoA, 2015) are required to

> provide potential and current trainees and the public with accurate information on the program and on program expectations. This information is meant to describe the program accurately and completely, using the most up-to-date data about important admissions, support, and outcome variables, and must be presented in a manner that allows applicants to make informed decisions about entering the program. (p. 105)

The public materials for most APA CoA–accredited internship programs can be found either directly on the internship webpage or within the internship training program brochure, which should also be available on the internship webpage. Accredited training programs are required to update public materials on an annual basis and often release updated brochures in early fall. These will include information such as minimum intervention and assessment hours required for application, financial benefits, and other minimum criteria used in the initial screening process (i.e., U.S. citizenship if applying to a Veterans Affairs (VA) hospital/clinic, information regarding American Psychological Association or Canadian Psychological Association [CPA] training programs, background screening information, etc.). It is crucial for applicants to carefully review this information prior to submitting an application. Required public materials also include pertinent information that allows applicants to determine their "fit" with a program and, while not listed directly within the required tables, internship public materials will also provide general information regarding selection processes. Lastly, accredited internship programs are also required to provide information regarding initial postinternship positions including both postdoctoral and employment placements. While this last piece of information is general in nature and is likely to include the postinternship placements of both neuropsychology-focused and other clinical psychology trainees, it allows neuropsychology internship applicants an initial starting point to determine how successful a program is in placing neuropsychology interns into neuropsychology residency positions.

Tip 2: Review the program's specific materials. In addition to required public materials, most neuropsychology internship programs will provide detailed information regarding the nature of the training opportunities, and many internship sites may also provide applicants with the actual internship training manual. It is essential that neuropsychology internship applicants review these materials. While the importance of some training opportunities will vary across intern applicants and be related to their own self-assessment, factors an applicant might consider when reviewing these documents include:

- Does the program accurately describe their training opportunities within the context of the neuropsychology taxonomy?

- How are the neuropsychology tracks arranged? Is the training year divided into major neuropsychology rotations with minor psychotherapy rotations?

- What patient populations will the neuropsychology interns have access to?

- Are there opportunities for the neuropsychology interns to supervise externs/practicum students? Similarly, does the program have a post-doctoral residency in neuropsychology and will the neuropsychology intern have opportunities to work with the neuropsychology resident?

- Are there research/neuropsychology research opportunities and does the program provide protected time or research rotations?

- How are the didactics described in the training materials? Will the neuropsychology interns have access to both generalist didactics as well as neuropsychology-specific didactics?

- How are interns evaluated, and what are the minimum levels of achievement required to graduate from the internship?

- How many neuropsychology training staff will the interns have access to?

- Are there board-certified neuropsychologists within the training program?

Step 3: Decide Where to Apply

A number of different websites and resources are available to help one find and narrow down what at first appears to be an overwhelming number of internship sites. Some of the more common websites to begin compiling your internship wish list are listed below in the resource table (see Table 2.3). While looking through sites, it may be a good idea to create a spreadsheet that lists characteristics of the program, such as intensity of the neuro-psychology training (e.g., a Major Area of Study), accreditation status, start date, possibility of staying for a neuropsychology postdoctoral residency,

TABLE 2.3. Resources for the Internship Application Process

Organization	Acronym	Specifics	Website
American Psychological Association	APA	The go-to website for psychology in the United States	https://www.apa.org
Association of Psychology Postdoctoral and Internship Centers	APPIC	Lists all possible internship sites and can sort by location, accreditation, or program type	https://www.appic.org
Association for Internship Training in Clinical Neuropsychology	AITCN	Has a member program directory listing	https://www.aitcn.org
Association of Neuropsychology Student and Trainees	ANST	Provides a community of support and resources for trainees in neuropsychology	https://scn40.org/anst
Association of State and Provincial Psychology Boards	ASPPB	Assists with licensure and professional development	https://www.asppb.net
California Psychology Internship Council	CAPIC	CAPIC internships and fellowships are recognized by the CA board for licensure	https://capic.net
National Matching Services	NMS	Information on how the Match system works for applicants	https://www.natmatch.com/psychint
Neuropsychology listservs	n/a	Examples: PED-NP-SY, NPSYCH, AACN, etc.	n/a
The Society for Clinical Neuropsychology (APA Division 40)	SCN	Searchable database for neuropsychology internship and fellowship programs	https://www.scn40.org
Time2Track, PsyKey	N/A	Websites for tracking training hours	http://www.time2track.com http://www.psykey.com

stipend, and any training experiences that may interest you. Also, remember to ask your mentors, neuropsychology supervisors, and peers for sites they would recommend you consider.

Tip 1: Consider accreditation status. We believe that APA/CPA accreditation provides the most rigorous and highest quality of psychology training standards in the United States and Canada, and advocate that neuropsychology internship applicants limit their focus to these accredited programs. However, some applicants may be unable to attend an APA/CPA accredited internship for various reasons (e.g., lacking sufficient training hours to make them competitive for an APA/CPA accredited internship; only able to apply within a very restricted geographic area). In such cases we do recommend that an internship applicant refer to their self-preparation checklist and give serious consideration to potential implications of not attending an accredited program.

APA accreditation occurs through the APA CoA, which is recognized by both the secretary of the U.S. Department of Education and the Council for Higher Education Accreditation, as the national accrediting authority for professional education and training in psychology (https://www.apa.org/ed/accreditation/about/index). In addition to APA-accredited programs, applicants may consider applying to internship programs accredited through CPA, as well as internship programs offered through the California Psychology Internship Council (CAPIC). Please note that CAPIC is not an accrediting agency, per se, but rather a council with internship member programs recognized by the California Board of Psychology (as of 2019, CAPIC reports having 70 internship programs offering full- and part-time internship opportunities). However, of the 70 internship programs listed on the CAPIC website, only one is listed as being currently accredited by the APA. While it remains possible that some CAPIC internship programs might pursue APA accreditation in the future, neuropsychology internship applicants should be mindful of the internship accreditation requirements for board certification. For more information regarding board certification, the reader is encouraged to review Chapter 5 of this book. In brief, starting in 2020 the American Board of Professional Psychology (ABPP), the organization for Specialty Board Certification in Psychology, will require applicants to have completed an internship accredited by APA, CPA, or another accrediting agency recognized by the U.S. Department of Education (ABPP, n.d.).

Attending an internship that is not APA accredited may affect eligibility for licensure and limit employment opportunities. Licensure requirements vary by state, with some states having codified requirements about completion of an APA-accredited internship, whereas other states may allow for internship experiences that are not accredited. Be sure to check with your state licensing board and consider the portability of your license and training should you have to move in the future. The Association of State and Provincial Psychology Boards (https://www.asppb.net) is another resource regarding state licensure requirements. Finally, be aware that a nonaccredited internship may also limit opportunities for postdoctoral training and eventual employment. Completion of an APA-accredited internship is required for postdoctoral residency training at VA training sites and is also a requirement for employment as a psychologist within the VA system. That the VA remains the largest trainer and employer of psychologists only adds to the importance of completing an APA-accredited internship in the United States. Outside the VA system, competitive postdoctoral fellowship sites may require and will certainly prefer that applicants have completed APA- or CPA-accredited internships, and employers will consider the quality of both your internship and subsequent fellowship training.

Tip 2: Consider personal factors. Many personal factors may influence where you want to apply for internship. While we encourage flexibility, as that will allow you full access to all the programs that may fit your training needs, we also understand that factors such as family obligations and regional preferences are important to consider. For example, some applicants may restrict their potential internship sites to areas where it will be easy to return home quickly in case an ailing family member needs care. Also, if there is an area where you think you could never be comfortable due to the climate, then it may be worth narrowing down your search. However, in instances where a location may fit all your needs but may not have ideal weather, remember that internship is only one year and the training may be worth some short-term discomfort.

Outside of family and geographic restrictions, you may also want to consider whether the site has the option of a postdoctoral residency. The positives of staying in the same location for postdoctoral training include potentially avoiding a costly household move, familiarity with a training site, and having the opportunity to take advantage of all of the training opportunities your site has to offer. Another important factor to consider when thinking about whether to stay in the same location for internship and postdoctoral training is where you ultimately want to find employment. If your internship is in New York and you want to work in California, it may be wise to apply to California postdoctoral residencies, so that it is easier to network and job hunt when the time comes. However, you may also want to consider a different site for your postdoctoral residency in order to expand your network of colleagues, peers, and mentors. Having contacts in a variety of locations may help when looking for future employment as they may be able to alert you of specific job opportunities.

Step 4: Submit Your Application

So now that you have pored over and combed through the past 4+ years of your life, inventoried the experiences you have had and the ones that you hope to have, and identified several sites that seem to fit the bill, how do you decide how many sites to apply to?

That magic number: Many applicants wonder what the perfect number of sites to apply to is, and in reality, there is no straightforward answer to that question. It is going to be applicant-dependent and will depend on factors such as finances, strength of your application, and personal preferences. For example, if you are restricted to a particular geographical location due to family or personal interest, or just that you can't imagine living anywhere else, then the number of applications you submit is likely to be low (i.e., fewer than five), but ideally you will apply to more sites. If you come from a graduate program that has a strong neuropsychological background, a variety of neuropsychological practicums and externships, strong letters of recommendation, and have been productive in research, you will most likely be safe in applying to approximately 15 sites. However, if you are a student who decided later in their graduate career to pursue neuropsychology and are feeling as though you are scrambling to catch up, came from a graduate program that does not have a neuropsychology-specific track, or did not have as many externships available in your area, then perhaps consider applying to more than 15 sites. For each person, the number of sites to apply to will be different. We advise against applying to more than 20 programs, as there is a diminishing return in terms of time and attention spent per application. As always, consult with mentors and peers (particularly ones who just recently went through the process) to get different perspectives on how many sites to consider applying to.

Tip 1: Be familiar with all application components. Your internship application includes the AAPI, a well-written cover letter, a polished curriculum vitae (CV), your essays, a letter from your director of clinical training (DCT), and strong letters of recommendation. Tips on completing your AAPI have already been covered in this chapter. This section provides guidance on how to write a polished cover letter, CV, and essays. There are several excellent resources available both in book and online format on how to write the various components of the application. One source we recommend is *Internships in Psychology: The APAGS Workbook for Writing Successful*

Applications and Finding the Right Fit (Williams-Nickelson et al., 2019). In addition, reach out to your mentors and peers for examples of their application materials, as well as to have them review and proofread your materials. Furthermore, think about your application as a complete body of work. As much as possible, you want to keep the same formatting, font, and spacing throughout all of your materials. It will help make your application look polished and put together. Last, remember that you may have reviewers and interviewers who represent other areas in psychology. Make sure cover letters, essays, and letters speak to knowledge and skills more broadly.

Tip 2: Complete your cover letter. The cover letter should be written in the format of a formal business letter. The beginning of your cover letter should include a heading that consists of the site's DCT and address, and you should always begin the body of your letter by addressing the DCT with an appropriate salutation (e.g., "Dear Dr. X and members of the Internship Selection Committee"). The body of the letter should include some key information. In the first paragraph, you want to indicate the program and the specific track you are interested in applying for. You also will want to specify the rotations or training experiences you want to pursue should you match with that program. Be careful with this, as some programs will explicitly state how you should note this information (e.g., bolded, bullets). In the next paragraph, be sure to indicate what your goals are, which may include becoming a board-certified neuropsychologist, the type of setting you plan to work in (best if your dream job site matches the type of site you are applying to), and the areas in which you want to gain training experience. Next, briefly describe your accomplishments; however, refrain from simply repeating your CV, as the selection committee will review the CV as well. Once you summarize your experiences, discuss your areas of growth and gaps in training and note specifically how the internship program can help you achieve those goals. Last, tie everything up in a neat bow by summarizing how your previous training, your goals for internship, and the training provided by the internship program are a match and indicate your enthusiasm for that specific program. Be sure to conclude the letter with an appropriate closing (i.e., Sincerely,) and signature line.

Tip 3: Polish your curriculum vitae. When preparing your CV, you want to make it readable and easy to quickly scan for information. Try to avoid going overboard with lots of bolded, underlined, or italicized fonts. By using these sparingly, you can direct your reviewers' attention to those parts of your CV that you want to highlight, such as your neuropsychology experiences. You might do this by creating a separate header just for your neuropsychology training or creating a more detailed or bulleted outline of the training experience. In your research section, make sure you are appropriately categorizing your work. If a paper is in progress or under review, do not list it under Publications, as that section should only be used for papers that have been accepted for publication. Similarly, avoid double dipping: if your poster presentation was also published as an abstract, only list one in your CV. You want to avoid giving the training committee the impression that you are trying to pad your CV. You should have someone proofread your CV to catch any typographical or grammatical errors or redundancies.

Tip 4: Write your essays. For some people, the essays can be a daunting task. It can be a challenge to balance (within the 500-word limit) enough personal information to help separate you from the pack, but not so much information that it seems as though you are oversharing. Luckily, there are lots of resources available to help you craft your best essays. The APA's website is a great place to start looking. On their website you can find links to articles (https://www.apa.org/apags/resources/internships) about what to include and not include in your essays, as well as additional resources to help you with your application. The Association of Neuropsychology Students & Trainees website also offers support and helpful links to additional resources (https://scn40.org/anst/). Just remember to have a few trusted people review your essays before submitting them to catch any typos and make sure your writing is effective.

Tip 5: Seek letters of recommendation. When requesting letters of recommendation, specifically ask if they would be willing to write you a strong letter. While this verbiage may feel awkward, it will help avoid a mediocre letter of endorsement. In addition to a letter from your graduate school mentor/advisor, you should have at least one or two letters from a neuropsychologist who can speak to your clinical skills. You may also want to consider asking for a letter from a supervisor who is familiar with your intervention skills. A range of letter writers is particularly helpful when applying to programs that advertise themselves as strong generalist programs. Make sure you are paying attention to your overall application timeline and giving your letter writers a sufficient amount of time (at least a month) to prepare a well-thought-out letter.

Step 5: Attend the Interview(s)

At this point, all of your application materials have been submitted and now it is time to wait for the offers to roll in. During this down period, use your time wisely by preparing ahead of time a rough outline, calendar, or spreadsheet of all of the possible interview dates each site might offer and deciding for yourself what the best-case scenario for interviews would be. You can find these potential interview dates in program brochures, on the APPIC.org website, or on online forums. This plan will help when you need to respond very quickly (sometimes within minutes!) to interview offers in order to try to get the most preferred date. However, if for some reason, you are unable to make the offered interview dates work in your schedule, it is okay to reach out to the training director or committee and ask for alternative interview methods. Internship sites understand that this is a challenging time and some sites may be willing to accommodate you by offering the opportunity to interview by phone or through a platform like Skype or Zoom.

Tip 1: Be familiar with the various interview formats. Internship sites will interview in a variety of different formats. Some sites will have individual interviews throughout the day with one or more faculty members and trainees, while others will interview in a panel format (i.e., one applicant and several interviewers). It is also possible that you may be interviewed in a group with other applicants. In other instances, some sites may offer an all-day open house option that allows you to tour the facility and interview or speak with several of the staff members and trainees. No matter what the format is, though, you want to portray the best professional version of yourself. You should dress in professional attire, which typically means some variety of a business suit. However, try to add a pop of color or something distinctive that will help your interviewers remember who you are. Besides dressing professionally, you also want to make sure that your verbal and nonverbal behaviors are equally as polished and professional. It is strongly recommended that you ask a supervisor or mentor to do a mock interview with you. This not only helps you practice responding to questions, but they can help identify any behaviors that may distract your interviewer from your well-thought-out answer.

Tip 2: Prepare yourself for a range of interview questions. Be sure to adequately prepare for a variety of interview questions, including but not limited to your credentials and clinical experiences, goals and interests, research experiences and dissertation progress, strengths and weaknesses, ethical decision-making, multicultural considerations, case conceptualization, knowledge about neuropsychological measures (e.g., which measure might you update, what type of measure might be most clinically useful or is your "favorite"), and your background and hobbies. You may be asked to talk about a therapy or assessment case you have seen; the interviewer will want to see if you can present clinical information in a concise and clear way, and may also be listening for clues about your case conceptualization skills, theoretical orientation, and general clinical knowledge. While you may find that much of what you prepare will be useful at multiple sites, some of your preparation needs to be site-specific. Before your interview, review notes that you took about the site. Familiarize yourself with why you were attracted to the site in the first place, the rotations you are interested in, and the mentors you would like to work with. You should make the case for the "fit" between your goals and interests, and what this specific site has to offer. Make sure you are also prepared with questions to ask your interviewers or the current interns or postdocs. Asking appropriate questions indicates to your interviewers that you have taken the time to review their brochures and are genuinely interested in their program. Questions to consider asking include:

- What type of supervision might you expect to receive?
- Are there opportunities for tiered supervision?
- What types of didactics are there?
- What is the ratio of time testing versus training?
- What is a typical day for an intern?
- Approximately how many neuropsychological reports are written per week?
- Is research time protected or even expected of interns?
- Does the site have a postdoc position?
- Does the site encourage preparation for eventual board certification?

After the interview day, write down as many notes and impressions for the day as possible. These will be invaluable to you when preparing your rank order list. Many sites tend to blur together by the end of the interview season, and notes may help distinguish one site from another.

Step 6: Rank Internship Programs and Wait for Match Day

The psychology internship process culminates in a formal "match" administered by the National Matching Service (NMS). In the beginning of February, both applicants and sites rank their preferences, and a computer algorithm uses this ranking information to place individuals into available positions, with Match Day occurring in mid-February. If you would like a better understanding of the match process, the NMS website (https://natmatch.com/psychint-landing.html) provides an illustrative example of how the matching algorithm works, important dates, and a list of common misunderstandings associated with the match.

Tip 1: Consider how you want to rank internship programs. After completing your interviews, the next step is to review your notes and experiences from the interview process while keeping your internship goals in mind. Specifically, it is important to consider whether your goals, priorities, and interests have remained stable or have changed during the application process. Reflect on what was most important to you regarding the training opportunities offered across the various sites and create a hierarchy of training needs. At this point in time, you should review the notes you took during your interviews to refresh your memory on the various programs' training opportunities, faculty members and trainees, and anything else that stood out to you as being particularly attractive or deterring. Since the decision process for ranking programs can be particularly challenging, it may be helpful to create a spreadsheet that compares and rates sites across a number of important factors, including training environment, reputation, training fit, quality of interactions with faculty and trainees, quality of supervision, board-certification preparation, postdoctoral fellowship options and support, research opportunities, location, work–life balance, and cost of living. Create a list of pros and cons for each site and qualitatively compare them to one another. It is important to rank the programs based on your own preferences, without consideration of how you think the programs have ranked you. After you have created your rank list, enter and certify these rankings to the NMS website several days before the deadline to avoid any unforeseen issues. Even after you certify your rankings, you can continue to edit and resubmit them until the deadline.

Tip 2: Endure the waiting game. The wait of a couple weeks between the ranking deadline and Match Day can be particularly grueling. It is recommended to avoid dwelling on your ranking choices and to continue your normal everyday life. If you find yourself ruminating, use your clinical skills to identify and challenge negative thoughts and engage in more adaptive ways of thinking. The night before Match Day, it is important to engage in self-care! This could include spending time with friends or family, being alone, eating comfort foods, binge-watching TV, meditation, or exercising. Remind yourself that no matter the outcome, everything will be okay!

Tip 3: Look for your results on Match Day. Phase I match results are released by 10:00 a.m. Eastern Standard Time (EST) through the NMS website and are also sent to the email address that applicants specify on their APPIC application. Be sure to check your spam folder if you have not received a notification by the specified time. Beginning at 11:00 a.m. EST, internship DCTs can contact their respective matched applicants, so be prepared to answer a phone call from your new DCT.

Tip 4: Be familiar with what to do if you do not match. If you have learned that you have not matched in the Phase I process, take a deep breath and remember that it is not the end of the world. Due to the competitiveness of the match process, each year many qualified graduate students are not provided with an internship offer on Match Day. Phase II of the Match begins at 11:00 a.m. EST, when a list of programs with available positions is released. Applicants who are eligible to participate in Phase II of the Match will be able to submit applications to available programs beginning at 11:00 a.m. EST, with deadlines typically set for the following week. After the specified deadline, a second phase of ranking and matching occurs, with a Phase II Match Day typically held approximately 1 month after the Phase I Match Day. Following the Phase II Match, APPIC hosts a Post-Match Vacancy Service to assist unmatched applicants and unfilled sites.

If at the end of this process you are without a site match, then you can reapply the following year. Take this extra year to reflect on the previous year's application process, identify and correct any problems or issues that may have occurred (e.g., too narrow focus of training sites), and to work towards increasing your competitiveness for the next year. This may mean defending your dissertation, seeking additional research experiences, and/or completing additional clinical practica. In some instances, it may be appropriate to reach out to training directors and ask for feedback regarding your application (keeping in mind that not all training directors are willing or able to give feedback). Overall, an additional year can be viewed as an opportunity to further develop and refine your clinical and assessment skills, as well as your research productivity, to help ensure that you are successfully matched the second time around.

CONCLUSION AND FUTURE DIRECTIONS

Applying for internship may feel like a daunting task, especially when you have so many other graduate school and life responsibilities to manage. However, we hope we've inspired you to avoid procrastination and given you a plan for organizing yourself and your search. Reviewing our suggested timeline will help you plan for the amount of time the internship application process will take and may help you stay on track and avoid unnecessary worry or anxiety in the future. Remember to reach out to your peers—both the ones going through the application process alongside you and those who were recently accepted to an internship program or are finishing up their internship. Your graduate school advisors and faculty members are also resources for you. They can assist with reviewing your essays, cover letters, and CVs, and may also be able to practice a mock interview with you.

You will make it through the application process—just remember to keep your overarching goals in mind, stay organized, avoid procrastinating, take time to reward yourself for completing steps in the process, and keep breathing.

REFERENCES

American Board of Professional Psychology (ABPP). (n.d.). *General requirements.* https://www.abpp.org/Applicant-Information/Degree-Requirements.aspx

APA Commission on Accreditation (APA CoA). (2015). Implementing regulations: Section C: IRs related to the standards of accreditation. Washington, DC: American Psychological Association. http://www.apa.org/ed/accreditation/section-c-soa.pdf

Association of Psychology Postdoctoral and Internship Centers (APPIC). (2021). *Integrated report.* https://www.appic.org/Internships/AAPI/Integrated-Report

Bieliauskas, L. A., & Matthews, C. G. (1987). American Board of Clinical Neuro-psychology: Policies and procedures. *Clinical Neuropsychologist, 1*(1), 21–28. https://doi.org/10.1080/13854048708520032

Hannay, H. J., Bieliauskas, L. A., Crosson, B. A., Harmneke, T. A., Hamsher, K. deS., & Koffler, S. P. (1998). Proceedings of the Houston conference on specialty education and training in clinical neuropsychology. *Archives of Clinical Neuropsychology, 13*(2), 157–158. https://doi.org/10.1093/arclin/13.2.160

INS/Division 40 Task Force. (1987). Reports of the INS/Division 40 task force on education, accreditation, and credentialing. *The Clinical Neuropsychologist, 1*(1), 29–34. https://doi.org/10.1080/13854048708520033

Keilin, G. (2017, February 13). *Applicant survey 2016 part 2.* Association of Psychology Postdoctoral and Internship Centers (APPIC). https://appic.org/Internships/Match/Match-Statistics/Applicant-Survey-2016-Part-2

Keilin, G. (2018, December 30). *Applicant survey 2018 part 1.* Association of Psychology Postdoctoral and Internship Centers (APPIC). https://appic.org/Internships/Match/Match-Statistics/Applicant-Survey-2018-Part-1

Ritchie, D., Odland, A. P., Ritchie, A. S., & Mittenberg, W. (2012). Selection criteria for internships in clinical neuropsychology. *The Clinical Neuropsychologist, 26*(8), 1245–1254. https://doi.org/10.1080/13854046.2012.727871

Sperling, S. A., Cimino, C. R., Stricker, N. H., Heffelfinger, A. K., Gess, J. L., Osborn, K. E., & Roper, B. L. (2017). *Taxonomy for Education and Training in Clinical Neuropsychology*: Past, present, and future. *The Clinical Neuropsychologist, 31*(5), 817–828. https://doi.org/10.1080/13854046.2017.1314017

Whiteside, D. M., Guidotti Breting, L. M., Butts, A. M., Hahn-Ketter, A. E., Osborn, K., Towns, S. J., Barisa, M., Santos, O. A., & Smith, D. (2016). 2015 American Academy of Clinical Neuropsychology (AACN) student affairs committee survey of neuropsychology trainees. *The Clinical Neuropsychologist, 30*(5), 664–694. https://doi.org/10.1080/13854046.2016.1196731

Williams-Nickelson, C., Prinstein, M. J., & Keilin, W. G. (2019). *Internships in psychology: The APAGS Workbook for Writing Successful Applications and Finding the Right Fit* (4th ed.). American Psychological Association.

3

PREPARING FOR AND OBTAINING A POSTDOCTORAL FELLOWSHIP

DOUGLAS BODIN

Postdoctoral training in neuropsychology is the final stage in preparation for independent practice or research in neuropsychology. During the postdoctoral phase, emerging neuropsychologists receive 2 years of intensive and structured clinical, research, and didactic training. It is also at this stage that students refine various professional skills, such as ethical, cross-cultural, supervisory, and interdisciplinary skill sets. Although not required for clinical practice in most states, a 2-year postdoctoral fellowship is required for board certification in clinical neuropsychology. The goal of this chapter is to provide a review of the history of postdoctoral training in clinical neuropsychology, as well as guidance on how applicants can navigate the selection process, such as identifying programs, completing applications, and interviewing for positions.

HISTORICAL CONTEXT OF THE NEUROPSYCHOLOGY POSTDOCTORAL FELLOWSHIP

Prior to the 1970s, postdoctoral training in neuropsychology was largely obtained through unstructured or semistructured apprenticeships. Students would find supervised postdoctoral experiences through word of mouth or

https://doi.org/10.1037/0000250-004
The Neuropsychologist's Roadmap: A Training and Career Guide, C. Block (Editor)

personal contact from their graduate school mentors. As the profession of neuropsychology became more widely recognized in the 1960s and 1970s, particular attention was given to developing training guidelines (Meier, 1998). The International Neuropsychological Society (INS) formed the Task Force on Education, Accreditation, and Credentialing (TFEAC) in the 1970s to begin establishing education and training guidelines for neuropsychology. TFEAC published training guidelines at the doctoral, internship, and post-doctoral levels (INS-Division 40 Task Force, 1987). These guidelines became widely known at the INS/Division 40 Training Guidelines and defined the minimal qualifications to practice as a neuropsychologist as completion of a doctoral degree and an internship with at least 50% experience in neuro-psychology. As such, completion of postdoctoral training was not a requirement for independent practice under the INS-Division 40 guidelines. However, these guidelines defined postdoctoral training as designed to produce an advanced level of competence in neuropsychology. The TFEAC document essentially created two tiers of independent neuropsychologists: (a) those who met minimal qualifications and entered practice after internship and (b) those who met advanced competency by completing formal postdoctoral training.

In 1996, clinical neuropsychology was recognized by the American Psychological Association (APA) as a specialty. As part of this process, the Clinical Neuropsychology Synarchy (CNS) was developed to serve as a forum for specialty organizations to discuss issues facing neuropsychology. Members of the CNS began discussing holding a training conference to develop an integrated model of training in neuropsychology (Bieliauskas, 1998) and this discussion ultimately led to the Houston Conference on Specialty Education and Training in Clinical Neuropsychology held in September 1997 (Hannay et al., 1998). The delegates were tasked with creating an "aspirational, inte-grated model of specialty training in neuropsychology" across the doctoral, internship, and postdoctoral levels (Hannay et al., 1998). The Houston Conference Guidelines specify that completion of a 2-year postdoctoral train-ing program is necessary for independent practice in neuropsychology, an important departure from the INS/Division 40 guidelines. The Houston Conference Guidelines specify that postdoctoral training consist of 2 years of full-time clinical, didactic, and research training.

As clinical neuropsychology began to mature during the 1970s and 1980s, and somewhat simultaneous with the development of the above-mentioned training guidelines, formal postdoctoral training programs were developed. In 1988, a group of neuropsychology postdoctoral programs formed the Midwest Neuropsychology Consortium initially to promote the TFEAC training guidelines (Hammeke, 1993). In 1991, the American Board of Professional Psychology (ABPP) sponsored a conference on accreditation of postdoctoral programs in professional psychology that led to a call for specific specialties to develop national organizations of postdoctoral program directors. Following this call, the Midwest Neuropsychology Consortium hosted a meeting of 27 postdoctoral program directors, which led to the formation of the Association of Postdoctoral Programs in Clinical Neuropsychology (APPCN; Hammeke, 1993).

APPCN was incorporated in 1994 as a nonprofit organization with the mission to "foster the development of advanced postdoctoral education and training in clinical neuropsychology and the establishment of residency program standards designed to provide the competency necessary for specialized practice" (Boake et al., 2002). APPCN member programs complete a self-study that describes the program faculty, facilities, clinical activities, didactics, and research opportunities. Member programs include a program director who is board certified by ABCN; a minimum of 2 years of full-time training; and the provision of at least 50% clinical service, 10% didactic activities, and 10% research or scholarly activities. APPCN endorses the Houston Conference Guidelines, as well as board certification (https://www.appcn.org). APPCN has grown substantially as an organization since its inception and now has over 100 member programs. Member programs have access to several training resources including video didactic talks, mock oral exams, and a mock written exam. APPCN program directors also have access to an email listserv for discussing postdoctoral training issues.

Early in the history of APPCN, the organization planned to formally accredit postdoctoral programs in neuropsychology (Boake et al., 2002). However, in the 1990s the APA Council of Representatives tasked the Commission on Accreditation (CoA), to develop postdoctoral accreditation standards for professional psychology. APPCN worked with the CoA to develop specialty postdoctoral accreditation procedures that were eventually approved in 1992. The APA accreditation process for postdoctoral programs involves an extensive self-study document and a site visit from trained evaluators. Programs can apply for specialty accreditation in clinical neuropsychology and the first of such programs were approved in 2002 (Boake, 2008). APA accreditation at the postdoctoral level is not as widely adopted as is accreditation at the internship level. There are several reasons for this, including the fact that several states no longer require postdoctoral hours for licensure. Currently, 42 postdoctoral programs are accredited by APA in neuropsychology, with the majority being Veterans Administration (VA) hospitals (American Psychological Association, 2018). That said, the number of APA-accredited postdoctoral programs in neuropsychology has steadily increased over the past decade and will most likely continue to rise.

Recent developments in the education and training of neuropsychologists that are important to be aware of are the movement towards competency-based education and the creation of a taxonomy to described training opportunities (Smith, 2018). The competency-based movement in education and training specifies functional and foundational competencies that should be achieved during training (Rodolfa et al., 2005). This competency movement was first applied to neuropsychology by Rey-Casserly et al. (2012) and was specifically applied to the postdoctoral stage of training by the CNS (Smith, 2018). These specific competency areas can be used by postdoctoral training programs to design curriculum and evaluate fellows' progress towards training goals. The taxonomy document (Sperling et al., 2017) was developed to assist training programs and trainees in describing the intensity of specific training experiences by defining terms such as Exposure, Experience, and Major Area of Study (Sperling et al., 2017). Applicants to postdoctoral training programs should become familiar with the taxonomy document when describing specific training experiences in their CVs and other application materials.

POSTDOCTORAL FELLOWSHIP PROGRAM STRUCTURE

Consistent with the Houston Conference Guidelines and the APA Commission for the Recognition of Specialties and Subspecialties in Professional Psychology taxonomy, postdoctoral programs in neuropsychology consist of 2 years of full-time clinical, research, and didactic experiences. The majority of neuropsychology postdoctoral programs are hospital or medical center based and tend to be either adult-focused or pediatric-focused, although there are several programs that offer a lifespan experience for trainees. There is quite a bit of variability in terms of how different programs structure their training experiences. Students are advised to closely study program brochures and websites when they are considering applying to different programs. Since postdoctoral training is specialty-focused, students should expect that all experiences outlined in the programs will be neuropsychology-focused. As such, neuropsychology should be the major area of study at this training stage, not merely an exposure or an experience (Sperling et al., 2017).

As discussed elsewhere in this book, general and specialty specific competencies are becoming the focus of many neuropsychology training programs (Rey-Casserly et al., 2012). Most programs offer a combination of outpatient and inpatient experiences. Some programs have specific rotations based on clinical populations (e.g., epilepsy rotation, traumatic brain injury rotation), whereas other programs are structured to provide access to different clinical populations simultaneously throughout both training years. Supervision should be provided by a program faculty member for each case, either in individual or group formats. Regularly scheduled didactics are an essential component of postdoctoral training. As such, applicants are encouraged to only consider programs that offer formal structured didactics. Didactics vary between programs but might include activities such as neuropsychology seminar, neuroanatomy courses, brain cutting, epilepsy surgery conference, brain tumor board meetings, grand rounds, and research presentations. Students should expect some research or scholarly component of their postdoctoral training. In fact, many programs require a formal research project. This commonly involves collaborating with a faculty member using existing data or it could involve an original data collection project. Attendance at professional conferences is encouraged at the postdoctoral level and is often financially supported, although this varies among programs. Finally, many programs offer experiences in learning how to supervise others as part of postdoctoral training.

A final note about postdoctoral program structure pertains to how postdoctoral trainees are titled by different programs. There is no universal agreement on this, as some programs refer to postdoctoral trainees as "residents" and some refer to postdoctoral trainees as "fellows." These terms are often used interchangeably when discussing postdoctoral training. For the sake of consistency with the rest of this text, we use the term "postdoctoral fellow." Presented below is each phase of the application and interview process, with helpful tips noted for each phase.

STEPS TOWARD SECURING A PREDOCTORAL INTERNSHIP IN NEUROPSYCHOLOGY

Step 1: Identify Programs of Interest

For most individuals, the timeline of obtaining a postdoctoral fellowship in clinical neuropsychology begins soon after they start internship (see Figure 3.1). I recommend that students join various student groups, such as the Society for Clinical Neuropsychology (APA Division 40) Association for Neuropsychology Students in Training (ANST), and have a trusted mentor to help guide them through this process. Additional steps and tips are noted in Table 3.1.

FIGURE 3.1. Timeline of the Postdoctoral Selection Process

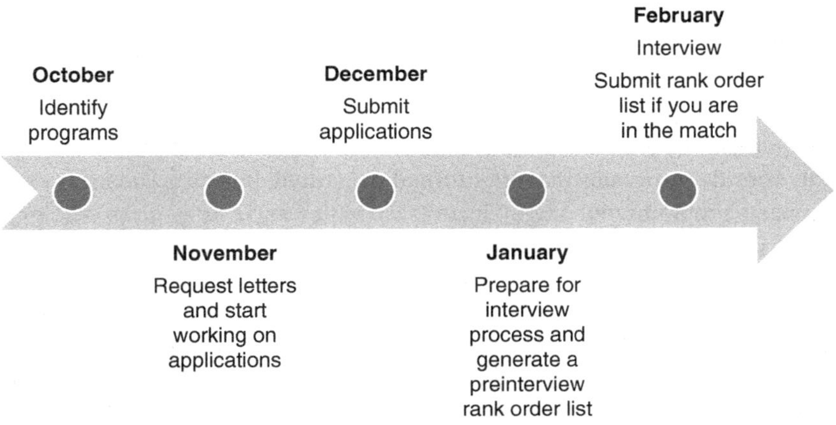

February
Interview
October Submit rank order
Identify list if you are
programs in the match
December
Submit
applications

November **January**
Request letters Prepare for
and start interview
working on process and
applications generate a
preinterview
rank order list

TABLE 3.1. Steps and Tips for Getting a Postdoctoral Fellowship in Neuropsychology

Step	Suggestion
1	Identify programs of interest.
	Tip 1: Start the process early.
	Tip 2: Look for program announcements.
	Tip 3: Join neuropsychology listservs.
	Tip 4: Talk with your mentor and consult other valued sources.
2	Prepare your application.
	Tip 1: Prepare and personalize a cover letter.
	Tip 2: Update your curriculum vitae.
	Tip 3: Identify (then de-identify) good sample reports.
	Tip 4: Request letters of recommendation.
3	Submit your application.
	Tip 1: Know the submission requirements for each program.
	Tip 2: Apply to enough (but not too many) programs.
4	Interview for fellowship programs.
	Tip 1: Secure time off to attend the INS North American meeting.
	Tip 2: Come prepared and be engaged.
	Tip 3: Meet with current fellows.
	Tip 4: Be familiar with match rules.
5	Select a fellowship program.
	Review the FAQs in this section of the chapter.

Note. INS = International Neuropsychological Society; FAQs = frequently asked questions.

Tip 1: Start the process early! The first step in obtaining a postdoctoral training position in neuropsychology is researching different programs to determine which programs have openings and are consistent with your interests and training goals. Students should expect to begin this process in October of their internship year (or the year in which they are applying).

Tip 2: Look for program announcements. This process can be more difficult than at the internship stage because there is no one universal list of available programs. Students have to explore several different websites or email listservs to find listings of available programs. Programs with specialty accreditation can be found on the APA accreditation page (https://www.apa.org/ed/accreditation/programs/specialty.aspx). Programs that are members of APPCN have listings at https://www.appcn.org that are updated annually to indicate which programs are actively recruiting. As mentioned in the previous section, not all programs are APA-accredited and/or an APPCN member, so know that these are not the only two sources of information that students should rely on. In fact, there are many excellent postdoctoral training programs that are not APA accredited or members of APPCN. The SCN maintains a listing of postdoctoral programs at https://www.scn40.org/training-directory. This listing is voluntary and may not include every potentially available postdoctoral position.

Recently, the Association of Psychology Postdoctoral and Internship Centers (APPIC) has become actively engaged in addressing this issue by creating a Universal Psychology Postdoctoral Directory (UPPD) that includes voluntary listings of APPIC member and nonmember postdoctoral training programs in multiple specialties. The UPPD can be found at https://www.appic.org/Postdocs/Universal-Psychology-Postdoctoral-Directory-UPPD and can be searched by specialty and location. Unfortunately, not all neuropsychology programs have adopted the UPPD, though this listing may become the preferred source of program listings in the future.

Tip 3: Join neuropsychology listservs. In addition to the previously mentioned websites, postdoctoral program directors frequently post announcements for available positions on various email listservs. Unfortunately, there is no one source of information out there on which neuropsychology listservs are active and how to subscribe to them. For students, a good start would be to subscribe to the listserv offered by the SCN ANST. Instructions for joining the ANST listserv can be found at https://www.scn40.org/anst/anst-listserv/.

Tip 4: Talk with your mentor and consult other valued sources. Talking with mentors about other active listservs and getting information about current subscription procedures is strongly encouraged. Personal contact and word of mouth are also good ways of hearing about post-doctoral programs that are recruiting. Joining student groups such as the SCN ANST is also strongly advised to provide support and additional resources. Finally, many postdoctoral programs are housed at institutions that also have doctoral internship training programs. Researching places that you applied to for internship to determine if they also offer postdoctoral training could be an additional valuable source of information. Once you have a list of programs that fit your interest and training goals, share it with colleagues and mentors so that you can begin preparing application materials and eliminating programs that may not be a good fit for you.

Step 2: Prepare Your Application

Applying to postdoctoral programs in neuropsychology is also not as straight-forward as applying at the internship stage. Because position announcements or listings are commonly publicized in October of each year, students need to start thinking about the application process shortly after many internships have started. Application deadlines vary but typically occur in December or January. There is no universal application for postdoctoral training like there is for doctoral internship.

Tip 1: Prepare and personalize a cover letter. Application materials will vary from site to site, but students should expect to prepare a cover letter for each site specifying your interest in the program and outlining how you are a good fit for their training program. This is important as programs tend to receive applications from more students than they will be able to interview. Do not just use the cover letter as a means to repeat what you have listed in your CV. Instead, use your cover letter as an opportunity to "stand out" in some noticeable way. You can do this by briefly highlighting relevant training and defining how you are a good fit—as well as highlight areas of need in your training that a particular program happens to offer. You should plan on personalizing your cover letter to each program. Cover letters should be no longer than 1 to 2 pages in length, maximum.

Tip 2: Update your curriculum vitae. Another typical application component is an updated curriculum vitae (CV). Your CV should highlight relevant graduate experiences and rotations that you have not yet completed on internship (remember that programs will be looking at your materials early in your internship year). If you have a scheduled internship rotation later in the year that has a neuropsychological focus, you should list that on your CV.

Tip 3: Identify (then de-identify) good sample reports. Typical post-doctoral fellowship applications require two to three sample neuro-psychological evaluation reports that candidates have conducted either in graduate school or internship. Work with your mentor(s) to identify and select good representative reports. If possible, sample reports should be similar to the populations available to each program to which you are applying. For example, if you are applying to pediatric neuropsychology programs, choosing child and adolescent cases would be most appropriate. If possible, choose medical populations for your sample reports if the programs to which you are applying are hospital-based. Sample reports should be redacted to exclude any protected health information (PHI) such as patient names, referral names, dates, and so on. Carefully proof-read to eliminate unintentional inclusion of PHI in your sample reports! This includes (but is not limited to) all names, medical record numbers, social security numbers, account numbers, telephone and fax numbers, and addresses.

Tip 4: Request letters of recommendation. Most programs will also require two to three letters of recommendation from professionals who are familiar with your work. Programs will typically specify the number of letters of recommendation required for the application. If a program does not specify a number, three letters would be enough to provide a good perspective on your previous work. Ideally, these letters should be from neuropsychologists who are familiar with your clinical or research work. That said, if one letter is from a nonneuropsychologist who can say good things about your work, then it is safe to use this letter. You do not have to have letters from famous neuropsychologists! Given the December/January application deadlines, you should approach your letter writers sometime in October or early November to ask them if they will write a letter for you. What this means is that you may have only worked with an internship supervisor for a month or two before you ask them for a letter. Fear not! Your mentor(s) should be used to this, and they can still talk about the work you have done (and will continue to do) on internship. You do not have to ask for a letter from your internship director if you have other letter writers who can better speak to your neuropsychology training. Most applicants also ask for letters from a graduate school mentor and/or practicum supervisor. You are not required to ask your dissertation advisor or graduate school mentor for a letter if you think that other individuals can provide more relevant letters. Again, asking for advice from colleagues and other mentors would be helpful to your individual situation.

Step 3: Submit Your Application

Tip 1: Know the submission requirements for each program. Now that you have assembled your application materials, you will need to determine how each program wants you to submit your application. Currently, most programs will likely request some form of electronic application submission. That said, there may be a few programs that still prefer that applicants mail hard copies of their applications materials. If this is the case, make sure that you have the materials ready and mailed so that they arrive in time for the deadline. Pay attention to any holidays that might delay the mail! Many programs will want you to electronically submit applications by email directly to the training director or to an administrative staff member. Just make sure that you are scanning in and attaching the correct documents for each application. It makes applicants look careless if they send a cover letter to program A but it is worded for program B. Double-check!

Several programs have begun to use an internet-based application service offered by APPIC called the APPIC Psychology Postdoctoral Application Centralized Application System (APPA CAS). There is a monetary fee for submitting each application but there are several advantages to using APPA CAS, such as having letter writers submit letters directly to the system and being able to track the status of your application materials. This process is very similar to the APPIC Application for Psychology Internships online submission that you did for internship (AAPI OnLine). The difference is that most postdoctoral programs have not yet adopted the APPA CAS. Chances are, you will email some applications directly to programs and some via APPA CAS.

Tip 2: Apply to enough (but not too many) programs. Students frequently ask for advice on how many programs they should apply to. Each year, there is an imbalance, in that there are more applicants than there are programs. Applying to only a few programs could lessen your chances of finding a postdoctoral program. If you are not geographically restricted, you will increase your chances of finding a position by applying to more than just a few programs. How much is enough? There is not a hard and fast rule but most candidates apply to anywhere from eight to 12 programs. Again, having a trusted mentor who knows your circumstances will be valuable in helping you decide on the number of programs to which you will apply.

Step 4: Interview for Fellowship Programs

Tip 1: Secure time off to attend the INS North American meeting. The interview process for neuropsychology postdoctoral training is structured around the timing of the North American meeting of the INS. Historically, most programs have chosen to interview postdoctoral applicants at the INS conference, which is typically held in early to mid-February. Programs should specify if they plan on interviewing at INS. Some programs prefer to do either on-site or virtual interviews prior to the INS meeting, but the majority do interview at INS. As a result, you should request permission from your internship director (if you are applying during your internship year) well in advance to attend the INS meeting.

Typically, many programs reserve the Tuesday of INS week (the meeting starts on Wednesday) as their day to interview applicants. This is commonly called "INS interview day." You should plan to arrive at the conference city on Monday and stay for as long as allowed. The bulk of your interviews might be on Tuesday, but you may have interviews spread throughout the rest of the conference. Interviewing at INS is an interesting and busy experience to say the least. While very efficient, the downside is that you do not get to see the training site itself and have limited time for each program. So you need to be prepared! You will likely meet with several different programs in a relatively short period of time. Interviews might range from 30 minutes to 90 minutes and could include multiple faculty members or just one.

Tip 2: Come prepared and be engaged. For each of your interviews, have prepared notes handy for each program listing specific experiences or faculty that stand out as a good fit for you. Bring copies of your CV in case interviewing faculty members do not have one available. Having one copy of other application materials would be sufficient. Also, have questions that you would like to ask ready (even if you think you already know the answer; see Table 3.2 for sample interview questions). When applicants do not have many questions, interviewers often interpret that as lack of interest. Jot down notes during your interviews. If you are meeting with multiple programs in one day, you will quickly get the different programs and faculty mixed up in your head without notes. This also happens to faculty, who are sometimes interviewing 12 to 15 applicants in one day.

Tip 3: Meet with current fellows. In addition to meeting with program faculty, it is crucial to meet with existing postdoctoral trainees at each program. They can provide you their perspective on the training program, site, and faculty. Many programs arrange for times for existing trainees to be available during the INS meeting. Alternatively, they can be reached by email and telephone. Regardless of whether or not these meetings are simply informational, come as prepared and engaged as you would to any of your faculty interviews. Be yourself, but be your best self. Current fellows may not play a direct role in ranking candidates, but training faculty do

TABLE 3.2. Sample Interview Questions

Domain	Sample questions
Asked by interviewer(s)	✓ How did you become interested in neuropsychology?
	✓ What sort of populations have you worked with? Which do you enjoy most?
	✓ What are your goals for fellowship? After fellowship?
	✓ What would you like to know about our program?
	✓ What are your research interests?
	✓ What is the current status of your dissertation?
	✓ Tell us about a recent neuropsychological case you've seen. How did you arrive at your final diagnosis? What would you have done differently?
	✓ Tell us about an ethical dilemma that you faced. How was this resolved?
Asked by candidate	*To faculty:*
	✓ What do you consider your program's strengths and weaknesses?
	✓ Can you describe a typical week for a fellow?
	✓ Do you anticipate staffing and/or rotation changes in the next two years?
	✓ Where have previous fellows ended up?
	✓ What characteristics do successful fellows in your program have?
	✓ How does the program help prepare fellows for board certification?
	✓ Do fellows have productivity expectations for billing?
	✓ Do fellows receive training in how to deal with insurance companies?
	To current trainees:
	✓ How are fellows treated by faculty and staff?
	✓ What do you like best about this site? Least?
	✓ Did anything surprise you about this program?
	✓ Has this program been consistent with what was advertised?
	✓ What is your typical week like?

listen to their input when considering candidates. If you are presenting at the INS meeting, be aware that program faculty or existing fellows might go to your poster session and ask questions.

Tip 4: Be familiar with match rules. After completing your interviews, you may or may not be contacted directly by the programs for follow-up talks. You should not assume that programs that do not contact you in the days following interviews are not interested in you. It is acceptable to email program faculty to ask follow-up questions or to thank them for meeting with you. You also are permitted to ask about the general status of your application (i.e., if you are in their top group or no longer being considered as a candidate). You cannot ask for specific rank information, however.

Step 5: Select a Fellowship Program

The selection process for neuropsychology postdoctoral positions is not without controversy and can be stressful for applicants. A brief history is provided here with a description of the current selection process; there is a small but recent literature describing in more detail the postdoctoral recruitment and selection process (Belanger et al., 2013; Bodin et al., 2018). Prior to 1994, there was no organized process for making and accepting offers for postdoctoral training in neuropsychology. Programs had various application deadlines and timelines for extending offers. In 1994, the APPCN organized a uniform notification date (UND) where participating program directors would call applicants and make offers based on a preferential rank order. This process was somewhat of an improvement, but was still considered stressful and problematic (Boake et al., 2002). In 2001, the APPCN partnered with National Matching Services (NMS) to operate a computerized match for neuropsychology postdoctoral training. The APPCN-NMS postdoctoral match for neuropsychology continues to operate to this day. Students should be aware, however, that not all postdoctoral programs participate in the match. The pros and cons of having a computerized match and the current controversy regarding this is beyond the scope of this chapter. The interested reader should review recent publications addressing recruitment and selection (Belanger et al., 2013; Bodin & Grote, 2016a, 2016b; Bodin et al., 2015, 2018; Nelson et al., 2016).

APPCN member programs are required to participate in the match, and independent programs can participate in the match provided that their training meets the Houston Conference Guidelines. As mentioned earlier, there are many excellent independent postdoctoral programs in existence. Some of these independent programs participate in the match and some do not. Anecdotally, it seems that most pediatric focused neuropsychology postdoctoral programs participate in the match. In addition, there seem to be fewer programs in the Northeast and West Coast that choose to participate in the match. What these means is that you may apply to several "match programs" and several "nonmatch" programs. Many independent programs operate on a similar timeline as the APPCN programs, in that they have deadlines in December and January and invite applicants to interview at INS. However, some independent programs choose to interview candidates before INS. Independent programs will sometimes make offers of acceptance either before or during INS. This can be stressful for candidates because they have to make a decision to accept or decline this offer before they have finished interviewing with other programs. Be prepared for this possibility if you apply to both "match" and "nonmatch" programs. Be familiar with NMS match rules and guidelines (https://natmatch.com/appcnmat). Answers to some frequently asked questions regarding program selection and matching follow.

FAQ 1: What do I do if I receive a nonmatch offer prior to the rank order list deadline for the match? You can ask for further information from the match programs on your list about where you stand with them. Note that if your nonmatch offer comes during INS, the match programs are still interviewing and may not be able to provide you with definitive information. Have a mental ranking of the programs to which you applied based on all the information that you have, and think about where that program is in your preferential ranking. If that program is your top choice based on your personal and professional preferences, then it could make sense to accept the offer and withdraw from the match. If you do this, communicate your decision to other programs on your list.

FAQ 2: What happens if I receive an offer from a nonmatch program that is not at the top of my list of preferences? Or, what happens if I receive a nonmatch offer before I have the chance to interview with other programs? This is where the process can be quite difficult to manage. You could ask the program for more time, but there is no guarantee of this being granted. You could decline the offer and proceed with the match. Alternatively, you could accept this offer and withdraw from the match. Having a trusted mentor "on-call" to help problem-solve in the event of this situation is recommended. This mentor could be a previous or current supervisor who is familiar with your individual circumstances.

FAQ 3: How do I make my rank order list? I strongly recommend having a trusted mentor or colleague on-call and available to process this decision, if you decide to apply to match and nonmatch programs. This should be a neuropsychologist (or trainee who has gone through the process) who knows your personal circumstances (i.e., geographic restrictions, family factors, professional interests/goals) and can help you think through nonmatch offers and make a decision on how to proceed. If you apply to only match programs, the process will be more like what you experienced for internship. I recommend generating a preinterview rank order list of programs based on your preferences prior to the interviews. After finishing your interviews, speaking with existing postdoctoral trainees, and reviewing each program's training experiences, you will generate a final rank order list based on your preferences. You will likely have both personal and professional factors in mind when generating this list. It is important to consider both of these factors because it is not uncommon for neuropsychologists to end up taking their first job at the institution where they did their postdoctoral training. Again, having a trusted mentor or colleague to help think about your rankings is advised. The match dates and deadlines vary each year, but typically the rank order list has deadline is 7 to 10 days after the conclusion of the INS meeting. Make sure you accurately enter and certify your rank order list. After the rank order list deadline, there is typically a 1- to 2-week wait before the match results are released. You will be notified by email of your match.

FAQ 4: What if I do not match? Unfortunately, every year there are more applicants than available positions in the match. Qualified applicants sometimes do not match. This is more likely to happen if you are geographically restricted and only rank two or three programs. If you do not match, do not give up! NMS releases a listing of available positions after the match at noon Eastern Time on Match Day. In addition, there are some really good postdoctoral programs that become available after the match because of new funding sources or positions that were pending budget approval that occurred after the match. Keep your eye on the listservs. Talk with mentors; they may know someone who has an open position. Students sometimes decide to wait a year and go through the process again. As disappointing as this sounds, you could use that year to bolster areas of your CV that would increase chances of matching.

CONCLUSION AND FUTURE DIRECTIONS

Postdoctoral training in neuropsychology has evolved over the relatively young history of the specialty. This evolution will likely continue to occur. Postdoctoral training programs will need to develop competency-based models of training, including creating ways to measure successful attainment of specified competencies. Given changing demographics, a focus on multicultural competency has been and will continue to be an important focus of training. With the ever-changing health care landscape, postdoctoral trainees will need to be educated on how the health care system works, how to advocate for neuropsychology services, and how to shift practice in response to the health care environment. For example, taking neuropsychology out of the testing room and into interdisciplinary settings has been and will continue to be important. Obtaining and completing postdoctoral training in neuropsychology is a significant accomplishment. Essential clinical and research skills will be solidified and you will learn how to be a professional independent neuropsychologist!

REFERENCES

American Psychological Association. (2018). *APA-accredited programs.* http://www.apa.org/ed/accreditation/programs/specialty.aspx

Belanger, H. G., Vanderploeg, R. D., Silva, M. A., Cimino, C. R., Roper, B. L., & Bodin, D. (2013). Postdoctoral recruitment in neuropsychology: A review and call for inter-organizational action. *The Clinical Neuropsychologist, 27*(2), 159–175. https://doi.org/10.1080/13854046.2012.758780

Bieliauskas, L. (1998). History and background of the conference. *Archives of Clinical Neuropsychology, 13*(2), 167–168. https://doi.org/10.1093/arclin/13.2.167

Boake, C. (2008). Clinical neuropsychology. *Professional Psychology, Research and Practice, 39*(2), 234–239. https://doi.org/10.1037/0735-7028.39.2.234

Boake, C., Yeates, K. O., & Donders, J. (2002). Association of postdoctoral programs in clinical neuropsychology: Update and new directions. *The Clinical Neuropsychologist, 16*(1), 1–6. https://doi.org/10.1076/clin.16.1.1.8333

Bodin, D., & Grote, C. L. (2016a). Commentary: The postdoctoral residency match in clinical neuropsychology. *The Clinical Neuropsychologist, 30*(5), 641–650. https://doi.org/10.1080/13854046.2016.1199737

Bodin, D., & Grote, C. L. (2016b). Rebuttal to Nelson et al. 'Response to Bodin and Grote regarding postdoctoral recruitment in clinical neuropsychology'. *The Clinical Neuropsychologist, 30*(5), 660–663. https://doi.org/10.1080/13854046.2016.1199738

Bodin, D., Roper, B. L., O'Toole, K., & Haines, M. E. (2015). Postdoctoral training in neuropsychology: A review of the history, trends, and current issues. *Training and Education in Professional Psychology, 9*(2), 99–104. https://doi.org/10.1037/tep0000057

Bodin, D., Schmidt, J. P., Lemle, R. B., Roper, B. L., Goldberg, R. W., Hill, K. R., Perry-Parrish, C., Williams, S. E., Kuemmel, A., & Siegel, W. (2018). Recruitment and selection in health service psychology postdoctoral training: A review of the history and current trends. *Training and Education in Professional Psychology, 12*(2), 74–81. https://doi.org/10.1037/tep0000181

Hammeke, T. A. (1993). The association of postdoctoral programs in clinical neuro-psychology (APPCN). *Clinical Neuropsychologist, 7*(2), 197–204. https://doi.org/10.1080/13854049308401522

Hannay, J., Bieliauskas, L., Crosson, B. A., Hammeke, T. A., Hamsher, K. deS., & Koffler, S. P. (1998). Proceedings of the Houston conference on specialty education and training in clinical neuropsychology. *Archives of Clinical Neuropsychology, 13*(2), 157–250. https://doi.org/10.1093/arclin/13.2.160

INS-Division 40 Task Force. (1987). Report of the INS-Division 40 task force on education, accreditation, and credentialing. *The Clinical Neuropsychologist, 1*(1), 29–34. https://doi.org/10.1080/13854048708520033

Meier, M. (1998). Developmental milestones in the specialty of clinical neuro-psychology. *Archives of Clinical Neuropsychology, 13*(2), 174–176. https://doi.org/10.1093/arclin/13.2.174

Nelson, A., Bilder, R. M., O'Connor, M., Brandt, J., Weintraub, S., & Bauer, R. M. (2016). Response to Bodin and Grote regarding postdoctoral recruitment in clinical neuropsychology. *The Clinical Neuropsychologist, 30*(5), 651–659. https://doi.org/10.1080/13854046.2016.1188990

Rey-Casserly, C., Roper, B. L., & Bauer, R. M. (2012). Application of a competency model to clinical neuropsychology. *Professional Psychology: Research and Practice, 43*(5), 422–431. https://doi.org/10.1037/a0028721

Rodolfa, E. R., Bent, R. J., Eisman, E., Nelson, P. D., Rehm, L., & Ritchie, P. (2005). A cube model for competency development: Implications for psychology educators and regulators. *Professional Psychology, Research and Practice, 36*(4), 347–354. https://doi.org/10.1037/0735-7028.36.4.347

Smith, G. (2018). Education and training in clinical neuropsychology: Recent developments and documents from the clinical neuropsychology synarchy. *Archives of Clinical Neuropsychology, 34*(3), 418–431. https://doi.org/10.1093/arclin/acy075

Sperling, S. A., Cimino, C. R., Stricker, N. H., Heffelfinger, A. K., Gess, J. L., Osborn, K. E., & Roper, B. L. (2017). *Taxonomy for Education and Training in Clinical Neuropsychology*: Past, present, and future. *The Clinical Neuropsychologist, 31*(5), 817–828. https://doi.org/10.1080/13854046.2017.1314017

4 PROFESSIONAL LICENSURE AND CREDENTIALING

JOSEPH ACKERSON AND CADY BLOCK

You've now had that very, very satisfying and well-deserved walk across the stage as the recipient of a doctoral degree. You may have even framed your diploma already. However, as the infomercials often say: But wait! There's more! Graduation means the end of formal coursework but the beginning of professional licensure and credentialing. You have mastered jumping through hoops and overcoming obstacles, so with a little guidance and direction, you can complete the process to becoming a fully licensed, practicing neuropsychologist. By following this section of your guidebook, you can navigate the potential perils of obtaining (and maintaining) your psychology license and understand the potential benefits of pursuing advanced credentials in your chosen specialty.

The United States takes the well-being of its citizens seriously, and as a result, psychologists and neuropsychologists are required to go through a rigorous licensure process to prove their qualifications for professional practice. Licensure occurs at the state level, primarily overseen by a given state's psychology board—a group of individuals authorized through state law to regulate the standards and practice of psychology. The licensure process can vary from state to state, meaning that applicants must be cognizant of

https://doi.org/10.1037/0000250-005
The Neuropsychologist's Roadmap: A Training and Career Guide, C. Block (Editor)

the particular requirements and procedures required of the state in which they wish to practice. That being said, individuals who work in colleges, universities, state institutions, or federal institutions may be exempt from licensure.

Regardless of state or position, there are a few common elements of the licensure process: (a) application review and approval by the State Board of Examiners to ensure that the applicant meets the state's requirements for education, training, and moral character (e.g., criminal background check, letters of reference, reporting of training rotations and cumulative hours); (b) study and complete the (national) Examination for Professional Practice in Psychology (EPPP); (c) completion of the state's specific examination on its laws and licensure issues, which in some states may entail an additional written or oral ethics/jurisprudence examination; and (d) license granted.

STEPS TOWARD LICENSURE AND CREDENTIALING

People seek licensure for a variety of reasons. You may plan to practice clinically full time; alternatively, you may plan to work in an academic setting but wish to engage in part-time clinical work. Since each state can vary in their licensure requirements and procedures (e.g., requiring an ethics/jurisprudence examination or not, or whether such an examination is completed in written or oral format), a thorough review of the topic is simply not possible. However, we can impart some very important preparatory steps to ensure that you can work through the process quickly and successfully. Best of all: these are steps (summarized in Table 4.1) that you can start today, no matter your training level.

Step 1: Prepare for Licensure Well in Advance

Tip 1: Start a nest egg to cover licensure costs. Early on in your training, begin to plan for licensure costs by setting aside some funds, and contributing over time. Like most other aspects of your education and training, the licensure process can be expensive. Licensure requirements for each state can range anywhere from $500 to well over $1,000. This represents the culmination of fees for the application for licensure and for any additional examinations that may be required (e.g., ethics or jurisprudence examination). The Association of State and Provincial Psychology Boards (ASPPB) does have a handy online guide, *EPPP Candidate Handbook* (2020), that outlines the fees associated with licensure across all states, provinces,

TABLE 4.1. Steps and Tips for Getting Licensed and Credentialed

Step	Suggestion
1	Prepare for licensure well in advance.
	Tip 1: Start a nest egg to cover licensure costs. Tip 2: Research educational requirements and make sure you meet them. Tip 3: Collect your education, training, and professional records. Tip 4: Consider credentials banking.
2	Apply for licensure.
	Tip 1: Know the licensure requirements for position application. Tip 2: Know the test requirements for licensure application. Tip 3: Be thorough and accurate in your licensure application.
3	Study and take the EPPP.
	Tip 1: Learn about the EPPP. Tip 2: Prepare appropriately for the EPPP. Tip 3: You can (and should) talk to recent test-takers. Tip 4: Formulate a realistic study plan. Tip 5: Study smart, not necessarily hard. Tip 6: Plan ahead for the day of the test.
4	Remember that the early bird gets the worm.
	Tip 1: Take the EPPP as soon as possible. Tip 2: Allow sufficient time for credentialing.

Note. EPPP = Examination for Professional Practice in Psychology.

and territories (https://cdn.ymaws.com/www.asppb.net/resource/resmgr/eppp_2/10_2020_eppp_candidate_handb.pdf). You may also check out various state psychology board web pages to get a sense of the fees associated with licensure in that particular state.

Tip 2: Research educational requirements and make sure you meet them. As early as graduate school, begin exploring the web pages of various state psychology boards so you can get a general sense of the education and training requirements (e.g., number and type of courses, number and type of rotations, hours of direct clinical contact and/or supervision), documentation requirements (e.g., syllabi, copies of your graduate, internship, and fellowship certificates or even verification letters from your various directors of training), test requirements (e.g., your EPPP score), and the general timeline for licensure (i.e., how many steps are involved, how often the state psychology board meets to review applications, what sort of fees may be involved).

At a minimum, state licensing boards require completion of a doctoral degree program in psychology accredited by the American Psychological Association (APA) or Canadian Psychological Association (CPA). All states require completion of an APA-accredited predoctoral internship, and a sizeable portion also require completion of a postdoctoral fellowship. Aside from the training level required for licensure, there may also be requirements with regards to coursework. Some states are stricter than others in terms of educational requirements (e.g., some states require a higher number of hours of direct client contact, or differ in required supervision hours), so it is important to peruse the psychology board websites for a few different states to make sure that you're getting all the credit hours you need to be eligible for licensure (e.g., enough credit hours in ethics). If you're quickly nearing (or already in) the process of applying for licensure and realize your coursework may fall short of the license requirements of your state, check with the board on what options are available to you. There may be ways to make up for missed credits via approved independent study, continuing education, or workshop-based learning courses.

Tip 3: Collect your education, training, and professional records. To make the licensure process as easy as possible, be extra conscientious when it comes to maintaining documentation over the years. Create a professional dossier of sorts. During graduate school, save a digital copy of all syllabi. From graduate school until the end of fellowship, carefully record all of your clinical hours, supervision hours, and support hours (e.g., report writing time). Track your training rotations, and the names and credentials of all supervisor(s) for each. For all levels of training, be sure to photocopy your diplomas and transcripts (master's and doctoral degree), certificates (internship, fellowship, board certification), and any state licenses (if you were previously licensed in any other states). All of this documentation will come in very handy when applying for licensure, credentialing, and when applying for any jobs—now and in the future.

Tip 4: Consider credentials banking. While you could certainly maintain all records yourself, it can be very useful to "bank" or store this information for long-term use. This means that you, the applicant, would use a web-based portal to enter all information relevant to your graduate coursework (e.g., course titles, number of credit hours, syllabi), clinical training (e.g., graduate, internship, and fellowship certificates, as well as number of hours for direct client contact and supervision). This can provide you with the peace of mind that all of your most important professional documents are safely stored. It can also facilitate *licensure mobility*, meaning that these documents and your information remain accessible whenever you relocate or expand your practice to a new state or territory. Many people are surprised to know that credentials banking can begin as early as the first year of graduate school.

You have several possible options for credential banking services. One such option is a credentials bank sponsored by the National Register of Health

Service Psychologists (https://www.nationalregister.org). While there is usually a fee to apply for this service, the National Register does offer annual scholarships that waive this fee. Any psychology doctoral students, interns, postdoctoral fellows, or early career psychologists (within 10 years of degree completion) are eligible to apply for this scholarship.

ASPPB also sponsors a credentials bank (https://www.asppb.net/page/TheBank), which has a mobility component that allows you to transfer information and documents to new states or territories; however, this does come at an additional cost. Further, some states are in the ASPPB's Psychology Licensure Universal System (PLUS) program, an online system that uses the information and documentation already banked toward applications for licensure, certification, or registration in any state, province, or territory in the United States or Canada currently participating in the PLUS program. PLUS also enables application for an Interjurisdictional Practice Certificate (IPC), which grants you temporary authority to practice in another state for at least 30 work days without obtaining full licensure in that state. PLUS also enables application for a Certificate of Professional Qualification in Psychology (CPQ), which documents that the certificate holder has met a specific set of requirements in licensure, education, training, and examination without any history of disciplinary action. ASPPB is also currently developing an e-Passport program that will facilitate licensed providers to practice telehealth services across jurisdictional lines.

Step 2: Apply for Licensure

Overall, the process of licensure breaks down something like this: You apply to a state psychology board, which involves a credentials review. The credentials review involves verifying your education and training, including your degree(s) and internship. For those who attended APA-approved programs this part is a breeze. If you did not, this can be challenging but is doable, as long as the graduate program and internship you attended meet APA-established criteria. Your application will require you to report any criminal history (anticipate a possible background check), along with any prior ethical violations or board sanctions. You will provide a written statement where you delineate your intended area of practice that will be compared with your training and education background. Finally, the board may contact references (provided by you) to verify your ability to practice psychology.

Tip 1: Know the licensure requirements for position application. Before identifying your target state(s), you must know what your potential position will require. Licensure requirements will fall into one of three categories: (a) the job does not require a license (e.g., working as faculty within a college or university), (b) the job requires a license in the state in which you intend to practice (e.g., most clinical positions), or (c) the job simply requires a license—regardless of whatever state it comes from (e.g., federal positions such as those within the Veterans Affairs system of hospitals).

While most positions don't necessarily require licensure as early as the time of application, some strongly prefer it, so having your license squared away in advance can be to your advantage. It can also be challenging to know where you may land professionally for your first position, but you may at least have a general sense of the region in which you desire to live. Use that as a springboard from which to begin.

Tip 2: Know the test requirements for licensure application. "Test requirements" refers to the specific examination requirements in the state(s) you are targeting for licensure. All states will require completion of the EPPP. However, there are some specifics that will vary by state: Do they require an oral examination? A written examination? Or is it a state that requires both? Is the examination pertinent to general knowledge, ethics, state psychology rules/laws, or all of the above? One fantastic resource is the PsyBook sponsored through ASPPB, which outlines requirements of all member jurisdictions (https://www.asppb.net/page/psybook). An additional benefit: by reviewing this information well in advance, you can ensure that all of your training can be better tailored to meet the total hour requirements for licensure.

The timeline for licensure in a given state is also important to know. After submitting your application for licensure, the state psychology board convenes to review all submitted applications before approving them to proceed to the examination. Not all state boards meet on a monthly basis, some meet every other month or less—so you have to know the timeline to be able to map out your application process, and start your future job on time.

Tip 3: Be thorough and accurate in your licensure application. As we noted earlier, a number of components are required for your licensure process to be successful. This all starts with the application you submit, and allows you to sit for your state's written and/or oral examination(s). We offer some advice here, based on common mistakes made by applicants. First and foremost, read the instructions for your state. All done? OK, now read them a second time. Be clear on what is required, and contact the board if you have any outstanding questions. It's better to submit a well-prepared application than to find out one or more months later that your application was incomplete or insufficient.

Second, keep in mind that an application for licensure typically requires professional references. Make sure your references meet that state's criteria. Typically, you should include people from all phases of training (graduate, internship, and fellowship) who know your clinical work. This step could entail that your references produce a free-form original letter, or conversely involve them completing a form email sent by the board. Similarly, the board may require that past training directors complete degree verification forms. Whether letters of reference or degree verification forms, let your writers know in advance what they can expect so that they can plan accordingly (and ensure that nothing important falls victim to an email spam filter).

Third, please do not stretch the truth when completing your application. Beyond being a major ethical "no-no," lying on your application can justify the board never granting you a license. Further, know that you'd likely be caught. Many states also incorporate a background check into the licensure process, and since many now use federal databases, you should assume that the background check will be thorough and prior offenses (if any) will be discovered.

Fourth and finally, states often require that you complete a specialization statement as part of the licensure process. This is intended as a declaration of your area(s) of practice (e.g., neuropsychology). When competing your specialization statement, do not list areas of intended practice that fall outside of your previous training. Overstating one's competencies often serves as a red flag for the board reviewers to dig even deeper, and may delay your acceptance. Remember, if you have any questions, contact the board directly.

Step 3: Study and Take the EPPP

Licensure is accomplished in part through completion of a culminating psychology examination: the EPPP. After your application is reviewed and approved by the board, you are now ready to take this test. You may be groaning internally and thinking: Another test? What if I don't pass? I took some of these courses 5, 7, even 10 years ago. And the process for registering and taking my licensure exam seems so . . . complicated. What do I do? Where do I start? Sound familiar? First of all: take a deep breath. Make it a diaphragmatic breath. If you understood what that term meant, congratulations! You just got your first test item correct on the EPPP.

Tip 1: Learn about the EPPP. Knowledge, as they say, is power. The EPPP is developed and owned by ASPPB, but proctored by a company called Pearson. For many years, the EPPP was a one-step general knowledge examination. In the near future, candidates taking the EPPP may also be required to pass a second portion involving a practice component. Licensure jurisdictions across states will have the choice of using the Part 1 examination, or the newer Part 2 examination. Each part is briefly reviewed here, but the interested reader is referred to the ASPPB website for more information (https://www.asppb.net).

Part 1 of the EPPP is the general knowledge examination. This part covers eight content areas, each covering a certain percentage of the examination through a range of topics (see Table 4.2). It is a computerized examination, proctored at one of more than 270 testing centers in the United States and Canada (pro tip: you can choose to take the EPPP at any of these locations). There are 225 multiple-choice test items, only 175 of which actually count toward your final score (the other 50 are exploratory items for use in future exam iterations). Candidates are allowed 4 hours and 15 minutes to complete the examination, with scratch paper and pen provided. Test results are provided on the day of the examination. Pass rates vary between states, but in general a score of 500 or above (indicating 70% of items correctly answered) falls within the passing range.

Part 2 of the EPPP is the practice examination, the "show how" counterpart to Part 1's "know how" questions. Part 2 covers six content areas, each representing a certain percentage of the examination through a range of topics (see Table 4.3). It is also a computerized examination, proctored again at one of more than 270 testing centers in the United States and Canada. In this part of the EPPP, the test format is much more varied. It contains scenarios, exhibits, multiple choice items, and matching items, but not essays. Similar to Part 1, test results are provided on the day of the examination.

Tip 2: Prepare appropriately for the EPPP. First, remember that you've taken many tests before, and have gotten this far. Your education and training have prepared you well; in fact, the average first-time pass rate for the EPPP exceeds 80%. You can do it—we believe in you! After your application for licensure is reviewed and approved by the state board, you may then register and pay for the EPPP. This starts the clock—you now have 90 days to schedule and take the EPPP through an approved testing center (https://home.pearsonvue.com/asppb). Once scheduled, you may have to pay an additional exam sitting fee. On the day of the examination:

- Arrive to the testing center 30 minutes early with two acceptable forms of identification, such as driver's license, passport, or other picture identification.

- Take the EPPP Part 1 or Part 2, depending on the guidelines specified by your state psychology board.

- Receive your EPPP test score.

At this point, that's all the information you need to know. If you have a burning thirst to learn more about the EPPP, you will find unbiased and

TABLE 4.2. Examination for Professional Practice in Psychology Part 1 Content Areas, Percentage of Examination Items, and Sample Topics

Content area	Sample topics
Biological Bases of Behavior (10%)	✓ Neuroanatomical and genetic correlates of psychological disorders ✓ Psychopharmacology classifications and mechanisms of action ✓ Drugs of abuse
Cognitive-Affective Bases of Behavior (13%)	✓ Intelligence theories and models ✓ Principles of learning and memory ✓ Theories and models of emotion
Social and Cultural Bases of Behavior (11%)	✓ Theories and models of social cognition ✓ Personality theories and models ✓ Identity diversity and intersectionality
Growth and Lifespan Development (12%)	✓ Development across the lifespan ✓ Development risk and protective factors ✓ Diversity and identity development ✓ Disorders impacting development
Assessment and Diagnosis (16%)	✓ Psychometric theories ✓ Organizational assessment ✓ Constructs of epidemiology and base rates of psychological disorders ✓ Psychopathology theories and models
Treatment, Intervention, Prevention, Supervision (15%)	✓ Interventions for individuals, couples, families, and organizations ✓ Health promotion, risk reduction, resilience, and wellness approaches ✓ Models of supervision
Research Methods and Statistics (7%)	✓ Sampling, data collection methods ✓ Design of case, correlational, quasiexperimental, and experimental research ✓ Statistical interpretation
Ethical, Legal, and Professional Issues (16%)	✓ APA Ethics Code ✓ Laws, statutes, and judicial decisions affecting psychology ✓ Identification and management of potential ethical issues

TABLE 4.3. Examination for Professional Practice in Psychology Part 2 Content Areas, Percentage of Examination Items, and Sample Topics

Content area	Sample topics
Scientific Orientation (6%)	✓ Select and critically review relevant research literature ✓ Acquire and disseminate knowledge in accord with scientific and ethical principles
Assessment and Intervention (33%)	✓ Apply knowledge of individual and diversity characteristics in assessment and diagnosis ✓ Administer and score instruments ✓ Interpret and synthesize results from a variety of sources ✓ Formulate and communicate diagnosis and recommendations effectively ✓ Apply and modify interventions
Relational Competence (16%)	✓ Integrate and apply theory, research, professional guidelines, and personal understanding about social contexts to work with diverse clients ✓ Work effectively with individuals, groups, families, communities, and/or organizations ✓ Demonstrate respect for others in all areas of professional practice ✓ Identify, manage interpersonal conflict
Professionalism (11%)	✓ Identify and observe boundaries of competence ✓ Critical self-evaluation via self-reflection and seeking of feedback from others
Ethical Practice (17%)	✓ Promote values and behaviors commensurate with ethics codes, laws, regulations ✓ Accurately represent and document work in professional practice and scholarship ✓ Establish and maintain a process that promotes ethical decision making
Collaboration, Consultation, Supervision (17%)	✓ Demonstrate interdisciplinary collaborations ✓ Create and maintain an environment that provides effective supervision for trainees and other professionals

nonemotionally charged information on the ASPPB website (http://www.asppb.net). Try to refrain from visiting any of the blog or discussion forum sites (e.g., Student-Doctor Network). These can heighten anxiety in some prospective test-takers, and in other instances provide misinformation about the test itself.

Tip 3: You can (and should) talk with recent test-takers. Ask whether they have recommendations for EPPP study materials—including any used materials that they would be willing to lend or share. Speaking with recent test-takers can help give you an idea on how often or how intensive you should be in your study routine. Often, prospective test-takers "track" their scores across practice exams during the course of their EPPP preparation; by knowing this information, you as a prospective test-taker now have a point of reference in knowing whether you are advancing your studies appropriately. As a general rule, prospective test-takers who consistently achieve a score of 70% or higher on practice exams are ready to take the EPPP.

Tip 4: Formulate a realistic study plan. To help you develop a realistic study plan, you should understand your own personal learning style. That way, you can procure study materials and construct a study schedule that are likely to enhance your chance for success. Ask yourself the following questions:

- *What's my learning style?* Are you more of an auditory learner a visual learner, a haptic learner, or a combination of these styles? Auditory learners will likely do better by focusing on audio files for studying (e.g., those provided by third party services like the Association for Advanced Training in the Behavioral Sciences [AATBS]), while visual learners may benefit more from flashcards. If you're a multimodal learner, you could incorporate elements of each into your routine.

- *What is my study schedule?* Remember that spaced practice is better than massed practice (seriously, cramming only on weekends just doesn't work for most people). You'd do better studying a short amount each day. However, you know your current schedule best. Take the time to print off a week's calendar. Write down all of your obligations for each day of that week. Where do you have free time? What can you reasonably afford for study time each day? Are you overcommitting yourself anywhere? Is there anything you can reprioritize?

- *What kind of study environment do I prefer?* Do you need absolute quiet? Or do you prefer a bit of "background buzz" when you study? Again, experiment with different situations: a library, a coffee shop, or at home. Do a self-check afterwards: what was your level of distractibility? What was your level of frustration? How much work did you get done? This will help indicate which type of study environment works best for you. If you need a bit of background noise, there are any number of free websites and apps to play during your study sessions (even "coffeehouse noise" via http://www.coffitivity.com).

• *Do I need personal accountability?* Do you need to study alone? Or, do you study more efficiently and learn better when working with a partner— or even a small group? Alternatively, do you just prefer to have a person that you can report to, so you can stay accountable for your study time? At a bare minimum, do some self-monitoring (we all know that's the key for behavior change anyway). Create an Excel spreadsheet where you can log the date of study sessions, content studied, practice exams completed and scores (if applicable), and the total time logged each day.

• *Have I communicated my goal to everyone I know?* Above all else, I recommend communicating that you're studying for this important test to everyone you know—and asking for some understanding and flexibility on their part. Have your partner take the kids or pets out for a while, so you can get some study time in. Turn your phone's ringer off. Close the computer window(s) or app(s) containing your social networking sites. Tell others you may be socially unavailable for a period of time.

Tip 5: Study smart, not necessarily hard. It's now time to actually sit down and study for the EPPP. Breathe easy! Again, APA statistics indicate that over 80% of test takers pass the EPPP Part 1 their first time around. Remember the key here is to study smarter, not harder. Frankly, it would be incredibly challenging to learn and retain all of the information necessary for acing the EPPP. Rather than learning to identify the correct response for all test items, the goal here is to train yourself to whittle down your possibilities and make an educated guess. So, you want to hit that zone of studying *just enough*.

But how to study? This is probably the most important question of all. We have heard the gamut of study approaches, ranging from only using practice tests to attending a workshop. A large part will depend on the materials you use to study. Determining what sort of materials you need goes back to what kind of learner you are. Depending on whether you are primarily a visual or auditory learner, this will help you decide what modality to emphasize. That being said, you should consider multimodal studying. By presenting the material across modalities, you're honing your mind to think about the concepts and terms in different ways. This means using a combination of the following: individual, paired, or group review using a mixture of practice exams, a good old psychology 101 textbook, audio files, and/or mobile quiz/flashcard apps (e.g., AATBS and MedPreps [http://www.medpreps.com/practice-tests/eppp]).

One question often asked by prospective test-takers is how old test materials need to be. The beauty of the EPPP Part 1 is that you can use older materials and still do fine, because much of the test is based on seminal psychological theories. The downside to purchasing used materials is that they are so expensive to begin with that most folks are looking to recoup their costs, and thus discounted materials may still be pretty pricey. Whenever you consider preparing for the EPPP, know that people sell their old materials online all the time. Or just ask people you know who have taken (or are studying to take) the EPPP Part 1, as you may be able to get materials for free or at reduced cost If you're taking the EPPP Part 1 during fellowship specifically, sometimes programs cover the cost of the study materials, so that is a good place to start, if you haven't already taken the exam.

Now that you've decided on your test materials, consider your approach to studying. Begin your studies by assessing what you already know, and what you don't. Based on your training, you'll be stronger in some areas than others. Visit the ASPPB website and check out their listing of average EPPP scores from students in your doctoral program. Depending on how high the scores are from your program, you can then determine how much time you may need to allot for studying. If the scores were high, you can know that your program's curriculum does a good job of preparing you for the exam. You should start with at least one practice exam to judge where you are before any studying takes place, which will also help you to determine your knowledge level. For a fee, you can take 200 retired exam questions through the ASPPB website or through a testing center.

Now that you've conquered your first practice exam, focus on strengthening your areas of weakness. This means putting down the practice exams (for now). Either solo or in a study group, review exam material and take notes along the way. You can supplement this with audio files and/or mobile study apps. Then return to the practice exams. We advise this approach rather than studying using exams alone, which runs the risk of being inefficient and time-consuming. Once you're consistently achieving above a 70% score, you are likely in good shape to pass the EPPP Part 1. That final week before your exam, hit each day hard with practice exams and flashcards.

One final question asked by many prospective test-takers is how much time one should allot for EPPP studies. While this will certainly depend on your areas of weakness and program preparation, there are some ways you can anticipate how much time to allot for studying. Anecdotally, most people report that they allowed for 2 to 4 months of study time. APA statistics show that there is a point of diminishing return somewhere around the 200-hour mark (Clay, 2012). Overall, most people spend an average of 70 to 100 hours studying. Over the course of 2 months, that breaks down to about 12 hours per week.

Tip 6: Plan ahead for the day of the test. In the final week before the EPPP, familiarize yourself with the testing center location. Perhaps even drive there ahead of time, just to be familiar with the route. Review the testing rules and requirements, and make sure you have the two forms of required identification (and that they are both up-to-date). Meanwhile, don't forget self-care! It can be very easy to skip eating healthily for junk food or caffeinated products. You must resist! And by all means, take the day before the test off. You earned it. And feel confident that you will pass with flying colors.

Step 4: Remember That the Early Bird Gets the Worm

Tip 1: Take the EPPP as soon as possible. If we may impart one final piece of wisdom to you, it is this: be proactive and start this process as early as possible. In many (but not all) states, you can apply for licensure at the master's level and, once approved, take the EPPP; the drawback here is that you will then have to later reapply for licensure at the doctoral level, but the good news is that you do not have to retake the EPPP. At the very latest, we advise you to take the EPPP before the end of December in the second year of your postdoctoral fellowship (keeping in mind the time required to apply and register for the EPPP, which can range from 3 to 6 months). The sooner you get the EPPP done, the quicker you can move through the licensure process. The quicker you move through the licensure process, the faster onboarding will be at your job.

Tip 2: Allow sufficient time for credentialing. For those of us in the clinical realm, the hiring/onboarding process entails becoming credentialed with various insurance panels. This means that after you are hired on at a hospital or other institution, your institution will submit applications on your behalf to various health care insurance "panels" or companies (e.g., United, Cigna, Humana, Medicare, Medicaid); once accepted, you are then able to bill these health care companies for services rendered. Hospitals and similar organizations have a legal responsibility to verify your identity, education, work experience, professional liability history, and license verifications to protect patients from unqualified providers or poor care.

One major entity in which providers are credentialed in the United States is the Centers for Medicare/Medicaid Services (CMS). Here, you or your institution will apply for a National Provider Identifier (NPI), a unique 10-digit code that is assigned to a provider and is subsequently used on all claims forms submitted by the provider or health care organization as part of the Health Insurance Portability and Accountability Act (HIPAA). You apply for an NPI through the National Plan and Provider Enumeration System (NPPES) pages on CMS's website (https://www.cms.gov/Regulations-and-Guidance/Administrative-Simplification/NationalProvIdentStand/apply). Typically, after receiving an NPI you are then able to become paneled with other health care insurance companies.

The caveat here is that insurance credentialing can only begin *after* you are fully licensed. The process of credentialing could take a number of months, and much longer if any mistakes are made in the application process. So, if you are supposed to start your first clinical job in August, do not wait until June to take your EPPP or obtain licensure. If you cut your timeline too short, you run the risk of delaying the credentialing process (and starting your first day of work having already annoyed your department's leadership).

CONCLUSION AND FUTURE DIRECTIONS

You now have the basic building blocks of knowledge that will see you through the EPPP and licensure process. These are important bridges to your first professional job. While the EPPP and licensure can seem overwhelming, a little bit of preparation and organization can go a long way in making the process less stressful and daunting. Take advantage of the advice contained here, and of the abundant resources available to help you successfully navigate each of these steps. And by all means, celebrate the fact that you are that much closer to achieving professional independence!

REFERENCES

Association of State and Provincial Psychology Boards (ASPPB). (2020). *EPPP candidate handbook: Examination for professional practice in psychology*. https://cdn.ymaws.com/www.asppb.net/resource/resmgr/eppp_2/10_2020_eppp_candidate_handb.pdf

Clay, R. A. (2012). *Are you studying too much for the EPPP? Research suggests that more than 300 hours can backfire*. [Blog post]. American Psychological Association Career Center. https://www.apa.org/gradpsych/2012/11/eppp-myths

The Health Insurance Portability and Accountability Act of 1996 (HIPAA). 45 C.F.R. Part 160 et seq. https://www.hhs.gov/hipaa/for-professionals/privacy/index.html

5 BOARD CERTIFICATION IN NEUROPSYCHOLOGY

CHRISTOPHER GROTE, JASON R. SOBLE, AND ADELINE LEÓN

Those who have successfully navigated 4 years of high school, another 4 of college, 4 to 7 years of graduate school, a year of internship, 2 more years of a postdoctoral fellowship, and then finally the psychology licensing exam may justifiably think, "Finally, no more tests the rest of my life. Hallelujah!" But, there is still *board certification* to consider, this being a voluntary process that demonstrates your commitment to showing competence in a specialty area of practice, in this case, neuropsychology. As illustrated in the text that follows, this is a step beyond licensure, which is required by states or local jurisdictions to engage in the practice of clinical psychology.

Why, one might ask, would one sign up for another exam when they have already taken more tests than most of the general population? We present in this chapter our reasons: In short, board certification is good for the neuropsychologist, for our profession, and most important, for the general public! We review the specifics of the advantages of pursuing this milestone through a brief exploration of the history of board certification in neuropsychology and in other professions, the benefits and reasons to achieve certification, an overview of the process in neuropsychology, and finally ways in which one can prepare for the examination process. This chapter examines in depth the

https://doi.org/10.1037/0000250-006
The Neuropsychologist's Roadmap: A Training and Career Guide, C. Block (Editor)

standards and procedures used by the American Board of Clinical Neuropsychology (ABCN), which operates under the auspices of the American Board of Professional Psychology (ABPP). The focus on ABCN in this chapter, versus other board-certifying bodies within the specialty, is a natural one in that this is the board certification pursued by the authors. Additionally, one of the authors is a former member of the board of directors for both ABCN and its allied organization, the American Academy of Clinical Neuropsychology (AACN).

WHAT IS BOARD CERTIFICATION, AND WHY IS IT IMPORTANT?

All board-certified neuropsychologists are licensed psychologists, but not all licensed psychologists are board certified. That is, each state determines the criteria by which an individual is eligible to obtain a state-issued license to engage in the practice of clinical psychology. These criteria typically include that the licensure candidate (you) possess a relevant doctoral degree (i.e., PhD or PsyD), obtained sufficient training, which would include a 12-month internship and frequently supervised postdoctoral clinical experience, and successfully pass the Examination for Professional Practice in Psychology (EPPP). The issuance of a license to practice psychology allows the public to know that the license holder has met criteria for general practice. However, clinical psychology is a very broad field, and no one individual can claim specialized knowledge of all its specialized areas of practice, including (but is not limited to) pediatric psychology, health psychology, psychotherapy, clinical neuropsychology, geropsychology, and rehabilitation psychology, among others. Often, an individual's interests may lead them to one of these specialized areas of study and practice, sometimes to the point that they end up practicing exclusively within that subfield of clinical psychology. The board certification process allows you to demonstrate to the public that your knowledge and skill of a specialized area meets the criteria for this designation. This occurs through a series of qualifying steps and examinations designed to demonstrate that an individual has proficiency in the specialty area of clinical neuropsychology.

It is estimated that fewer than 5% of licensed clinical psychologists are board certified, compared with more than 80% of physicians (Cassel & Holmboe, 2008). This is obviously a striking difference, and the reason for this disparity is not clear but perhaps can be attributed to at least two reasons. First, board certification in medicine started earlier. The American Board of Ophthalmology was incorporated in 1917. This later fell under the auspices of the American Board of Internal Medicine, which was incorporated in 1936, and now has 24 member boards. Thus, the second possible reason that relatively few clinical psychologists pursue board certification might be one of culture. Using a "carrot and stick" analogy, many academic medical centers and other health care organization require physicians to be board certified in order to obtain or renew medical staff privileges, but the same is rarely true for psychologists. In fact, the authors are aware of some medical centers whose medical staff reappointment procedures exempt only psychologists from a requirement to be board certified. This might be viewed as a "lowered bar" for psychologists, especially when one hears the specific objections of nonboarded colleagues in psychology as to why board certification, or at least its pursuit, should not be required as a condition of employment. This objection does not accurately reflect the high ambitions and standards of organized psychology. These reasons often include the cost, energy, and time needed to take the exams, and not seeing a benefit that would outweigh these factors. Thus, boarded psychologists must be advocates both to those who might become candidates for certification, as well as to hospital and organizational managers as to why board certification should be valued and perhaps required.

Overview of the American Board of Clinical Neuropsychology

ABPP[1] was established by the American Psychological Association (APA) and incorporated in 1947. ABPP now has 15 member boards, one of which, ABCN, was established as a member board in 1983. ABCN is the organization charged with examination of candidates for the diplomate in clinical neuropsychology. Those who successfully complete the ABCN examination process then become members of AACN, a separate organization charged with advocacy for neuropsychology. The rate of growth of candidacy for diplomates in clinical neuropsychology is astonishing. The first ABCN diplomate was awarded in 1984, after which 20 years passed before the 500th was awarded in 2004. However, it only took an additional 10 years before another 500 individuals passed the exam (2014) and over 300 more have passed the exam in the following years (Stringer et al., 2019). As of 2019,

---

[1]ABPP is just one of many board certification bodies in neuropsychology. While page limits prohibit a full review of all possible options, readers should know that other options include the American Board of Professional Neuropsychology (ABN) and American Board of Pediatric Neuropsychology (ABPdN). For more information, readers are encouraged to visit the respective websites of these board certification bodies.

more than 1,300 individuals have passed the ABCN examinations necessary to earn the diplomate in clinical neuropsychology. Indeed, the rapid increase in the number of candidates has at times challenged the abilities of institutions that have hosted the oral exams (Rush University Medical Center from 1991 to 2012; the University of Illinois at Chicago from 2013), but to date, necessary space has been procured for each exam. It is difficult to estimate what percentage of "neuropsychologists" are board certified because the phrase "clinical neuropsychologist" is not usually protected, and it is impossible to know how many clinicians consider themselves neuropsychologists and/or have necessary specialty training in that area. However, 25% or more might be considered a reasonable estimate, knowing that there are about 4,000 members of the Society for Clinical Neuropsychology and about 3,000 in the National Academy of Neuropsychology. This would appear to be a much higher rate when compared to other ABPP member boards. The reason for this relatively high rate of attainment again might be attributed to "culture" within neuropsychology, in which the increasing number of individuals who are ABCN-certified then encourage their peers and trainees to pursue this process. Further, the Houston Conference Guidelines (Hannay et al., 1998) laid out training models that include board certification, which are then adhered to through the ABCN process.

Benefits of American Board of Clinical Neuropsychology Certification

There are additional reasons that pursuit of ABCN certification seems to increasingly be becoming the norm (Stringer et al., 2019). Decades ago, even in academic medical centers, having a board-certified neuropsychologist on staff might have been the exception. Today, one might be surprised if a practicing neuropsychologist, at least one who has graduated from a 2-year fellowship in recent years, is not board certified or at least pursuing this goal. If one has been able to be accepted into and graduated from a 2-year postdoctoral fellowship, it would seem to naturally follow that one would want to demonstrate to others the benefits of this advanced training by obtaining board certification. Indeed, as only Louisiana protects the title "neuropsychologist," clinicians value the attainment of a diplomate as a way of demonstrating to the public, your colleagues, and yourself that you indeed have demonstrated a level of knowledge and competency that merits this distinction.

Other reasons for ABCN certification are outlined by Armstrong et al. (2008). These include the potential for higher income, as board-certified clinical neuropsychologists employed by the Veterans Administration or the U.S. military are eligible for higher salaries or bonuses.

Additionally, the most recent salary survey by Sweet et al. (2015) shows that ABCN-certified neuropsychologists earn, on average, a "gross psychology income" of $161,600 per year compared with $125,300 for those who are not ABCN board certified. At least part of this income differential might be attributable to opportunities to engage in forensic consultation, given that attorneys may well prefer presenting an expert who is board certified, over one who is not, to a judge or jury. Of course, there are nonmonetary benefits to becoming ABCN certified, including taking understandable pride in achieving this goal. Additionally, ABCN certification might facilitate licensure reciprocity and a streamlining of credentialing either for medical staff or licensure purposes. That is, board certification can be used in lieu of more extensive documentation to obtain licensure in another state or in attaining hospital or medical staff privileges. Finally, perhaps the most important reason to achieve board certification is that it will facilitate additional learning on the part of the candidate. No matter the education or training you have, preparation for certification will help you discover gaps in your knowledge and skill base.

OVERVIEW OF THE BOARD CERTIFICATION AND EXAMINATION PROCESS

This section details the process for becoming board certified in clinical neuropsychology by the ABCN from start to finish. A flowchart is also included to serve as a quick reference guide and checklist (see Exhibit 5.1). Before proceeding, two important caveats are in order. First, this reflects the process, procedures, and requirements as of this writing. Given that these are periodically updated, you are encouraged to consult the ABPP/ABCN *Board Certification Guidelines and Procedures: Candidate Manual* (ABPP/ABCN, 2020) for the most current information (https://abpp.org/BlankSite/media/Clinical-Neuropsychology-Documents/ABCN-Manual.pdf). Second, although the process is fairly linear and prescribed, proactive planning often goes a long way to avoid unnecessary delays. Many of the steps, such as the written and oral examinations, are only offered a few times per year and have registration/submission deadlines months before the actual exam. As such, not being aware of or staying abreast of this information can result in a much longer-than-anticipated candidacy.

EXHIBIT 5.1. American Board of Professional Psychology Clinical Neuropsychology Board Certification Process Flowchart

Application/Credential review

✓ Fee: $125 ($25 if done through ABPP Early Entry Option)

Step 1: ABPP General Application

☐ Application.

☐ Psychology licensure.

☐ Official transcripts.

☐ Internship completion certificate.

Step 2: ABCN Specialty Application and Credential Review

☐ Application.

☐ Completed 2-year neuropsychology fellowship.

☐ If fellowship is <u>not</u> APA-accredited or an APPCN member: supporting documents that demonstrate didactic experience in the eight core knowledge areas.

Examination process

Step 3: Written examination

✓ 125 questions, 100 of which count toward the final score

✓ Score of 70% or higher required to pass

✓ Administered at local PSI Premier Testing Centers in three 2- to 4-week windows per year

✓ Fee: $590 ($300 registration, $290 testing seat fee)

Exam window in which you plan to sit for the written examination: _____

Deadline for written examination registration: _____

Step 4: Practice sample submission

✓ Practice sample materials uploaded/submitted via the ScholarOne submission portal

✓ Fee: $250

Practice Sample 1:

☐ De-identified report

☐ Data/Norms summary sheet

☐ Scanned raw data/test summary sheet

Practice Sample 2:

☐ De-identified report

☐ Data/Norms summary sheet

☐ Scanned raw data/test summary sheet

Step 5: Oral examination

✓ Three components: Ethics/Professional Practice, Case Defense, Fact Finding (each examination component lasts for 50 minutes and is administered by a board-certified clinical neuropsychologist who has undergone extensive training to be a board examiner)

✓ Administered at the University of Illinois (Chicago, IL) twice per year

✓ Fee: $450

Exam window in which you plan to sit for the oral examination: _____

Deadline for submission of practice samples: _____

EXHIBIT 5.1. American Board of Professional Psychology Clinical Neuropsychology Board Certification Process Flowchart (*Continued*)

Step 6: Maintenance of certification (MOC)

✓ Required of all ABCN specialists awarded board certification after January 1, 2015

✓ Renewed every 10 years

✓ Those board certified early are advised to opt in

✓ Grid system of credits in five categories:

- Research

- Collaborative clinical consultation

- Teaching

- Training

✓ Details at https://theabcn.org

Note. ABPP = American Board of Professional Psychology; ABCN = American Board of Clinical Neuropsychology; APA = American Psychological Association; APPCN = Association of Postdoctoral Programs in Clinical Neuropsychology.

APPLICATION AND CREDENTIAL REVIEW

The board certification process begins with an application submission and review of credentials, including your doctoral degree, internship, and psychology license. Applications are submitted electronically via the ABPP website (https://www.abpp.org). There are three application options: (a) regular, (b) senior for those practicing for 15 years or more, and (c) early entry for those who are currently in a doctoral program or who have graduated but are not yet licensed for independent practice. Given the focus of this book, only the regular and early-entry options are detailed here. As part of the regular application process, candidates must meet both the ABPP general requirements (Step 1) and the specialty-specific application requirements (Step 2). The early-entry option closely mirrors the regular application, except this option allows for banking of credentials (see Chapter 4) as they are acquired and has a discounted application fee of $25 (instead of the standard $125). As of September 1, 2017, ABPP has partnered with the Association of State and Provincial Psychology Boards (ASPPB) to allow early-entry applicants to upload and store their credentials through ASPPB Credentials Bank, which are then sent to ABPP for review once completed. Thus, students/trainees may wish to begin banking credentials early for eventual ABPP applications (and state licensure) as this allows for banking of credentials along the way as they are completed (e.g., internship). Candidates may access the credentials bank at https://www.asppb.net/page/TheBank.

Step 1: General Application Requirements

General requirements are outlined on the ABPP website (https://www.abpp. org/Applicant-Information/Degree-Requirements.aspx). They require that you (the candidate) possess a doctoral degree from a professional psychology program accredited by APA, the Canadian Psychological Association (CPA), or listed in the *Academic Program Requirements for ABPP and ABGP* document (ABPP, 2016) at the time that the degree was awarded; complete an accredited internship program (or 1 year equivalency of supervised experience); and are independently licensed for practice in a jurisdiction in the United States and U.S. territories or Canada. As of 2018, the general requirements specifically state the academic program from which the applicant's doctoral degree was awarded must have been accredited by APA, CPA, or an accrediting agency recognized by the U.S. Department of Education at the time of completion. As supporting documentation, you are required to submit official transcripts sent directly from the degree-awarding institution and documentation of internship completion (e.g., a copy of the internship completion certificate or a letter from the internship training director verifying completion). As of this writing, the application fee is $125.

Step 2: Specialty Application and Credential Review

Following approval of the general requirements, ABPP forwards applications to the ABCN Credentials Committee to determine specialty specific eligibility. The ABCN specialty-specific application requirements can be found online at https://theabcn.org/ and are designed to document an applicant's didactic and experiential training in clinical neuropsychology. This section exclusively discusses the requirements for those graduating after January 1, 2005, which follow the Houston Conference Guidelines (Hannay et al., 1998). In brief, applicants must demonstrate didactic experience in the following eight core knowledge areas: (a) basic neurosciences; (b) functional neuroanatomy; (c) neuropathology; (d) clinical neurology; (e) psychological assessment; (f) clinical neuropsychological assessment; (g) psychopathology; and (h) psychological intervention that was obtained at any time during your graduate, internship, or postdoctoral training via formal coursework and/or other didactic training (e.g., brain cuttings, case conferences, grand rounds). Additionally, completion of a 2-year postdoctoral fellowship (or equivalent of 2 full years if done on a half-time basis) in which at least 50% of time is spent in neuropsychology-related training activities is required. The primary focus of the fellowship must be training, and it must involve structured clinical and didactic experiences, as well as supervision of clinical cases. While most applicants will have had neuropsychological training on internship prior to fellowship, it is not specifically required. Moreover, it is not required that an applicant's postdoctoral fellowship be accredited; however, applicants who complete a specialty program in clinical neuropsychology that is either (a) APA-accredited or (b) a full member program of the Association of Postdoctoral Programs in Clinical Neuropsychology (APPCN) are allowed to skip several items on the specialty application that require a detailed accounting of training in the eight core knowledge areas.

Following credential approval, the applicant has 7 years to complete the entire board certification process, including all written and oral examinations. If the entire process is not completed within this 7-year window, applicants must reinitiate the application and credential review process.

THE EXAMINATION PROCESS

The examination process for board certification in clinical neuropsychology is detailed below and reflects current policies and procedures. Prior to initiating the process, the reader is also encouraged to visit the ABPP website for further information (https://abpp.org/Applicant-Information/Specialty-Boards/Clinical-Neuropsychology/Certification-Exam-Process.aspx), including any updates or revisions to the examination process or procedures.

Step 3: Written Examination

Following credential review and approval, you are invited to sit for the written examination, which assesses your knowledge of neuropsychological assessment, basic and clinical neurosciences, behavioral neurology, and general clinical psychology. The exam consists of 125 questions, 100 of which count toward the final score, whereas the remaining 25 "pretest items" are used to gather psychometric data for future exam questions. You are not told which 25 of the 125 examination questions do not count toward your final score. The written examination is administered electronically by PSI Premier Testing Center, which can be done locally. It is presently offered in three 2- to 4-week examination windows during each calendar year with a registration deadline that closes about 2 months prior to the examination window. The current written exam fee is $590, which includes that ABCN registration fee ($300) and the PSI testing seat fee ($290). Candidates are allowed 2.5 hours to complete the exam and must earn a score of 70 or higher to pass. Candidates are informed whether they passed or failed

3 to 4 weeks after the exam window closes. Those who passed are invited to proceed to the next step of the certification process, the practice sample submission. Those who did not pass are allowed to retake the written examination up to three times during their 7-year candidacy period. If a candidate fails the exam three times, they are not eligible to take it again under their initial candidacy period and must instead reinitiate the certification process by resubmitting their application for credential review.

Step 4: Practice Sample Submission

After you (the candidate) successfully pass the written examination, you are invited to submit two practice work samples for double-blind peer-review by ABCN board-certified clinical neuropsychologists who are trained as practice sample reviewers. These practice samples are meant to demonstrate your competency in clinical neuropsychological practice and reflect the range of your normal clinical practice. Practice samples must be cases that you evaluated while practicing independently as a licensed psychologist. Cases completed while you were in internship or postdoctoral training are not acceptable, nor are cases completed by a student trainee under your supervision. You do not have to wait until you pass the written examination to begin selecting and preparing practice samples. Therefore, having your cases selected and prepared to submit as soon as you are informed that you passed the written exam may help to move the process more expeditiously. You are required to submit three sets of documents for each sample: (a) the de-identified neuropsychological evaluation report, (b) a data sheet that includes a summary of all test scores and identifies which norms were used for tests, and (c) scanned copies of the raw data/test protocols. You are also allowed to submit an optional supplementary document if you wish, to provide the reviewers with additional context related to your clinical practice or further highlight or clarify any aspects of your practice samples (e.g., test/norms selection, decisional issues) that may not have been appropriate to include in the evaluation report. The maximum length of this supplementary document is three double-spaced pages. Practice samples and supporting materials are submitted electronically to ABCN via the ScholarOne submission portal. The current practice sample submission fee is $250. Following submission, practice samples are reviewed by three ABCN specialists who render an opinion as to whether the practice samples can be reasonably defended at oral examination. Two of the three reviewers must rate the practice samples as acceptable for you to pass to the oral examination. If accepted, you will be notified of your eligibility to sit for the next oral examination. If practice samples are rated as unacceptable, you will receive specific feedback detailing the issues raised by the reviewers and instructions on how to resubmit new practice samples.

Step 5: Oral Examination

Following acceptance of the practice samples, candidates typically are invited to sit for the next oral examination. There are two oral examination periods annually, one in the fall and one in the spring. The exam currently is held in Chicago, Illinois, and is hosted at the Neuropsychiatric Institute at the University of Illinois at Chicago. The current exam fee is $450. The oral exam consists of three, one-hour components: (a) Ethics and Professional Practice, (b) Practice Sample Defense, and (c) Fact Finding (see Table 5.1). Prior to the commencement of the exam, you are provided with your specific examiner team and given the opportunity to articulate any potential conflict(s) of interest. You will also sign a confidentiality agreement that precludes you from discussing specific content of the oral exam or the identity of any other candidates present. After the conclusion of all three components, examiners meet to evaluate your performance and to vote on

TABLE 5.1. Board Certification Oral Examination Components

Component	Description
Ethics and Professional Practice	Candidates are presented with a brief vignette and asked to identify relevant issues that may emerge (e.g., informed consent; practicing within the scope of one's competence; use of appropriate assessment procedures).
	Candidates are also asked to articulate their professional identity as a neuropsychologist (e.g., discuss how they stay abreast of the literature; describe professional activities in which they engage, such as training interns/fellows).
Practice Sample Defense	Candidates are asked to present their two sample cases, in order to demonstrate a reasonable, rational, and defensible approach to evaluation, treatment, report writing, and intraprofessional communication.
Fact Finding	Candidates evaluate a neuropsychological clinical referral *de novo*, selecting either an adult or pediatric case.
	Candidates are provided a brief clinical vignette of a real case, and asked to elicit all relevant information (e.g., history, test results, impressions) to demonstrate case conceptualization and conclusion formulation.

whether or not to award board certification. It should be noted that the final decision is based on your performance across the *entire* oral examination—you do not pass/fail individual exam components. Candidates who pass are notified by ABPP and ABCN that they have been awarded board certification. Candidates who are not awarded board certification are provided with summary feedback from the ABCN Central Office and are allowed a second and, if necessary, third attempt to retake the oral examination during their 7-year candidacy. If board certification is not attained after the third attempt, the candidate must reinitiate the process beginning with an application/credential review.

Step 6: Maintenance of Certification

ABCN/ABPP recognizes that those who receive board certification should not necessarily use this distinction for the rest of their career to espouse competence without some sort of demonstration that they have engaged in continued study and other efforts to maintain competence. As such, Maintenance of Certification (MOC) is now required of all ABCN specialists who were awarded board certification on or after January 1, 2015. Those who obtained certification earlier are encouraged to opt in. MOC does not require re-examination but instead requires evidence that the boarded individual has continued to engage in professional activities and self-evaluation. The details can be found at the ABCN website (https://theabcn.org), and are organized as a "grid system" of credits obtainable in five categories of professional activities, including research, collaborative clinical consultation and teaching, and training. The MOC must be renewed every 10 years.

PREPARING FOR THE BOARD CERTIFICATION AND EXAMINATION PROCESS

This section provides guidance and resources to help you prepare for each step involved in the process of becoming board certified in clinical neuropsychology. As a reminder, below are the general stages of the process: (a) application and credential review, (b) written examination, (c) practice sample submission, and (d) oral examination (see Table 5.2). Although you have 7 years to complete the evaluation process after the initial credential review, this is well beyond the amount of time that is typically needed, which is closer to 1 1/2 to 2 years.

TABLE 5.2. Preparing for the Board Certification and Examination Process

Step 1: Preparing for the application and credential review

- Gather all the necessary supplementary materials:
  - Official graduate school transcripts
  - Internship completion certificate
  - Updated curriculum vitae
  - Psychology license (excludes early entry applicants)
- Complete the application form and document necessary information based on the latest *ABCN Candidate Manual*.
- Outline didactic experiences demonstrating competency in the eight core knowledge areas: basic neurosciences, functional neuroanatomy, neuropathology, clinical neurology, psychological assessment, clinical neuropsychological assessment, psychopathology, and psychological intervention (truncated for those who complete postdoctoral fellowship at an APPCN site).

Step 2: Preparing for the examination process

Written examination	• Commit to a study routine and create accountability: - Join a study group. - Connect with a board-certified neuropsychologist. • Review comprehensive study resources: - Be Ready for ABPP in Neuropsychology (BRAIN; https://theaacn.org/board-certification) - Clinical Neuropsychology Study Guide and Board Review (Stucky et al., 2020) • Attend continuing education workshops covering board certification preparation at neuropsychology conferences.
Practice sample submission	• Choose 2 practice work samples for double-blind review: - Exclude cases seen during training - Pick challenging, but not overly complicated, cases • Cases should be disparate enough in terms of age, diagnoses, symptomatology, and neuropathology. • Cases should demonstrate skills in assessment, brain-behavior relationships, differential diagnoses, and formulation of recommendations. • Mentors can be helpful during this stage to comment on strengths and weaknesses of potential practice samples. • Carefully redact identifying information prior to submission.
Oral examination • Ethics & Professional Practice • Practice Sample Defense • Fact Finding	• Practice regularly with others, including with a study group, mentor(s), and/or colleagues. • Form a study group, if not already done during preparation for the written exam. • Review APA's *Ethical Principles of Psychologists and Code of Conduct* (https://www.apa.org/ethics/code). • Have mentors and study group members critique cases and come up with questions that may be posed during the exam. • Focus on efficient time management for Fact Finding portion. • Practice, practice, PRACTICE!

Note. APPCN = Association of Postdoctoral Programs in Clinical Neuropsychology; APA = American Psychological Association.

Step 1: Preparing for the Application and Credential Review

The purpose of the credential review is to demonstrate to ABCN that you have met all the necessary prerequisites for board certification in clinical neuropsychology. Again, only candidates who graduated from (or for early-entry candidates, are enrolled in) a professional psychology doctoral degree program accredited by APA, CPA, or an accrediting agency recognized by the U.S. Department of Education are eligible. At least 1 month prior to submitting your applications, you will need to gather all the necessary supplementary materials: official graduate school transcripts, internship completion certificate, updated curriculum vitae, and psychology license (excluding early-entry applicants). This would also be a good time for you to ask for two to three letters of support from references familiar with your clinical training and skills. Preferably, at least one of the references should be board certified by ABCN. Recent graduates are strongly encouraged to obtain at least one letter from a supervisor involved in your training, such as the postdoctoral fellowship program director.

Next, you will need to document information required to complete the application form (https://abpp.org/Applicant-Information/Application-Process.aspx). You should carefully read through the entire *ABPP/ABCN Candidate Manual* (ABPP/ABCN, 2020), which has the latest information on clinical neuropsychology requirements for board certification (https://abpp.org/BlankSite/media/Clinical-Neuropsychology-Documents/ABCN-Manual.pdf). The most time-consuming aspect of this part of the process involves outlining all of the didactic experiences one has completed to attain competency in the eight core knowledge areas (i.e., basic neurosciences, functional neuroanatomy, neuropathology, clinical neurology, psychological assessment, clinical neuropsychological assessment, psychopathology, and psychological intervention). These didactic experiences may include formal coursework, as well as attendance and participation in brain cuttings, case conferences, grand rounds, for instance. However, this process is shortened for candidates who completed postdoctoral fellowship at an APPCN training site.

Once the application and credentials are approved, this starts the 7-year time clock. It is worth reiterating here that the candidacy period is much longer than the amount of time needed to complete this process. In order to avoid losing momentum at this stage, you will want to set a date for when you plan to take the written exam.

Step 2: Preparing for the Examination Process

After your credentials have been accepted, you will need to prepare for the next steps in the process: the written examination, the practice sample submission, and the oral examination (for any updates to procedures since this writing, please refer to: https://abpp.org/Applicant-Information/Specialty-Boards/Clinical-Neuropsychology/Certification-Exam-Process.aspx). Preparing for the written examination typically requires several months of studying to feel adequately prepared. For the next step, you will submit two practice work samples for double-blind peer review that you evaluated while practicing independently as a licensed psychologist, *not* as a trainee (i.e., graduate student, clinical intern, or postdoctoral fellow). Lastly, you are advised to practice with others to prepare for the oral exam, which consists of three sections: Ethics and Professional Practice, Practice Sample Defense, and Fact Finding.

The Written Examination

Preparing for the written portion of the examination will likely be the most demanding stage of the ABCN certification process. While the written exam is certainly challenging (there is a 60% to 70% pass rate) most candidates feel comfortable with the exam content following 4 to 6 months of active studying (https://www.abpp.org/Applicant-Information/Specialty-Boards/Clinical-Neuropsychology/FAQs.aspx). A concrete deadline is one of the best ways to ensure you maintain a consistent study practice, so commit to a study routine that will allow ample time to study prior to your exam date.

Another effective way to create accountability during this process is to join a study group. Study group members can divide up the tasks of organizing subjects and creating notes to outline the exam topics, which can be an arduous task for one person alone. Ideally, the group would be made up of members with distinct specializations. Group members should meet every week, either in person or virtually, to discuss topic areas, progress, and barriers encountered. For those candidates who know peers in their geographic area who are also preparing for the exam: excellent! For those who do not know of anyone in their vicinity, there are still ways to connect with others, locally or not, who are interested in forming a study group. One resource to connect with others is through the AACN Board Certification Promotion Committee (https://theaacn.org/board-certification).

Candidates may also contact the promotion committee to be connected with a board-certified neuropsychologist to mentor them through the certification process. Unlike other standardized tests, like the GRE or the EPPP, there are no official study materials available for the ABCN exam. However, there are several comprehensive resources available to help you prepare, some of which are free. The *Clinical Neuropsychology Study Guide and Board Review* (Stucky et al., 2020) provides an overview of the process, helpful resources, study tips, and practice questions. The written exam assesses content areas identified by Section VI of the Houston Conference Guidelines (Hannay et al., 1998; found online at https://theaacn.org/wp-content/uploads/2015/11/Houston_Conference.pdf) which covers the foundational knowledge bases for neuropsychologists: (a) general psychology, (b) general clinical psychology, (c) general psychopathology/neuropathology, (d) brain–behavior relationships, and (e) practice of neuropsychology. Questions may cover such topics as ethics, culture/diversity, and professional issues in neuropsychology (https://theabcn.org/wp-content/uploads/2020/08/ABCN-Candidate-Manual-08-20.pdf).

An additional resource worth highlighting is BRAIN, which stands for Be Ready for ABPP in Neuropsychology. BRAIN is a network with a wealth of information to facilitate ABCN exam preparation: study notes organized by topic, flashcards, mock exams, textbook recommendations, and connection to other candidates looking to form study groups. It is worth perusing the website for the study notes alone, which cover such topics as aphasia syndromes, cerebral hemispheres and vascular supply, disconnection syndromes, endocrine disorders, models of frontal lobe functioning, somatosensory pathways, and test construction, among many others. These study materials were generously provided by board-certified neuropsychologists who volunteer their time to maintain the website (https://brainaacn.org).

Another way to prepare for the exam is attending a continuing education (CE) workshop. Annual conferences of the major neuropsychological associations (i.e., American Academy of Neuropsychology, National Academy of Neuropsychology, International Neuropsychological Society), often include a CE workshop that outlines the steps involved in board certification and strategies for how to prepare. Attending one of these workshops gives you the opportunity to ask questions about the process and has the added benefit of counting toward your continuing education credits to maintain licensure. Unfortunately, even after studying for the exam some candidates will not initially pass this stage of the process. As discouraging as this may be, aside from reaching out to mentors, you can seek advice and support from others through the BRAIN network's Survivor Support Group. Those who do pass the written exam will go to the next stage: the practice sample.

The Practice Sample Submission
Candidates who reach this phase of the examination process are surely breathing a sigh of relief. The practice sample is your first opportunity to demonstrate how you approach the actual practice of neuropsychology. When choosing which two practice samples to submit for review, you will

need to ensure that the cases are varied enough to display your clinical acumen and breadth. As ABCN (2019) puts it,

> Clinical neuropsychology is not merely the administration, scoring and reporting of neuropsychological evaluation techniques in a clinical setting; rather, it is a specialty practiced by a psychologist who can demonstrate to ABCN the integrated application of the broad range of neuropsychological, neurological, and allied clinical and research literature and concepts required of the practitioner in this field.

Identifying which cases meet the above standards can be a challenge. Aside from choosing cases that are disparate enough in terms of age, diagnoses, symptomatology, and neuropathology, the practice samples need to demonstrate your skills in assessment, brain–behavior relationships, differential diagnoses, and formulation of recommendations (Armstrong et al., 2008). Choosing cases that are either too straightforward or too complicated may have consequences, as the former will not give you an opportunity to showcase your clinical strengths, and the latter may generate additional questions that can be difficult to support during the oral examination. Mentors can be especially helpful during this stage, so you should seek out their opinions regarding strengths and weaknesses of potential practice samples. After choosing which cases to submit, you will need to prepare the reports for submission (refer to Step 4 under the Examination Process section of this chapter). It would be terribly unfortunate to fail this stage due to a careless oversight, so before submitting the samples, you must ensure that you have carefully redacted all identifying information in all of the documentation submitted. You can refer to the AACN Study Guide (AACN, 2015) for additional guidelines about navigating this stage of the application process.

The Oral Examination

Once the reviewers have accepted the practice sample submissions, the samples are then used to generate questions for the oral exam. Again, this phase consists of three components: (a) Ethics and Professional Practice, (b) Practice Sample Defense, and (c) Fact Finding (see Table 5.1). You are evaluated based on performance, rather than written materials, so the benefit of practicing with others—a study group, colleagues, and/or mentors—cannot be overemphasized. For those who have not formed a study group or connected with a mentor by the time they have reached this stage, now is a good time to do so via AACN or BRAIN.

The first two segments of the oral examination are reasonably predictable. To prepare for the ethics portion, you will want to spend time reviewing APA's (2017) *Ethical Principles of Psychologists and Code of Conduct* (https://www.apa.org/ethics/code). Reviewing vignettes illustrating ethical dilemmas would also be beneficial, as this would closely mirror what you will be asked to do during the exam. For the practice sample defense, you will have the advantage of being extremely familiar with the cases. The caveat to this, of course, is that the bar is set much higher during this section, so you need to ensure that you have exhaustive knowledge about anything even remotely related to your cases, including differential diagnoses, underlying neuropathology, and psychometrics of the assessments used. Therefore, it is essential that you have mentors and study group members critique your cases and come up with questions that may be posed during the oral exam. Refer to Armstrong et al. (2008) for an extensive description of how to prepare for this stage of the process.

The final component of the oral examination is the Fact Finding exercise. You can choose either an adult or pediatric case, and are asked to evaluate the neuropsychological clinical referral *de novo*, that is, with no prior knowledge about the case. A brief clinical vignette is provided, and you are asked to elicit all relevant information (e.g., history, test results, impressions) to demonstrate case conceptualization and conclusion formulation. It is important that you "think out loud" during this portion to demonstrate your deductive reasoning when asking questions about the case. For instance, instead of asking, "Does the patient report any changes in sleep behaviors?" the candidate may pose the statement as the following:

> The history so far makes me concerned about the possibility of Lewy body dementia, and this condition is often associated with changes in sleep behaviors, so I would like to know the patient and family members' perceptions about the patient's sleep and if there have been any changes.

The Fact Finding portion of the exam only lasts one hour, so it is imperative that preparation focus on efficient time management. You may choose to take a few minutes to write down your questions, and create an outline to organize your thoughts. It is suggested that you then use approximately 25 minutes to ask questions of the examiner to gather necessary details to form your case conceptualization. Once you have completed your questions and gathered enough information, you can request the neuropsychological test scores in writing. Finally, when you are ready, you should plan on taking about 10 minutes to discuss your case conceptualization and present impressions and recommendations. When presenting the conclusions, you will need to demonstrate your knowledge by explaining your rationale and reasoning; even if they are accurate, you should expect to be challenged about your conclusions and questioned about your knowledge base related to the case.

This is likely the most talked about segment of the exam, as it tends to invoke anxiety in many candidates. The good news is that—unlike the multiple-choice, right/wrong format of the written exam—reviewers during the Fact Finding portion are just as interested in the process by which candidates arrive at conclusions as they are in the conclusions themselves. It is essential that candidates practice doing Fact Finding exercises multiple times prior to the exam day. You will want to develop and practice the techniques you will use, and integrate history and test data (Armstrong et al., 2008) so that it will be automatic when test day arrives. For an in-depth resource specific to the Fact Finding process, you can refer to *The Neuropsychology Fact-Finding Casebook: A Training Resource* (Stucky & Bush, 2017).

CONCLUSION AND FUTURE DIRECTIONS

Board certification is a multistep peer-review process that requires you (the candidate) to demonstrate achievement of the highest standard of competency in clinical neuropsychology. The board certification process involves successful completion of an application/credential review, written examination, practice sample review, and oral examination. Although the process itself may seem daunting at first blush, there are abundant resources available, both in terms of published materials as well as profession- and peer-support networks, to help candidates successfully navigate the requirements. While some may pass all components of the board certification process on the first attempt, it is not uncommon for individuals to hit a roadblock during the process (e.g., failing the written or oral exam; practice samples not being rated as acceptable for passage to the oral examination). In fact, many qualified candidates do and many board-certified neuropsychologists have hit such roadblocks! Nonetheless, it is important to stick with the process so that you can experience the professional benefits and personal fulfillment that often accompany successful completing of board certification in clinical neuropsychology.

REFERENCES

American Academy of Clinical Neuropsychology (AACN). (2015). *AACN study guide.* https://theaacn.org/wp-content/uploads/2015/10/aacn_studyguide.pdf

American Board of Clinical Neuropsychology (ABCN). (2019). *Practice sample submission.* https://theabcn.org/practice-sample-submission

American Board of Professional Psychology (ABPP). (2016). *Academic program requirements for ABPP and ABGP.* http://legacy.abpp.org/files/page-specific/3357%20Group/15_Certificate_Procedures_ABGP_20161216.pdf

American Board of Professional Psychology/American Board of Clinical Neuropsychology (ABPP/ABCN). (2020). *Board certification guidelines and procedures: Candidate's manual.* https://abpp.org/BlankSite/media/Clinical-Neuropsychology-Documents/ABCN-Manual.pdf

American Psychological Association. (2017). *Ethical principles of psychologists and code of conduct* (2002, Amended June 1, 2010, and January 1, 2017). http://www.apa.org/ethics/code/ethics-code-2017.pdf

Armstrong, K. E., Beebe, D. W., Hilsabeck, R. C., & Kirkwood, M. W. (2008). *Board certification in clinical neuropsychology: A guide to becoming ABPP/ABCN certified without sacrificing your sanity.* Oxford University Press.

Cassel, C. K., & Holmboe, E. S. (2008). Professionalism and accountability: The role of specialty board certification. *Transactions of the American Clinical and Climatological Association, 119,* 295–303. https://www.ncbi.nlm.nih.gov/pmc/articles/PMC2394686/

Hannay, H. J., Bieliauskas, L. A., Crosson, B., Hammeke, T., Hamsher, K. D., & Koffler, S. P. (1998). The Houston conference on specialty education and training in clinical neuropsychology-policy statement. *Archives of Clinical Neuropsychology, 13*(2), 160–166. https://doi.org/10.1093/arclin/13.2.160

Stringer, A., Bobholz, J., & Vanderploeg, R. (2019). *Preparing for the ABPP board certification examination in clinical neuropsychology: Everything you wanted to know but didn't know who to ask–policies and procedures* [Paper presentation], 17th Annual AACN Conference, Chicago, IL. https://doi.org/10.1080/13854046.2019.1595155

Stucky, K. J., & Bush, S. S. (2017). *The neuropsychology fact-finding casebook: A training resource.* Oxford University Press.

Stucky, K. J., Kirkwood, M. W., & Donders, J. (Eds.). (2020). *Clinical neuropsychology study guide and board review* (2nd ed.). Oxford University Press.

Sweet, J. J., Benson, L. M., Nelson, N. W., & Moberg, P. J. (2015). The American Academy of Clinical Neuropsychology, National Academy of Neuropsychology, and Society for Clinical Neuropsychology (APA Division 40) 2015 TCN professional practice and 'salary survey': Professional practices, beliefs, and incomes of U.S. neuropsychologists. *The Clinical Neuropsychologist, 29*(8), 1069–1162. https://doi.org/10.1080/13854046.2016.1140228

6

FINDING A JOB

Clinical Careers in Neuropsychology

HEATHER G. BELANGER, JASON R. SOBLE, EDWARD PECK III,
PATRICK ARMISTEAD-JEHLE, MARK BARISA,
LUCIEN ROBERTS III, AND MIKE R. SCHOENBERG

A clinical career in neuropsychology can be both a rewarding and a lucrative path. In this chapter, we discuss the primary settings in which neuropsychologists pursue clinical careers. It is important to note, however, that many clinicians may choose to pursue clinical work in addition to administrative, research, and other roles. In addition, patient populations served can vary substantially, even within the same setting. For example, some neuropsychologists who have an independent practice may focus almost exclusively on forensic work, while others may specialize in seeing certain disorders, while still others may be more generalists. Neuropsychologists may work in independent practice, the Veterans Health Administration (VHA), the Department of Defense (DoD), in an academic medical setting, or some combination of these settings. In this chapter, we discuss each of these settings, as well as offer advice on how to land a job in that setting, the relative advantages and disadvantages of that setting, and how to succeed.

Before proceeding, we offer three key considerations to best utilize the information in this chapter. First, while each section contains general information relevant to that particular clinical setting, there can be considerable variability within individual settings. Second, the advantages/disadvantages

https://doi.org/10.1037/0000250-007
The Neuropsychologist's Roadmap: A Training and Career Guide, C. Block (Editor)

listed for each setting are relative and need to be considered within the context of one's preferences. For example, one professional may gravitate toward the more well-defined VHA duty tour, whereas another may find it too restrictive. Third, despite common perceptions, the perfect job is a myth, especially when considering one's first position. The reality is that no employment setting is likely to have it all, and compromise to strike a balance between pros and cons often is necessary.

VETERANS HEALTH ADMINISTRATION

The VHA is the largest employer and trainer of psychologists in the United States. As such, it is a sensible place to seek employment as a neuropsychologist.

Factors to Consider and Finding a Job

Possibly the best way to find a job there is to train there. One must be a United States citizen to train and/or be hired by the VHA. Interns and postdoctoral residents who complete their training there undoubtedly have an advantage in seeking employment within VHA (assuming of course that they were perceived favorably), although previous experience within VHA is not a prerequisite of employment. Prior training must be accredited by the American Psychological Association (APA) or the Canadian Psychological Association (CPA). Jobs can be found online (see https://www.usajobs.gov). Sometimes bureaucracy can cause delays and glitches in online applications, so it is recommended that job applicants also send their curriculum vitae (CV) directly to the chief of psychology at the VA location at which they hope to work. Jobs can open up within VHA at any time.

It is definitely advantageous to have already obtained one's psychology license when seeking employment within VHA, as psychologists who begin work without one are disadvantaged financially and do not start their federal service "retirement clock." Specifically, unlicensed providers must be supervised and are designated not as staff, but rather "graduate psychologists," which involves temporary appointment for a period not to exceed 2 years. Failure to obtain licensure during that period is justification for termination of the temporary appointment. Because VHA is a federal system, psychologists can be licensed anywhere in the United States, though holding licensure in a different state than one's VHA facility limits one's ability to engage in outside clinical work (e.g., private practice). It is also advantageous to have completed postdoctoral training, as these years count as experience that allows the new hire to start at a higher level/salary.

The VHA salary and promotion system is based on years of experience beginning at the postdoctoral level. Those who complete one year of postdoctoral training start their VHA career at General Schedule (GS) 12 (i.e., Grade 12), while those who complete 2 years of fellowship begin at Grade 13 (a roughly 18% higher salary). There are 10 steps between each grade, with increases based on longevity and acceptable performance (waiting periods of 1 year at Steps 1–3, 2 years at Steps 4–6, and 3 years at Steps 7–9). It normally takes 18 years to advance from Step 1 to Step 10 within a single GS grade, if an employee remains in that single grade, though specialty step increases (Special Advancement for Achievement; SAAs) can be earned for specified activities/accomplishments (e.g., ABPP board certification). There is variability within the VHA system as to how much can be negotiated when offered a position. For job applicants right out of training, there is not much room for negotiation when it comes to salary, as starting salaries in VHA are dictated by years of experience. Conversely, people offered a VHA job coming from some prior clinical job may have some ability to negotiate salary, though there are still some limitations based on the ceiling of the GS pay scale. Regardless of when entering the VHA system, some negotiable aspects of the job might include starting date, test supplies (e.g., neuropsychological or psychological tests, research equipment, etc.), reimbursement of continuing education and other professional expenses, relocation expenses (only if listed in the job announcement), tour of duty (or work schedule), and sometimes the ability to telecommute (less likely for strictly clinical positions than for administrative or research positions).

Advantages and Disadvantages

Most psychologists who work in VHA primarily do clinical work. However, some do exclusively research or administration, and some do a mixture. Because it is a large, national health care system, the VHA has many leadership and training opportunities that can help with advancement opportunities. Working within such a large health care system can be advantageous for those who wish to pursue careers with a greater mix of responsibilities and opportunities to advance. And once within the system, there is an ability to transfer to other facilities.

Although VHA salaries are competitive with private practice salaries in the first 5 years of clinical practice, private practice salaries generally far exceed institutional salaries over time (Sweet et al., 2015). However, as is

TABLE 6.1. Advantages and Disadvantages of Becoming a Veterans Health Administration Neuropsychologist

Advantages	Disadvantages
✓ Fewer limitations on services provided (i.e., services based on patient needs)	✗ Increased pressure to enhance productivity and efficiency (i.e., see more patients faster) to enhance access
✓ Common mission of serving veterans	
✓ Rewarded quickly with salary in early years	✗ Restricted patient population
✓ Large system, can transfer within the system	✗ Different hiring class than physicians (limits pay and stature, particularly in mid-to-late career)
✓ Predictable salary and work schedule	✗ Large, inflexible system that can be slow to hire staff
✓ Possible step increases for achievement (based on accomplishments outside job description)	✗ Rigid work schedule (must be on site during tour of duty)
✓ Generous vacation time, particularly after 15 years of consecutive service	✗ Lack of monetary incentives for career success
✓ Opportunities to do research, administrative work, and training in addition to clinical work	✗ Negative media focus/taxpayer funded
✓ Trainees and psychometricians at many sites	
✓ Free continuing education credits (more likely at VAs with a training program)	
✓ Electronic records and other infrastructure	
✓ National listservs, other resources	

Note. VAs = Veterans Administrations.

the case with academic medical centers, taking on administrative roles is one way to increase one's income (e.g., clinical program director). Additionally, some VHA neuropsychologists supplement their income with private practice work on weekends and other off-duty times. Please see Table 6.1 for more about the advantages and disadvantages of working within the VHA.

DEPARTMENT OF DEFENSE

DoD provides unique opportunities for neuropsychological training and employment.

Factors to Consider and Finding a Job

There are three distinct routes to working in the DoD as a neuropsychologist: (a) active duty (AD) service member (SM), (b) GS civilian employee, or (c) civilian contractor. A brief overview of each will be provided, in addition to related advantages and disadvantages.

Active Duty

The United States Army, Navy, and Air Force employ AD psychologists for a range of positions. While the primary duties of these officers relate to maintaining the psychological readiness of the fighting force, these SMs are engaged in all aspects of AD service. Most commonly AD psychologists complete internship training with the Army, Navy, or Air Force. Each of these branches of service participates in the Association of Psychology Postdoctoral and Internship Centers (APPIC) internship matching program and has several training sites across the United States. With acceptance of internship training, there is an obligation of AD service that typically runs 3 years. At the end of this period, the psychologist may choose to separate from AD service or continue service with an additional contract. With further service, postdoctoral training as a neuropsychologist is available in the form of a 2-year fellowship. At the time of publication, fellowship training is available at the Walter Reed National Military Medical Center (Army) and the San Antonio Military Medical Center (Army and Air Force). Both of these programs are APA accredited and members of the Association of Postdoctoral Programs in Clinical Neuropsychology (APPCN). In addition, the Navy allows completion of postdoctoral training at civilian institutions. With fellowship training, the psychologist will incur an additional AD obligation of approximately 4 years.

General Schedule Civilian Employee

One may also work for the DoD as a GS employee. Here, the neuropsychologist would work for the Defense Health Agency and provide neuropsychological care to SMs, family members, and/or retirees. Work in this capacity has much in common with VHA neuropsychology positions, with postings advertised on https://www.usajobs.gov. However, the population served will be slightly different than the VHA, in that the focus will be on AD SMs. Neuropsychology positions with the DoD are typically at the grade of GS-13 or GS-14 and, depending on the site, can include administrative, teaching, and research opportunities, though the emphasis for most positions is clinical care. Unlike in VHA, developmental positions are very rare. One needs to be licensed prior to being considered for any psychology position and credentialing requires internship training at an APA-accredited program. Moreover, in order to be credentialed at a military treatment facility (MTF), one's education and training must be consistent with the Houston Conference Guidelines (Hannay et al., 1998).

Civilian Contractor

Beyond being a GS employee, a number of neuropsychologists work for the DoD as contractors. For instance, the Traumatic Brain Injury Center of Excellence (TBICoE) has many contracted neuropsychology positions at various MTFs within and outside of the continental United States. In short, several of these positions mirror the clinical duties of GS providers, but depending on the specific position can allow for more dedicated research time. There are also a number of research specific neuropsychology positions in TBICoE that are contract in nature.

Advantages and Disadvantages

Active Duty

Advantages to pursuing training and employment as a neuropsychologist while on AD status include the exceptional quality of fellowship training. Moreover, pay is based on military rank and not training status. Consequently, salary and benefits are substantially higher than nonuniformed service positions for trainees. A primary disadvantage of this career path is the lengthy route to becoming trained as a neuropsychologist. One usually comes on AD in their final year of graduate training as an intern and then must serve a 3-year tour prior to application for neuropsychology fellowship training. Moreover, there is no guarantee that one will be selected for fellowship training after internship, and thus, for those who know prior to internship that they absolutely want to obtain neuropsychology-specific fellowship training, this path has added risk. Next, after fellowship training, there is no guarantee that subsequent duty assignments will be related specifically to neuropsychology, as SMs are assigned based on the needs of the military. Table 6.2 summarizes these advantages and disadvantages.

Other factors to consider, that could be advantageous or disadvantageous depending on one's desires, relate to the AD lifestyle. This includes changes in duty stations (usually once every 3 years) and probable combat deployments. Moreover, Uniformed Services medical providers (neuropsychologist or otherwise) function as military officers and thus require the training necessary to meet these requirements. These experiences include basic

TABLE 6.2. Advantages and Disadvantages of Becoming a Department of Defense Neuropsychologist

Advantages	Disadvantages
Government Service:	*Government Service:*
✓ Generous vacation and retirement benefits	✗ Slow and deliberate hiring process that can take months
✓ Possible relocation, retention, retirement bonuses	✗ Limited monetary incentives for successful performance
✓ Possible travel funds for continued education, conference attendance	✗ Rigid work schedule (must be on site during tour of duty)
✓ Predictable salary with set schedule for step increases	✗ Limited focus/time and value for outside professional activities
✓ Possible opportunities for research, administration and training	✗ Ever-increasing pressure for higher productivity (i.e., more patient contacts)
Active Duty:	*Active Duty:*
✓ Excellent quality of fellowship training	✗ Obligated military service
✓ Pay based on military rank for internship and postdoctoral fellowship training (i.e., much higher than average)	✗ No guarantee of fellowship opportunities after finishing internship
✓ Guaranteed employment via military service while under contract	✗ May ultimately work outside neuropsychology
✓ Military benefits (i.e., insurance, retirement)	

physical fitness and weapons training, as well as education on military structure and logistics.

General Schedule Civilian Employee

Many of the advantages of GS employment as a neuropsychologist in the DoD match those of the VHA. The benefits packages for insurance, vacation, and retirement are highly competitive. Pay is also rather predictable with a set schedule for increases. In addition, there is the possibility of bonuses for recruitment and relocation when a position is initially filled and for retention bonuses annually. These can range from 5% to 25% of base salary and can be negotiated depending on the position, but are by no means guaranteed. Initial step level is set prior to starting the position and there can be room for negotiation, with previous experience and salary playing important roles. Those straight out of postdoc should not expect to have much negotiating power; however, those who have experience at non-GS positions could reasonably argue for a salary roughly commensurate to those positions. In addition, the federal system has historically had various student loan repayment programs available to new employees, and this could be broached with initial negotiations. It is important to understand that when accepting a GS position, all negotiations for step level and bonuses happen up front. Once the final offer is accepted there is typically limited opportunity to revisit these issues. Even with lateral transfers to a different position within the same grade, step levels are not open to increase. Consequently, it is to the employee's benefit to negotiate the best possible package (e.g., step level, recruitment/relocation, and/or loan repayment program) prior to starting the position. The same is true of VHA positions. An additional benefit is the historic availability of travel funds to attend professional conferences (though this too is not guaranteed and can vary from year to year). Finally, depending on the position there is potential for administrative/leadership opportunities, research, and training. However the focus of most such positions will be clinical in nature.

Disadvantages of this career path include the initial navigation of a slow hiring system that can take months to complete the necessary background checks and credentialing. Another disadvantage relative to private practice, is that salary is generally rather fixed and engaging more clinical work does not typically result in increased pay. Salary can be supplemented by "off-duty employment" but this requires approval from MTF leadership and has restrictions. The focus of job duties for most DoD neuropsychologists is clinical care, and while research and training opportunities can be available, there is a limited degree of value placed on other professional activities (e.g., involvement with professional organizations, journal editing or reviews, etc.). That is to say, such activities will typically not be included in performance standards, and will thus not be actively reinforced/rewarded or afforded much time to engage. Arguably, these activities are more valued in the VHA and without question, of greater value within academic medical centers.

Civilian Contractor

The main difference in contract versus GS employment comes with compensation. Contract employees work for the contracting company, and thus negotiate for salary and benefits with this company and are not subject to the federal GS pay scale. In general, take home pay for contractors can be more lucrative than for GS employees; however, benefits tend to be less competitive and job protection/security is somewhat diminished.

ACADEMIC MEDICAL CENTERS

As noted in Chapter 7, academic medical centers (AMCs) are institutions that emphasize the education of future health care professionals, state-of-the-art patient care delivery, and cutting-edge research as part of their core mission.

Factors to Consider and Finding a Job

There is not one prescribed trajectory to obtain an AMC position; however, some specific aspects of training and experience can strengthen one's application. For example, board certification is often needed within 2 to 3 years of hire for many positions, and obtaining board certification early can also make an application stronger. There is an increasing trifurcation of AMC positions: (a) positions that are clinically focused, (b) the more traditional positions that include a major research component, but also include teaching and clinical practice, and (c) careers more focused on student education and clinical practice. At the training level, practicum/externship, internship, and postdoctoral placements can provide valuable experience providing services in this setting, and may be viewed favorably in selecting applicants. Increasingly, AMC positions with a research component seek applicants with prior experience in obtaining grant funding (see Chapter 7, this volume, for greater detail on research careers). Thus, selecting a graduate program that offers explicit training in obtaining research funding may make a trainee more competitive for an eventual AMC position (see Chapter 13 for more on grantsmanship). The emerging clinical educator positions commonly entail a strong component of student education. In medical schools, the focus is on medical school education, but some AMCs may also highly value education of undergraduate students in the neurosciences, as well as graduate program education. While more limited, students interested in this career avenue may seek to develop their experience supervising undergraduate students, interns, or junior residents/fellows. Another avenue would be developing education research programs that evaluate education processes or outcomes, which may be obtained from national foundations or federal agencies involved in education (e.g., National Center for Education Research; see https://ies.ed.gov/ncer).

In terms of locating positions, it is important to note that unlike the federal system, which utilizes https://www.usajobs.gov/, there is not an analogous website where all AMC positions are posted. Thus, it is critical for applicants to be vigilant about postings on listservs, at professional meetings and organizational websites, and third-party websites (e.g., Indeed.com). Professional networking is beneficial for identifying potential job opportunities, as not all positions may be posted. Additional factors to consider when applying are that some institutions will require an in-person interview and/or one-hour job talk based on one's program of research or clinical focus. (Your job talk can involve reviewing a clinical case or discussing your research line. Tailor your job talk to the institution, and by all means practice well in advance.) In contrast to the federal system, which has well-defined guidelines that dictate starting salary, AMC applicants typically have more flexibility to negotiate their salary and other benefits (e.g., relocation expenses, sign-on bonus, testing materials). The salary survey (Sweet et al., 2015) is a particularly useful reference for understanding job characteristics across types of work settings, and potentially for use in advocating and negotiating one's salary. Another resource is the Association of American Medical Colleges (AAMC) annual faculty salary report (https://www.aamc.org/data-reports/workforce/report/aamc-faculty-salary-report).

This report provides the salaries of physicians and nonphysician doctoral faculty employed full-time in the participating medical colleges across the United States by academic rank, department/specialty, school ownership, and region. Further, unlike federal agencies, which do not require licensure in one's state of practice, those seeking AMC employment have to obtain licensure in the state in which they will be practicing, which often involves additional expenses (e.g., transfer fees, new licensure applications). However, sometimes the costs of licensure can be negotiated as part of one's compensation package.

Advantages and Disadvantages

AMCs offer a variety of career pathways. Accordingly, this setting is often appealing for those who want a diverse professional portfolio. Clinically, AMCs vary widely in terms of populations served and services offered, such that they may offer more latitude to tailor clinical activities to match one's interests/expertise. For instance, some neuropsychologists are housed in highly specialized programs (e.g., comprehensive epilepsy programs, movement disorder centers, cancer centers), whereas others are located in larger academic departments (e.g., neurology, neurosurgery, or psychiatry) and receive referrals from across the medical center and, often, the community at large. Many AMCs offer a wide referral base across outpatient and inpatient settings, given the numerous specialties found in most large medical centers.

Moreover, AMCs can offer viable employment for those who identify as pediatric and/or lifespan neuropsychologists. Within the course of normal clinical duties (and under the auspices of one's employing institution), some AMCs also allow neuropsychologists to partake in forensic work, including forensic evaluations, independent medical examinations, and providing deposition and trial testimony (Schwarz et al., 2009).

For those interested in establishing a program of research, AMCs are an appealing setting in that many will encourage neuropsychologists to have a portion of their salary supported through external grants (see Chapter 7). AMCs also regularly facilitate collaboration/mentorship with medical colleagues conducting research in areas in which aspects of cognition and/or behavior are a primary or secondary outcome measure. In addition to obtaining one's own grants, it is not uncommon for neuropsychologists to be coinvestigators or subinvestigators on other faculty members' grants, which also fund a portion of their salary. Teaching/training is another professional activity many neuropsychologists engage in at AMCs. For some, this can become a major source of salary support. For others, particularly for faculty funded primarily by research or clinical services, education may reflect a small portion of their faculty assignment. Most typically, education activities involve providing clinical supervision for psychology trainees at various levels of training, and lecturing about aspects of neuroanatomy or the clinical assessment of cognition/mood for medical students and for neuroscience focused residents/fellows. There are typically ample opportunities to attend lectures and seminars where one can obtain continuing education credit for licensure at no cost.

There are also advantages to AMC employment in terms of professional benefits. Per the most recent salary survey (Sweet et al., 2015), the mean salary of clinical PhDs (which include neuropsychologists) was $119,700 (academic-affiliated hospital) to $129,000 (primary university hospital) with a range of $50,000 to $425,000 (primary university hospital) and $50,000 to $500,000 (academic-affiliated hospital). Salary ranges vary widely due to several factors, including years in practice, academic rank, academic department, and level of duties (e.g., higher administrative positions). Some positions also allow for supplementation of base salary through other activities. For example, some neuropsychologists also operate part-time private practices, provided their institution does not contractually prohibit doing so. Other AMCs may allow for and financially incentivize forensic work through one's clinical appointment. In addition to salary, many AMCs operate on a productivity model such that neuropsychologists do not necessarily have rigid work schedules, provided they meet their productivity requirements, which can be appealing for those who value greater work flexibility. Finally, for those who seek to take on more of a professional leadership role, AMCs can provide avenues of advancement via administrative roles at various levels in the medical center.

Despite the many positive aspects of AMC employment, several potential disadvantages and/or limitations are noteworthy. First, there has been an increasing demand that individual professional activities cover the cost of the compensation plus overhead charges. For some, this has resulted in increased clinical productivity demand that can reduce engagement in other professionally rewarding activities, such as education or unfunded clinical research. In some settings, failure to meet productivity expectations can further result in decreased annual income (Sweet et al., 2015) or the position being closed/terminated. Second, in the current economically driven, integrated health care market, one's productivity and earning potential is intricately tied to third-party reimbursement, the largest of which is the Centers for Medicare and Medicaid Services (CMS). In general, CMS has a requirement to control health care expenditures, which can result in reduced reimbursement rates for specific procedures, which has led neuropsychologists to a broadening of the traditional, fee-for-service model of practice (Pliskin, 2018). Working with third-party payers also imposes limitations on certain training activities (e.g., testing done by student trainees cannot be billed to Medicare or Medicaid). In addition to declining reimbursement rates, some AMCs include contractual noncompete clauses that essentially prohibit outside clinical and forensic activities to supplement one's base AMC salary. Thus, annual salaries for institutional settings generally are lower than for private practice (Sweet et al., 2015). Moreover, unlike VHA, which includes a well-defined schedule for standard salary step increases, AMC salary increases can be more variable and there are rarely guaranteed increases, the exception usually being earning a promotion in academic rank. Further, salary increases may be tied to larger sociopolitical factors at some AMCs (e.g., state budgets for public institutions).

Another potential drawback for some is that promotion in academic rank (e.g., promotion from assistant to associate professor) often requires one to demonstrate evidence of outstanding/exceptional productivity/recognition within the field. Those with a prominent clinical faculty assignment must demonstrate regional recognition as a clinical provider for advancement to associate professor rank, along with professional contributions in the teaching and the institution. The demands for academic promotion can pose challenges for those who identify solely as clinicians or teachers. Job security in academic institutions has also changed, with faculty positions being less stable and increasingly dependent upon securing adequate funding. There are fewer tenure-track positions being offered, with some clinical departments choosing to discontinue offering tenure. Please see Table 6.3 for advantages/disadvantages of a clinical career within an academic medical center.

The career pathway in AMCs has been changing the past decade or more, and a new model of AMC faculty is emerging that is more diverse and competitive. The new model does not protect positions with tenure and many (if not all) AMCs have adopted financial modeling in which either individual faculty or academic divisions/sections/departments must financially

TABLE 6.3. Advantages and Disadvantages of Becoming an Academic Medical Center (AMC) Neuropsychologist (Clinical)

Advantages	Disadvantages
✓ Involvement in diverse professional activities (clinical, research, teaching, administration) with multiple avenues available to support one's salary	✗ Increasing clinical productivity demands to cover cost of one's salary plus overhead costs can result in less time to engage in other professional activities (e.g., unfunded research)
✓ Wide patient referral base from different programs and departments and often the larger community	✗ Failure to meet productivity requirements can result in decreased salary or position termination
✓ Ability to tailor clinical activities	✗ Clinical productivity largely tied to insurers/third-party providers and greatly affected by cost-cutting trends in the larger healthcare market
✓ Greater clinical opportunities for pediatric and/or lifespan clinicians	
✓ Opportunities for forensic work during normal clinical duties (and, in some AMCs, to earn supplemental income by doing forensic work)	✗ Third-party billing rules/regulations pertaining to student involvement may limit training opportunities
✓ Research collaboration and mentorship opportunities	✗ Salary increases are not guaranteed and can be erratic
✓ Ability to have some or all of one's clinical salary covered by external research grants	✗ Criteria for career advancement and academic promotion can be complex and require research productivity and/or recognition within the field above one's normal compensated clinical duties/productivity
✓ Abundant opportunities to teach and supervise psychology and medical students/trainees	
✓ Access to continuing medical education	
✓ Competitive salary prospects	✗ Less job security (particularly given dwindling tenure-track positions)
✓ Flexible schedule/hours	✗ Overabundance of professional activities can increase risk of over-commitment and academic burnout
✓ Opportunities for leadership, administrative positions	
✓ Funding opportunities to attend and present at professional conferences	

support themselves. There is also increasing recognition that not all successful faculty will obtain research grants, and there is a need for faculty to focus on clinical service provision to patients and others to teach students. These new career pathways can reflect a clinical education or clinical/scholar pathways and offer more focused models for career advancement and academic promotion.

INDEPENDENT PRACTICE

Many early career neuropsychologists look to independent private practice as a first option in employment following graduation and postdoctoral fellowship. While this certainly can be a great work environment with promises of flexible scheduling, assumptions of lucrative reimbursement, and minimal administrative control over clinical and other work activities, these expectations quickly get tempered by the stark reality of the time, money, and energy involved in starting or working in a private practice. The reader is referred to prior writings in this area by chapter coauthors (see Barisa, 2010; Peck, 2003; Peck & Roberts, 2019).

Factors to Consider and Finding a Job

There are several ways to set up an independent practice in neuropsychology. The more common models for independent practice include a traditional individual private practice; joining or starting a group practice; joining an independent or facility-based physician practice group; engaging in contract services through hospitals or other facilities on an as needed/hourly or regularly scheduled basis; or setting up a flexible, concierge practice with a select group of patients or referral sources. Blended models are also possible and these will be discussed as part of this general overview.

Traditional private practice, or a sole-proprietor model, is probably the most common scenario new professionals consider. Here, the clinician functions as a solo practitioner and may or may not incorporate as a professional limited liability company (PLLC) or sole proprietor limited liability company (LLC). This model can take multiple forms ranging from the stereotypical single office/single provider seeing patients referred from medical providers to a multifaceted practice with multiple referral streams, contracts with facilities/organizations, and multiple locations. In the early stages of a new practice, an independent practitioner may choose to rent space from a practice group or other office entity and set up their own clinical practice within the location. This is similar to a hairstylist renting a chair in a salon. The practitioner functions independently and manages their own practice in terms of legal aspects, scheduling, billing, etc. Rental may or may not include additional expense sharing such as receptionist, telecommunications, office supplies, test equipment, copy/fax devices, furniture, and so on.

Some new options have emerged for those venturing into independent practice, including day office rental and virtual office opportunities through companies like Regus, LiquidSpace, Servcorp, DaVinci, and others. These companies have large office suites in multiple locations with individual office rental available by the hour, day, week, month, year, or longer. They also have "virtual" office opportunities with a set mailing address, phone number, FedEx availability, receptionist, and other services provided, with office space available at hourly or daily rates as needed. This can be a great resource for those looking to dabble in independent practice or who are starting slowly, with opportunities to increase office hours as volume/need increases. This also allows for multiple practice locations with minimal additional cost.

Some independent practitioners look to join or start a group practice. Here the clinician joins a roster of other providers sharing space and some expenses. These can be structured formally, where the new clinician is hired on as a member of the group, paying a percentage of receivables to the head(s) of the group to help cover overhead and other costs. Percentage rates, salaries, and other models of payment can vary across and within groups and should be negotiated carefully prior to finalizing any agreements. Alternatively, the clinicians may have partnerships or other arrangements for equitable sharing of many expenses, but with each clinician maintaining an independent practice in terms of scheduling, billing, and reimbursement. Group practice membership can be quite variable depending on how the groups are structured, who has the controlling interest, and the various contracts that can be employed. However, this is sometimes an easy way to get into private practice with minimal startup costs, minimal up-front administrative requirements, more streamlined insurance credentialing, an established billing/reimbursement system, and an established referral base.

Another option for those looking to be part of a group practice is to join an independent or facility-based physician practice group. These contracts can be set up as a set salary, salary plus additional incentives for high productivity, or a straight percentage of reimbursement model with costs for practice management services on a percentage basis. This allows for direct referrals from within the practice group or from the supporting facility. Many of these are structured under an accountable care organization (ACO) where a large health system oversees and control the practice of providers across the inpatient and outpatient environments. Providers under an ACO agree to practice within the policies and procedures of the larger health care organization. While this can increase the number of referrals, it can also result in limitations in practice patterns through the oversight of the organization administrators.

It is possible to have an independent practice with nothing more than a virtual office address or PO Box, but with no formal office location. Practitioners with this type of arrangement can gain hospital privileges and engage in clinical or contracted services through hospitals or other facilities (e.g., nursing homes, skilled nursing facilities, rehabilitation units) on an as needed/hourly basis or with a professional billing model for patients seen within the facility setting. This could also include in-home or community agencies, again eliminating the need for a traditional office setting and the associated expenses. A concierge type of practice could also be developed where patients are seen in their home, personal office, or other location for assessment or therapy services on a more regular basis. Lastly, civil or criminal litigation opinions, disability, utilization reviews regarding medical necessity and projected charges, worker's compensation, or other medical record review services are common for such a virtual location, as no patient contacts are required. Practitioners who choose to use a virtual office might still consider Regus or another option to have office or conference room availability as needed for independent medical evaluations, depositions, family conferences, or other purposes. The practitioner will need some form of physical location for receipt of legal and other documents.

Advantages and Disadvantages

It is important to note that advantages and disadvantages are in the eye of the beholder, and this is very true for the case of independent practice. Entering into an independent or group practice, outside of the control and consistency of a facility-based practice, is not for everyone. Some practitioners prefer a solitary type of practice where they maintain total control of their work and have little time/value for collegial input/interactions. Others thrive in academic/collegial environments with set schedules and expectations that make the day more routine and predictable. Some enjoy the potential opportunities for new challenges and additional income or satisfaction from additional work, while others value the consistency and security inherent in a salary-based arrangement. Also, initial startup costs in independent practice can be quite high, including fees for incorporation and business licenses; malpractice and general liability insurance; application for Medicare and other payor panels; costs for credentialing assistance; fees for privileging applications for hospitals and other facilities; startup and monthly fees for electronic medical records (EMRs), scheduling/record storage services, billing services, and accounting assistance; business fax, phone, email, webpage, and other telecommunication needs; office equipment; basic office supplies; and, of course, test equipment and protocols. Table 6.4 provides some relative advantages and disadvantages that should be considered as "potential" advantages and disadvantages depending on perspective.

Future Trends

Independent practice will remain a viable option for neuropsychologists, but the rules for success will continue to evolve as health care policy, regulations,

TABLE 6.4. Advantages and Disadvantages of Becoming an Independent Practice Neuropsychologist

Advantages	Disadvantages
✓ Self-direction/self-determination	✗ Feast or famine
✓ Flexibility and control of schedule	✗ Variable income
✓ Personal autonomy	✗ No compensation during illness or vacation (but costs remain)
✓ Opportunity to learn new things	
✓ Contract negotiation, human resources, marketing, finance, office management, billing/reimbursement, budgeting, etc.	✗ No one to delegate nonclinical responsibilities when needed
	✗ Management of competition and marketing demands
✓ Decision-making control	✗ No continuing medical education, conference, educational, research, or other professional support
✓ Consistency in care and documentation	
✓ No surprise accreditation or other visitors	✗ Loss of collegial and professional relationships
✓ Focus can be on your practice rather than the needs of a larger organization	✗ Business budgetary activities
	✗ Management of supplies/maintenance
✓ Potential for higher financial return through practice management and high work ethic	✗ Startup costs can be high
	✗ Responsible for all expenses incurred
✓ Development of practice in areas of personal or financial interest	✗ Management of complaints/concerns
	✗ Maintenance of regulatory requirements
✓ No committee or administrative meetings	✗ No opportunity for advancement aside from practice growth
	✗ Loss of higher level resources to help in times of crisis

and reimbursement transition as a result of political, social, and economic forces. Opportunities will abound, but only for those who evolve, and only if neuropsychologists are able to demonstrate the added value of neuropsychology. We will need to objectively and repeatedly prove that our care creates better patient outcomes. There are opportunities for reimbursement increases if our profession is successful in advocating for inclusion in government-based outcomes and process documentation systems such as Merit-Based Incentive Payment Systems (MIPS), Advanced Alternative Payment Models (Advanced AMPs), or other quality/cost programs. However, declines in reimbursement levels will continue over the next 10 years, if our profession does not advocate effectively. We are moving away from per unit fees to global service fees. This is notable as the upper limit of allowable testing units decline, as Medicare and other payors increase the demand for computerized testing and, subsequently, decrease funding for our face-to-face integrated neuropsychological services.

As we look to the future of independent practice in neuropsychology, these changes will result in an even greater reliance on forensic and other professional services where fee structures are less regulated. This will also "make up" some of the lost revenue for those who continue to see Medicare and Medicaid patients. We also envision more neuropsychologists choosing to opt out of Medicare and work solely on a private contract arrangement with patients. The rise in concierge neuropsychology services is already a reality and has resulted in a paradigm shift to a fee-for-service model, as opposed to traditional billing through third party payors, for some, if not all, services for some practices. Many of the a la carte options typically offered to patients for free or little cost will need to transition to full fee expenses, so as to be able to operate at a profit versus loss for the time, talent, and effort involved. These items include (a) forms that the patient wants completed, (b) letters to document some element of care or diagnosis, (c) letters to document accommodation needs in school and work settings, (d) completion of disability or other administrative forms in relation to the clinical evaluation provided, and (e) other services that may not be billed to Medicare or other third-party payors. In the current model, these services are "nonbillable" and represent unreimbursed time taken by the provider.

Once Medicare and other insurance companies allow for services where the professional is not actually physically present onsite with the patient, the entire question of in-office testing will become moot. This is already happening. Research regarding the practical utility and reliability of neuropsychology through telemedicine is growing and the results are pointing toward implementation in regular clinical practice (see the detailed information regarding teleneuropsychology in Cullum & Grosch, 2013). Now that

EMRs have become more widespread, private practice neuropsychologists will need to adopt such technology. There will be many reasons for ultimate adoption, but simply being able to maintain record access from referral sources, maintain record security in accordance with HIPAA and other regulatory guidelines, and provide quick transmission and access of reports to other sources will become more critical. If we do not stay on par in terms of EMR technology with our physician referral sources, then the medical doctor could see the cost of their office having to copy or fax records to us as a financial disincentive for a referral. Additionally, active use of an EMR will be critical for involvement in MIPS and other payment incentive models, as submission of forms will be managed electronically through these systems.

SUCCESS AND SUSTAINABILITY FACTORS

Regardless of work setting, seeking the advice and counsel of others who have been successful in that setting is recommended. In independent practice, establishing relationships with medico-legal, disability, worker's compensation, vocational rehabilitation, or other non–insurance-based providers can be very beneficial early in the practice development as applications and requests are made for Medicare and managed care insurance panels membership.

Independent Practice

For those in independent practice, identification of early revenue streams is crucial. In general, as with any business, if the practice can manage the financial burdens of the first year, there is typically a good chance for financial success. Hiring an accountant is one excellent piece of advice; another is to recognize that many expenses are recurring (e.g., salaries, rent on the office, leases for equipment). See the comprehensive tables in Peck (2003), Peck et al. (2013), and Peck and Roberts (2019) for a review of expense categories and how these expenses determine when a reimbursed fee for service actually covers the cost of the service. It is also important to maintain a diversification of practice activities to include multiple revenue streams, including general clinical referrals and nonclinical activities such as disability/ utilization reviews, independent medical examinations, worker's compensation evaluations, immigration consultation, medico-legal referrals, and other nontraditional activities. Obtaining privileges at local hospitals can be helpful in increasing referrals and can provide additional monetary gains as well, and may allow for negotiated stipends or other payments to cover the costs of administrative, program development, or nonreimbursed care for their patients or departments. These contracts can provide some degree of stable income, while also strengthening the collaborative partnership with the facility and increasing overall referrals. Finally, practitioners in independent practice must remain cognizant of billing and reimbursement trends and their effects on evaluation length and reimbursement.

While the allure of independent practice is strong, it is not without its challenges. A recent survey of neuropsychologists revealed reversal of a prior trend toward increasing numbers of neuropsychologists working in private practice (Sweet et al., 2015). Since 2010, increasing numbers of neuropsychologists are working in institutional positions rather than private practice. With changes in health care law, large practices and institutions are becoming the favored employment setting.

Federal System

Within both DoD and VHA, learning about military culture is paramount. There are many writings on this topic (see Reger et al., 2008) and various edited books have been dedicated to military psychology (e.g., Kennedy & Zillmer, 2012) and military neuropsychology (e.g., Kennedy & Moore, 2010). Previous experience in the DoD or VHA as a GS employee, contractor, or AD SM is not necessary when applying for GS or contract jobs, but realistically it can provide for a more competitive applicant. Movement to higher GS grades will likely require additional administrative responsibilities and may require leadership duties with more generalized behavioral health involvement. With AD status, promotion to higher ranks will necessitate not only administrative duties, but success at military taskings outside of neuropsychological/psychological practice. Gaining administrative experiences might be accomplished through availing oneself of various local and national training opportunities, as well as volunteering for administrative tasks. Some examples might include working on self-studies for accreditation within psychology training programs, volunteering to serve on administrative review boards, creating databases for administrative or research purposes, working on process improvement projects, etc. Seeking opportunities for national exposure for one's program is another effective way to enhance one's credibility for a leadership position. For example, serving in leadership roles within professional organizations, joining VHA's national leadership organization (i.e., the Association of VA Psychologist Leaders), and publishing research are good ways to accomplish this goal. Since one can also advance to GS-14 and GS-15 positions via research service, one could secure independent funding and build a research portfolio.

Academic Medical Centers

In an AMC, focusing on one or two areas of research is important. An area of focus may initially be narrow (e.g., epilepsy and epilepsy outcomes, studying memory/learning, movement disorders, autism), but within these areas it is wise to cast your net broadly. It is often advantageous to capture multiple aspects of the behavior or cognitive function. Second, when beginning an academic career, it is important to collaborate with others. Agreeing to work as a coinvestigator on a research project of another faculty member can provide important experience. Third, it is often advisable to seek out new experiences/training in areas of care, teaching, or research that involve the same general clinical population/students but may be a completely different avenue or outcome measure. For example, a researcher interested in deep brain stimulation to treat movement disorders and Parkinson's disease might want to participate in a research project that has a cognitive secondary outcome that is studying the effect of a medication in treating Parkinson's disease. Some other factors that can contribute to success in academic medical centers include participating in academic grand rounds, teaching medical students, working with senior faculty within your area of interest, presenting consistently at national conferences in your area, and listening to/undergoing quality reviews of your work.

CONCLUSION AND FUTURE DIRECTIONS

There are many exciting career opportunities for neuropsychologists, many of them allowing for diverse experiences and skill sets to align with your particular clinical, research, teaching, programmatic, and/or administrative interests and passions. However, it is also important to remember that no career setting is likely to have it all (remember that the perfect job is a myth!), and it is quite normal for neuropsychologists to work in more than one setting as their professional careers evolve over time. Put another way, given that the average neuropsychologist's professional career spans several decades, it is unlikely that your first job will be your only job. Regardless of work setting, it is important to maintain work–life balance (see Chapter 16). Some strategies include keeping connected with colleagues and family, taking time to exercise and maintain hobbies, and seeking professional support when needed. Maintaining flexibility throughout one's career is advisable, as is keeping a sense of humor, and revisiting one's curiosity and enthusiasm for neuropsychology.

REFERENCES

Barisa, M. (2010). *The business of neuropsychology: A practical guide*. Oxford University Press.

Cullum, C. M., & Grosch, M. G. (2013). Special considerations in conducting neuropsychology assessment over videoteleconferencing. In K. Myers & C. Turvey (Eds.), *Telemental health: Clinical, technical, and administrative foundations for evidence-based practice* (pp. 275–294). Elsevier.

Hannay, H. J., Bieliauskas, L. A., Crosson, B. A., Harmneke, T. A., Hamsher, K. deS., & Koffler, S. P. H. J. (1998). Proceedings of the Houston conference on specialty education and training in clinical neuropsychology. *Archives of Clinical Neuropsychology, 13*(2), 157–158. https://doi.org/10.1093/arclin/13.2.160

Kennedy, C. H., & Moore, J. L. (2010). *Military neuropsychology*. Springer.

Kennedy, C. H. & Zillmer, E. A. (Eds.) (2012). *Military psychology: Clinical and operational applications* (2nd ed.). Guilford.

Peck, E. A. (2003). Business aspects of private practice in clinical neuropsychology. In: G. J. Lamberty, J. C. Courtney, R. H. & Heilbronner (Eds.), *The practice of clinical neuropsychology: A survey of practices and settings* (pp. 53–90). Swets & Zeitlinger.

Peck, E. A., & Roberts, L. W. (2019). Clinical neuropsychology practice and the Medicare patient. In L. D. Ravdin & H. L. Katzen (Eds.), *Handbook on the neuropsychology of aging and dementia* (2nd ed., pp. 105–130). Springer. https://doi.org/10.1007/978-3-319-93497-6_8

Peck, E. A., Roberts, L. W. & O'Grady, J. M. (2013). Clinical neuropsychology practice and the Medicare patient. In L. D. Ravdin & H. L. Katzen (Eds.), *Handbook on the neuropsychology of aging and dementia*. (pp. 121–134) Springer.

Pliskin, N. H. (2018). The economics of healthcare shape the practice of neuropsychology in the era of integrated healthcare. *Archives of Clinical Neuropsychology, 33*(3), 260–262. https://doi.org/10.1093/arclin/acy008

Reger, M. A., Etherage, J. R., Reger, G. M., & Gahm, G. A. (2008). Civilian psychologists in the Army culture: The ethical challenge of cultural competence. *Military Psychology, 20*(1), 21–35. https://doi.org/10.1080/08995600701753144

Schwarz, L., Schrift, M., & Pliskin, N. (2009). Forensic neuropsychological evaluations in an academic medical center. *Journal of Head Trauma Rehabilitation, 24*(2), 100–104. https://doi.org/10.1097/HTR.0b013e31819b0504

Sweet, J. J., Benson, L. M., Nelson, N. W., & Moberg, P. J. (2015). The American Academy of Clinical Neuropsychology, National Academy of Neuropsychology, and Society for Clinical Neuropsychology (APA Division 40) 2015 TCN professional practice and 'salary survey': Professional practices, beliefs, and incomes of U.S. neuropsychologists. *The Clinical Neuropsychologist, 29*(8), 1069–1162. https://doi.org/10.1080/13854046.2016.1140228

7

FINDING A JOB

Research Careers in Neuropsychology

YANA SUCHY AND MATTHEW J. EULER

This chapter focuses on describing academic research careers for neuropsychologists. Such careers can be found in a variety of settings and can offer stimulating and gratifying careers for those who are passionate about advancing the field through uncovering new knowledge. The following sections outline the various characteristics needed to succeed in a research career in neuropsychology and provide an overview of the distinguishing features and the pros and cons of the major settings in which research neuropsychologists work. In addition, the chapter gives practical guidance about how to navigate preparing and applying for, and ultimately succeeding in, research careers in neuropsychology.

However, before delving deeper into that topic, we want to acknowledge that there are a number of ways in which clinical neuropsychologists who are employed in clinical, not research, settings can also become involved in research. First, neuropsychology, unlike many other psychology specialties, inherently lends itself to research activities even within the context of a typical clinical practice. This is because neuropsychologists essentially collect data in the course of their daily clinical work. In fact, much neuropsychological research is based on such archival clinical data, with about 50% of

https://doi.org/10.1037/0000250-008
The Neuropsychologist's Roadmap: A Training and Career Guide, C. Block (Editor)

131

neuropsychologists reporting that they devote at least one hour a week to research activities (Sweet et al., 2021). Such research is inherently retrospective, but can nevertheless address a variety of important questions, including normative and cultural issues (Raudeberg et al., 2019), psychometric properties of neuropsychological instruments (Kuehnel et al., 2019; Messerly & Marceaux, 2020; Schroeder et al., 2019), patient recovery trajectories (O'Brien et al., 2020), or comparisons of diagnostic groups on test performance (Dorociak et al., 2018; Ruchinskas, 2019), to name a few. Investigations of this type are generally not associated with any formal reimbursement for research activities and these investigators are expected to meet their clinical productivity goals so as to earn their salary.

Second, neuropsychologists who hold clinical appointments within academic medical centers or Veterans Affairs (VA) hospitals can often become involved (typically as consultants, investigators, or coinvestigators) in research projects that are funded by federal or state funding agencies, private companies (e.g., pharmaceutical companies, testing companies), or foundations. In such scenarios, some portion of the neuropsychologists' salaries are covered by the funding entity for the duration of their involvement on the project. Although such projects may be headed by research-focused neuropsychologists, they perhaps even more often involve collaborations between clinically focused neuropsychologists and professionals from other disciplines. This is because neuropsychologists are frequently sought after for their expertise in evaluating cognition, which is a much-needed aspect of many clinical trials examining outcomes of medical or pharmacologic interventions.

In contrast to neuropsychologists whose primary role is to function as a clinician and whose research activities represent a minor (and in many cases unpaid) aspect of their jobs, some neuropsychologists do choose to pursue research as a primary career path. There are two main settings that comprise the majority of research careers in neuropsychology; these are (a) academic medical centers, and (b) psychology departments in university or college settings. Academic medical centers are institutions that combine, as their central mission, the education of future health care professionals, state-of-the-art health care service for patients, and cutting-edge research. Academic psychology departments, on the other hand, are primarily concerned with education of graduate and/or undergraduate students in conjunction with varying levels of research activities, typically without explicit clinical expectations. Importantly, among academic psychology departments, there can be considerable differences between colleges and universities, pertaining primarily to different expectations around research productivity relative to teaching, and whether one's teaching responsibilities primarily emphasize graduate versus undergraduate education.

ISSUES TO CONSIDER ABOUT A CAREER IN ACADEMIC NEUROPSYCHOLOGY

Before further detailing the unique aspects of different academic settings, we take up more general issues that pertain to research careers in neuropsychology in general: (a) determining whether a research career is a good fit for you, and (b) preparing for a research career.

Issue 1: Determining Whether a Research Career Is a Good Fit For You

In deciding whether a research career is a good fit for you, there are several issues to consider. The first is what might be thought of as the "wrong" reason to pursue a research career, namely, that somewhere along the way you have discovered that you dislike clinical practice and are hoping that a research career might allow you to avoid clinical work. There are two reasons why this approach is problematic. First, many research careers will still require that one engage in at least some clinical work, whether it be to supplement one's salary as a faculty member in an academic medical center, or to contribute to the clinical training of doctoral students as a faculty member in an academic psychology department (see Table 7.1). That said, satisfactory career paths do exist for trainees who find themselves questioning their commitment to a clinical identity and the associated responsibilities; such careers typically involve a faculty position in a psychology department that does not train clinicians (e.g., at a 4-year college, or in a nonclinical PhD program), in allied research fields such as psychometrics or cognitive neuroscience, in administrative roles, or in a variety of governmental (e.g., research scientist at the National Institutes of Health) or industry jobs (e.g., at a psychological test company).

Having addressed the "wrong" reasons, there are of course many affirmative reasons to pursue a research career in neuropsychology. The most important of these is that you have a true passion for research. If you are someone who is inherently drawn to identifying gaps in our knowledge and have the intellectual curiosity and generativity to come up with hypotheses and methods for addressing such gaps, then you have the first set of qualities needed for a career in research. Beyond having a clear passion for research and a deep intellectual curiosity, individuals who are successful in research careers typically also possess the following four characteristics.

First, because of the highly unstructured nature of day-to-day research activities, one needs to be highly self-motivated and able to independently identify and complete numerous tasks while constrained by few, if any,

TABLE 7.1. Overview of Salary Structure and Work Responsibilities in Different Research Settings

Domain	Academic medical center	Academic psychology (university)	Academic psychology (college)
Salary	12 months (soft money)	9 months (hard money)	
Tenure	Protection of job, but *not* protection of salary and job description (e.g., research vs. clinical)	Protection of job, salary, and job description	
Extramural funding	Crucial	Preferred	Not expected
Teaching	Grand rounds Occasional lectures	≤ four courses per year (graduate or undergrad)	Six to eight courses per year (graduate or undergrad)
Mentoring	Medical students Doctoral students Predoctoral interns Postdoctoral fellows	Doctoral students Predoctoral interns Postdoctoral fellows	Possibly under-graduate or masters-level students (but unlikely)
Clinical	Varies Optional or mandatory (may be mandatory if research funding is not secured)	Varies Usually optional (may involve private practice on side, training clinic, or combination)	Optional (may involve private practice)
Service	Departmental/university committees Regional/national/international service Community outreach		Departmental/college committees

Note. "Hard money" refers to positions where a faculty member's salary is guaranteed regardless of whether any, or what type of, grant funding is secured. "Soft money" refers to positions where a faculty member is expected to generate sufficient revenue so as to cover their salary either via continuous grant funding, or some combination of grant funding and clinical service delivery.

formal deadlines and little daily oversight. This flexibility is of course essential to creating an environment that encourages people to develop novel ways of solving problems, and to pursue projects that may have a low probability of generating immediate results.

Second, one needs to be able to not only generate broad research questions, but also identify and carry out an extensive set of subtasks that are necessary en route from the broad question to an actual scholarly product. In other words, a successful researcher must develop the ability to break large, somewhat amorphous goals into the discrete subtasks necessary for the ultimate goal attainment.

Third, as part of being able to provide your own structure, a successful research career also requires the ability to monitor many different ongoing projects and keep them all moving forward at once. Concretely, this may require a shift from a mindset that focuses almost exclusively on achieving successive milestones one at a time (as tends to be emphasized in graduate training, e.g., defend your master's thesis, pass your preliminary exam, propose your dissertation, etc.), to the longer-term view that is needed in pursuing a program of research. That is, while dividing a large project into a series of successive milestones is of course an important and effective strategy in general, developing and managing a research program essentially requires taking this skill and expanding it out to a much larger scope and timescale. For example, whereas an individual research project involves a series of smaller steps (i.e., secure funding, obtain institutional review board approval, begin data collection, prepare datasets for analyses, etc.), developing a program of research involves identifying an entire series of studies (and typically grants) that one would need to pursue in addressing the larger question. Thus, one needs to be able to transition relatively fluidly between different types of tasks over short intervals, as well as between projects at different stages of development. In any given week (or day), one might be involved in reviewing new literature for a grant application, finalizing manuscripts on older research projects, developing instruments or recruitment materials for upcoming studies, and reviewing a trainee's work on entirely separate topics.

The fourth requirement for a successful research career has to do with the ability to balance the demands of the job with your own personal welfare. Specifically, on the one hand, the unstructured nature of the research environment often translates into the need to devote time to projects on evenings and weekends, simply because various challenges and opportunities may arise at inopportune times but need be addressed in a time-sensitive way. On the other hand, research settings offer an unmatched degree of flexibility in pursuing your own interests and setting your own agenda and schedule, giving you tremendous freedom in determining how to balance personal needs and obligations with professional goals and demands. Within this context, one needs to possess the willingness and capacity to take breaks. In short, because the list of exciting opportunities that one might pursue is essentially limitless (and the more active you are in the discipline, the more opportunities will find you), it is important to be able to strategically recharge yourself to maintain the creativity required for generation of new knowledge.

Issue 2: Preparing for a Research Career

Successfully pursuing a career in research will require you to both have the profile necessary to get the job, and the skills to thrive in it. In order to be competitive, there are several things to attend to at each level of training (also see Chapters 1–6 of this volume). The most competitive candidates will be those who have completed their doctoral, internship, and postdoctoral training at sites where neuropsychology is a Major Area of Study, as defined by the recent *Taxonomy for Education and Training in Clinical Neuropsychology* (Sperling et al., 2017). In this respect, competency is competitiveness, in that attending sites with this designation will help ensure that you receive the didactic and clinical experiences needed at each developmental level to ultimately be an effective researcher, teacher, and supervisor. In brief, the guidelines that establish the Major Area of Study designation closely follow and expand upon the long-standing Houston Conference Guidelines for specialty training in neuropsychology (http://www.uh.edu/hns/hc.html) and consist of the following: (a) completing a minimum set of courses in neuropsychology and related topics during graduate training, in addition to multiple practica and a dissertation in neuropsychology; (b) spending at least 50% of your time during internship engaging in neuropsychology practice and neuropsychology didactics; and (c) at the postdoctoral level, having 2 full years of formal training in neuropsychology as described by the Association for Postdoctoral Programs in Clinical Neuropsychology (APPCN; http://appcn.org).

Postdoctoral Fellowship

The issue of postdoctoral training deserves further attention. Having completed their doctoral degree, many research-oriented neuropsychologists debate whether to pursue a clinical fellowship (also called a residency or a postdoc) in neuropsychology. It is important to know that clinical fellowships are not required for some research positions, and, in fact, positions within psychology departments may not even require one to be eligible for licensure (e.g., due to lacking sufficient postdoctoral hours). Nevertheless, such fellowships still serve an important purpose for research-oriented individuals, affording the opportunity to see a much greater diversity of cases and at a much faster pace than at prior levels of training. As a result, a fellowship is arguably the first real opportunity for trainees to see first-hand what it feels like to function as a practicing neuropsychologist. In our experience, it is often not until after completing their clinical fellowship that most trainees are in a position to look back and appreciate the professional growth and the additional depth of learning they gained in the process. In addition to these experiential benefits, the residency serves three important practical purposes for the research-oriented neuropsychologist.

First, if the residency you attend is a full member of APPCN, then upon successful completion you will be eligible for board certification in neuro-psychology (see Chapter 5). Critically, it has long been argued that board certification should be considered the minimum level of credentialing for representing oneself to the public as a practicing neuropsychologist, and accordingly board eligibility is often a threshold criterion when hiring neuro-psychologists, especially for positions in academic medical centers.[1]

Second, completing a clinical fellowship will not only allow you to gain board eligibility, but for those who go on to careers in psychology departments, it may be the last opportunity to see a rich variety of cases and to interact with colleagues in other disciplines. As such, it will furnish important clinical experience to draw upon in teaching neuropsychological assessment and related courses to graduate trainees.

Third, research activities are often an integral part of clinical fellowships and provide important opportunities for further developing your scholarly profile, particularly for those with more clinically-focused research.

Lastly, because board eligibility opens the door toward eventual board certification, this investment in one's clinical credentials also affords greater flexibility in future career choices, whether it be transitioning to a more clinically oriented position or developing a private clinical practice along-side your research career.

Publications
Obtaining the necessary education and clinical experiences outlined above represents the first key piece of being competitive for a research career in neuropsychology. In addition, the quality of your scholarly profile will be crucial. As a heuristic, if you are seeking a position in an academic medical center or an academic psychology department at a research university,

---

[1]Although eligibility for board certification is not a typical requirement for a job in an academic psychology department, it is still required by some search committees. Additionally, it is valued by departments that engage in clinical training, as it increases their prestige and contributes to positive evaluations by American Psychological Association accreditation reviews.

a good goal would be to publish at least two or three manuscripts per year throughout your training (including peer-reviewed articles published in well-respected journals), with at least a substantial minority of these being first-author contributions. Additionally, if you are seeking a career in an academic psychology department at a research university, your publication record should illustrate the beginnings of a program of research that you intend to pursue in the future.

Grant Funding

In addition to developing a strong publication record, it is increasingly common for doctoral and postdoctoral trainees to have experience in seeking grant funding, such as National Institutes of Health (NIH) National Research Service Awards (NRSA), NIH Career Development awards, and thesis and dissertation grants that are supported by various professional organizations in neuropsychology. Typically, competitive applicants at academic medical centers and research universities would have had several experiences with grant writing by the time they were seeking a faculty position, and likely one or more funded projects or awards.

Teaching

Successful applicants to faculty positions in academic psychology departments would ideally have taught at least one or two courses independently, in addition to having experience providing graduate student supervision. Notably, for jobs in academic medical centers, teaching experience is rarely considered, whereas search committees at 4-year colleges would naturally place a greater emphasis on teaching experience than on research productivity (see the Research Career Settings section for more detail).

Collaboration

Finally, obtaining a research career in academic medicine or in a psychology department will inherently involve working in a group setting, with colleagues who have different expertise and points of view. Thus, individuals who are highly collegial, conscientious, and value working in a team are apt to be the most successful and satisfied in these environments over the long term.

RESEARCH CAREER SETTINGS

There are two main settings in which neuropsychologists seek research careers: (a) academic medical centers, and (b) psychology departments in university or college settings. In this section, we describe requirements and work responsibilities, salary structure, and promotion practices in these settings, as well as some salient advantages of each setting.

Academic Medical Centers

The majority of research positions held by neuropsychologists are housed within academic medical centers.[2] These settings emphasize the education of future health care professionals and state-of-the-art health care delivery as key parts of their mission, making them highly attractive employment venues for research-oriented neuropsychologists. Consequently, although neuropsychologists holding research positions in such settings are expected to spend the majority of time on research activities, they are also expected to spend some time on other academic pursuits, including teaching and mentoring; service to the institution, the profession, and the community; and, in many cases, some small amount of clinical work. Specifically then, in addition to research activities, research neuropsychologists in academic medical centers may be expected to give grand rounds lectures (research or clinical colloquia, often housed within and presented to a specific department, e.g., neurology grand rounds) or contribute to a lecture series for medical students or medical residents, mentor postdoctoral fellows, attend faculty meetings, and demonstrate contributions to the profession by becoming involved in, for example, the governance of a professional organization or by contributing to the peer-review process.

Academic medical centers, by virtue of their affiliation with a university or a medical school (or both), observe strict rules with respect to academic rank (i.e., assistant, associate, or full professor). Such rules may specify the timeline within which one must be eligible for promotion, or the types of activities in which clinical versus research faculty must engage in order to qualify for promotion. Additionally, some academic medical centers differentiate between tenure-track and career-line (or nontenure track) positions, with only those hired as tenure-track being eligible to earn tenure. Importantly, while attainment of tenure is widely believed to represent a virtual guarantee of a job for life, this is a bit of a misconception when it comes to academic medical centers: specifically, intrinsic in most (though not all!) medical center research positions is the expectation that the faculty will

---

[2]Actual statistics are not available regarding how many positions in Academic Medical Centers are designated as "research" vs. "clinical," though nearly 40% of neuropsychologists employed in institutional settings work at academic medical centers (Sweet et al., 2021).

"earn" their salary by securing major extramural grant funding[3] (or combining extramural funding with revenues generated from clinical work). In many cases, lapses in grant funding will lead to a mandatory increase in clinical duties (to make up for lost revenue), although a handful of medical centers offer temporary stopgap salary in situations when grant funding does not come through. Regardless of the specific arrangements, what most research positions in academic medical centers ultimately have in common is the requirement that, over some predetermined period of time, faculty generate sufficient revenue so as to cover their salaries; in other words, faculty are funded by what is known as "soft money." As a result, while attainment of tenure may represent a guarantee of a job, it is not necessarily a guarantee that a faculty member will be able to keep the same job, nor is it a guarantee of the same income. For example, if a research neuropsychologist fails to secure grant funding, they may have to transfer to a clinical position; and if they fail to earn sufficient revenue from clinical work, their salary may eventually be proportionately reduced. However, because of the well-known capriciousness of the grant application process, most research positions in academic medical centers are designed from the get-go to offer some flexibility in the balance between research and clinical responsibilities. Additionally, many academic medical centers allow faculty to switch from, for example, a research professor position to a clinical professor position if needed.

As mentioned before, it is much more common for neuropsychologists to work in academic medical centers than in academic psychology departments (Sweet et al., 2021). There are several reasons for this. First, there are many more job openings in academic medical centers than there are in academic psychology departments. Second, as part of their training, neuropsychologists usually spend the last 3 years (internship and postdoc) before entering the job market in academic medical centers or similar settings; thus, they become familiar and comfortable with those settings, and are often guided by their mentors to stay in such settings. Third, academic medical centers offer unmatched access to a variety of clinical populations and medical technology. Fourth, many neuropsychologists fall in love with the fast-paced milieu of a medical center. And fifth, relative to academic psychology departments, salaries in academic medical centers tend to be

---

[3]Major grant funding here refers to grant funding that covers not only the cost of a given research project, but also some portion of the cost of the researcher's salary. "Extramural" refers to funding that is provided by someone other than the home institution.

somewhat higher (though this can often be accounted for by their 12-month, as opposed to 9-month, salary). Please see Table 7.2 for other advantages/disadvantages.

Academic Psychology Departments

As reported by Sweet et al. (2021), about 22% of neuropsychologists who work in institutions are housed in psychology departments. However, the majority of these are employed by the VA and other clinical entities, with only about 4% holding positions in departments of psychology within academic institutions of higher learning (Sweet et al., 2021). Similar to academic medical centers, academic psychology departments observe strict rules with respect to academic ranks (i.e., assistant, associate, or full professor). Such rules specify the timeline within which one must be eligible for promotion, often referred to as the "up or out" system, wherein one must attain promotion and tenure within 6 to 7 years of being hired in order to be retained and promoted to the next level. In addition, the types and relative amounts of activities (research, teaching, and service) in which one needs to engage are also explicitly specified. Similar to academic medical centers, some psychology departments have both tenure-track (a professor) and career-line (lecturer or instructor) positions. Although attainment of tenure may at times be associated with a greater scrutiny in academic psychology departments as compared with academic medical centers, it is also associated with considerably greater job security as compared to academic medical centers. This is because employment in academic

TABLE 7.2. Advantages and Disadvantages of Becoming an Academic Medical Center Neuropsychologist (Research)

Advantages	Disadvantages
✓ Opportunity to earn tenure and gain increased job security relative to nonacademic positions	✗ Attaining tenure does not guarantee that one will maintain their *exact* position and job description
✓ Excellent access to clinical populations and cutting-edge technologies for research	✗ Expectations to "earn" one's salary by securing major extramural grant funding or increasing one's clinical workload accordingly
✓ Greater availability of positions, and increased flexibility in geographical locations	✗ Year-round schedule
✓ Higher annual salary relative to university and college positions (12-month)	✗ Fewer opportunities to participate in classroom teaching and student mentoring

psychology departments is associated with what is known as "hard money," that is, the faculty salary is guaranteed regardless of whether grant funding is secured.

Academic psychology departments hold attractive advantages over academic medical centers. First, as mentioned earlier, attainment of tenure here is associated with unparalleled job security. Second, academic psychology departments offer unparalleled flexibility, not only because of the general nature of the job but also because of the academically liberal culture, marked by the principles of academic freedom. Third, this flexibility is further augmented by the 9-month length of the academic year, allowing unmatched freedom over the 3 summer months. Fourth, research universities typically offer a 6-month to 1-year sabbatical to their faculty every 7th year, often with full or nearly full salary. Lastly, psychology departments offer a highly intellectually stimulating environment, especially when housed in research universities. This is in part due to the structure of doctoral training, which offers frequent opportunities for faculty to discuss research and innovations in the field (e.g., in dissertation defense meetings). See Table 7.3 for an overview of advantages and disadvantages of academic psychology departments, and compare to Table 7.2 (advantages and disadvantages of academic medical centers).

Although neuropsychologists employed in academic psychology departments are virtually by definition expected to engage in research activities as part of their job description (e.g., novel data collection, publishing research, obtaining grants), there are considerable differences across institutions in

TABLE 7.3. Advantages and Disadvantages of Becoming an Academic Neuropsychologist (Research)

Advantages	Disadvantages
✓ Attaining tenure entails a virtual guarantee of one's position, salary, and job description	✗ Requirement to attain tenure within 6 to 7 years of being hired ("up or out")
✓ Unmatched freedom in determining one's research direction, highly stimulating intellectual environment	✗ Fewer positions available/limited choices regarding one's ultimate geographical location
✓ 9-month schedule; opportunities for sabbaticals	✗ Lower annual salary relative to academic medical centers or independent practice
✓ Highly flexible day-to-day schedule and liberal professional culture	✗ Fewer opportunities to see patients/reduced access to clinical populations for research

the percentage of time spent on research and the expectations about research productivity. Thus, when considering a job in an academic psychology department, one needs to understand the fundamental differences between research universities and colleges.

Research Universities

Research universities are typically PhD-granting institutions. Research expectations are fairly high, in part due to the fact that in order to train future PhD scientists, academic advisors need to have active laboratories with an active line of programmatic research. Research universities can be further divided based on Carnegie Classification System (http://carnegieclassifications.iu.edu) into Research 1 (*very high research activity*) and Research 2 (*high research activity*) universities. Whereas Research 1 universities have high research expectations of their faculty (in terms of rate of publication and securing of extramural funding), there tends to be a fairly wide range of expectations among Research 2 universities. Importantly, although research universities value research above other faculty contributions, it is nevertheless expected that faculty will engage in other scholarly activities, including graduate and undergraduate teaching, as well as service to the university, the profession, and the community. Thus, faculty employed in psychology departments should expect to spend some of their time teaching in a classroom, serving on departmental or university committees, and engaging in service on a national level. A typical teaching load at most research universities is three to four courses a year, though the actual number of courses taught is often fewer, as faculty may receive credit for other activities or may "buy out" of teaching by using salary support from their grants. Importantly, research universities tend to offer considerable support to their faculty to facilitate research, including research start-up funds when first hired, intramural pilot grants, lab space, grant preparation support, etc.

Colleges

In contrast to research universities, colleges tend to have considerably lower expectations of their faculty when it comes to research, but comparatively higher expectations with respect to teaching. It is important to keep in mind that there are several salient reasons why research activity is lower at colleges than at research universities: First, faculty have larger teaching loads and thus less time for research; second, faculty do not have doctoral students to help run their labs, since these tend to be 4-year colleges or master's programs; third, faculty receive less support for their research in terms of start-up funding, lab space, or intramural pilot grants. It is common for a teaching load at a college to range from six to eight courses a year (or more, if faculty choose to teach over the summer), though typically some of the courses are comprised of multiple sections of the same course and thus do not require extra prep time.

DECIDING WHICH PATH IS RIGHT FOR YOU

When deciding between an academic medical center, an academic psychology department at a research university, or a psychology department at a college, you should consider the following:

If you were in an academic psychology department would you . . .

- Have difficulty executing your research? In other words, does your research require access to certain resources (e.g., patients, imaging technology) that are only available in medical centers? If so, then an academic psychology department may still be a viable option, but you would need to limit your job search to research universities with a medical campus that is readily accessible and where you feel comfortable finding appropriate colleagues and collaborators.

- Miss seeing patients? If so, then an academic psychology department may still be a viable option, but you would need to limit your job search to departments that would allow you to see patients on the side, or that have a training clinic or an affiliation with a hospital/clinic.

- Miss the fast pace of the medical center? If so, a psychology department may not be a good fit.

- Hate teaching in a classroom? If so, a psychology department is definitely not a good fit.

Conversely, if you were in an academic medical center would you . . .

- Miss teaching in a classroom? If so, then an academic medical center may still be a viable option, but you would need to limit your job search to places that would allow you to partner with the psychology department and allow you to teach an occasional course. Sometimes, a part-time (e.g., 10%) position in a psychology department may allow you to scratch the teaching itch.

- Feel burdened by the need to always worry about earning your salary? If so, then academic medical centers are definitely not a good fit.

- Feel burdened by seeing patients? If so, an academic medical center is definitely not a good fit.

APPLYING FOR AND NEGOTIATING THE TERMS OF YOUR RESEARCH POSITION

When and Where to Apply

A number of useful resources exist for those seeking research positions (Chayer & Lehrmann, 2016; Hughes et al., 2012; Sternberg, 2003). When seeking such a position in academic medical centers, it is important to be vigilant, since there is no one "season" for job openings and advertisements can crop up at any time and in a variety of venues, including university websites, websites for neuropsychology organizations, or professional listservs, to name a few (see Table 7.4). In contrast, job openings in most academic

TABLE 7.4. Neuropsychology Training Materials and Other Resources

Organization	Website
Association of Neuropsychology Students and Trainees (ANST)	https://scn40.org/anst
Houston Conference Guidelines on Specialty Education and Training in Clinical Neuropsychology	http://www.uh.edu/hns/hc.html
Taxonomy for Education and Training in Clinical Neuropsychology	https://doi.org/10.1080/13854046.2017.1314017
Association for Postdoctoral Programs in Clinical Neuropsychology (APPCN)	http://appcn.org
Society for Clinical Neuropsychology (APA Division 40)	https://scn40.org
International Neuropsychological Society (INS)	https://www.the-ins.org
American Academy of Clinical Neuropsychology (AACN)	https://theaacn.org
The National Academy of Neuropsychology (NAN)	https://nanonline.org
Neuropsychology Listserv (NPSYCH)	https://jneuro.mrivner.com/index.php/2-uncategorised/86-npsych-home-page
Carnegie Classification of Institutions of Higher Education	http://carnegieclassifications.iu.edu

psychology departments are typically posted in the summer or fall, with application deadlines typically during the fall semester. Interviews, job offers, and negotiations then take place sometime during the late fall or early spring semester, with the job actually starting sometime during the summer. This means that you should have your application materials in order with this timeframe in mind, lest you may have to wait another year until positions open again.

In terms of deciding where to apply, this of course involves balancing professional and personal preferences. From a professional standpoint, you need to consider whether a given institution affords particular technologies, populations, collaborators, or other resources to which you will need access in order to conduct your research. From a personal standpoint, geographical location is important to consider, since quality of life involves factors such as closeness to extended family, access to recreational activities, and cultural fit (e.g., East Coast vs. Midwest vs. West Coast). However, it is important to consider that many more jobs typically exist for academic medical centers than for academic psychology departments. As a result, you can expect to have far greater leeway in deciding where to live when seeking a job in an academic medical center.

The Application Process

In terms of preparing your application package, any position will require you to submit a curriculum vitae and (usually three) letters of reference. Depending on the institution and the exact nature of the position, you may also be expected to submit (a) a research statement describing your past, current, and future research; (b) sample publications that are representative of your program of research; and (c) a teaching statement describing your teaching philosophy and your classroom teaching and supervisory experience. It is a good idea to develop these materials early and seek feedback from senior colleagues in revising them. Also, it may be a good idea to provide these with your application, even if the position announcement does not explicitly mention them, as you may be asked to provide them later in the process.

The Interview Process

After applying, you can expect to hear back about the status of your application within several weeks. If you haven't heard back for a month, it would be appropriate to send a brief, polite inquiry. If your application is deemed to be strong by the search committee, you can expect to first undergo a somewhat informal phone interview (or, if the timing is right, an interview at one of the major neuropsychology conferences). If all goes well, this first interview will be followed by an on-site visit, which will consist of 1 to 2 days of one-to-one or group interviews with potential colleagues, the department chair, and the dean; and one or more informal gatherings with potential colleagues (typically over meals). Remember that your visit is not just the opportunity for your potential future employer to learn about you, but is also an opportunity for you to learn about whether a given institution is a good fit for you. For that reason, be sure to ask any questions that are relevant to your ability to carry out your job (e.g., availability of relevant resources), and, during the less formal meetings (e.g., over meals), don't be shy to inquire about things that will be important for quality of life (e.g., recreation, weather, food).

In addition to formal and informal meetings, a typical interview visit will also require that you present one or more formal colloquia (i.e., your "job talk"). Across settings, a typical job talk would consist of a 45- to 60-minute colloquium (plus time for questions) in which the job candidate presents their research program to their prospective department. This typically involves framing the overall research area for the audience, detailing how your past studies have addressed specific subquestions in a way that illustrates your theoretical, methodological, (and often) clinical and teaching skills, and describing the future directions you will pursue in your prospective department. The relative emphasis on clinical and teaching skills depends on the setting (e.g., academic medicine vs. college or university), and if you are unsure about how to balance these, it is reasonable to ask the search committee about the typical balance of emphases for job talks in their department. Keep in mind that a good (or bad) talk can make or break a candidate. Be sure to have others review your slides and practice your talk multiple times.

A job talk for an academic medical center should also place a particular emphasis on factors like the clinical relevance of your work and its potential for securing the extramural funding that will be necessary to sustain it (e.g., if you conduct intervention research with a particular patient population, you might highlight how that area is a funding priority for a particular grant-funding agency). In contrast, job talks for academic psychology departments should emphasize the programmatic nature of one's research and future directions, although describing potential funding opportunities is also important for job talks in university psychology departments.

In addition, a good job talk is clear and compelling, speaks in a language that is understandable to nonspecialists (e.g., physicians, psychologists from other specialties, students), demonstrates the feasibility of conducting that work in that particular location, and often shows that the speaker has "done their homework" in terms of identifying the opportunities (and perhaps potential collaborations) that make that site particularly exciting.

Negotiating the Terms of Your Position

When you find yourself in the happy circumstance of being offered a job, the last task in the application process is to negotiate effectively. Numerous texts are available that address negotiation, but a key point of perspective is mentioned here. Namely, although you may be transitioning from being a trainee to your first "real" academic job, remember to approach the negotiation in a professional way, understanding that both you and your potential employer are invested in your success. In light of that, it is not only acceptable, but entirely appropriate, to ask for the resources you will legitimately need to be successful in your new position. This includes factors like your salary (will you need to hire expensive daycare? what is the cost of living in the area?), your start-up package (do you need funds to pay participants? special equipment or money for scans?), your teaching and clinical load (is there psychometrist support? funds to buy tests?), service expectations, and even moving costs. As part of the interview process, and especially during negotiation, be sure to also ask about any other relevant needs, such as parental leave policies and the like. Overall, keep in mind that the time when you negotiate for a new position is one of the few instances in your professional life when you are explicitly expected to advocate for yourself, and when potential employers (e.g., department chairs) are in a strong position to advocate on your behalf. Thus, while you should of course avoid being overly aggressive in negotiating with your prospective employer, advocating for yourself in a respectful but assertive way is expected and entirely appropriate.

THE TRAJECTORY AND SUSTAINABILITY OF A RESEARCH CAREER

Before closing, there are a few additional things worth considering for those who have transitioned into their first academic position. As noted earlier, research careers involve tremendous flexibility and little external structure, and while this freedom is a benefit, the prospect of developing a vibrant and mature research program on one's own in a new location can be quite daunting. A key here is to seek support from colleagues and mentors and avail yourself of their guidance and experience in both planning your research and responding to the inevitable setbacks that characterize research careers. Develop a planned trajectory for your work that will carry you out to your midtenure period. Diversify within your lab, such that your research portfolio contains both smaller projects that allow you to demonstrate your independence via early publications, as well as longer term, more ambitious projects that will allow you to demonstrate your ability to undertake complex and impactful work. Planning projects at different levels of complexity is also a good way to insure yourself against major setbacks and to build momentum while more ambitious projects take time to develop. Round out your portfolio by taking advantage of professional connections within your institution or elsewhere, establishing collaborations that allow you to supplement your primary research with smaller collaborative contributions. As part of this process, seek advice from trusted colleagues and mentors in evaluating your planned trajectory. And lastly, although you may feel that you are "on your own" at times, keep in mind that there are many others around you who are also looking for new connections, and that those who have gone before you and helped you get here remain invested in your success.

CONCLUSION AND FUTURE DIRECTIONS

A research career is one of the most stimulating and sought-after paths available to neuropsychologists. For those with the right mix of intellectual curiosity and self-directedness, it offers a great way to improve patient care and increase understanding of brain-behavior relationships, by working directly at the boundaries of our science. These efforts continually refresh the discipline and ultimately enhance the welfare of our patients and the public. We hope this chapter will be a guide and inspiration for those who are considering this route for themselves.

REFERENCES

Chayer, R., & Lehrmann, J. A. (2016). How to interview for a first academic position. In L. W. Roberts (Ed.), *The clinician educator guidebook: Steps and strategies for advancing your career* (pp. 35–42). Springer.

Dorociak, K. E., Schulze, E. T., Piper, L. E., Molokie, R. E., & Janecek, J. K. (2018). Performance validity testing in a clinical sample of adults with sickle cell disease. *The Clinical Neuropsychologist, 32*(1), 81–97. https://doi.org/10.1080/13854046. 2017.1339830

Hughes, A. K., Horner, P. S., & Ortiz, D. V. (2012). Being the diversity hire: Negotiating identity in an academic job search. *Journal of Social Work Education*, *48*(3), 595–612. https://doi.org/10.5175/JSWE.2012.201000101

Kuehnel, C. A., Castro, R., & Furey, W. M. (2019). A comparison of WISC-IV and WISC-V verbal comprehension index scores for children with autism spectrum disorder. *The Clinical Neuropsychologist*, *33*(6), 1127–1137. https://doi.org/10.1080/13854046.2018.1503721

Messerly, J., & Marceaux, J. C. (2020). Examination of the reliability and validity of the NAB Naming Test in a diverse clinical sample. *The Clinical Neuropsychologist*, *34*(2), 406–422. https://doi.org/10.1080/13854046.2019.1635647

O'Brien, S., Metcalf, K., & Batchelor, J. (2020). An examination of the heterogeneity of cognitive outcome following severe to extremely severe traumatic brain injury. *The Clinical Neuropsychologist*, *34*(1), 120–139. https://doi.org/10.1080/13854046.2019.1598501

Raudeberg, R., Iverson, G. L., & Hammar, Å. (2019). Norms matter: U.S. normative data under-estimate cognitive deficits in Norwegians with schizophrenia spectrum disorders. *The Clinical Neuropsychologist*, *33*(Suppl. 1), 58–74. https://doi.org/10.1080/13854046.2019.1590641

Ruchinskas, R. (2019). Wechsler Adult Intelligence Scale–4th edition digit span performance in subjective cognitive complaints, amnestic mild cognitive impairment, and probable dementia of the Alzheimer type. *The Clinical Neuropsychologist*, *33*(8), 1436–1444. https://doi.org/10.1080/13854046.2019.1585574

Schroeder, R. W., Martin, P. K., Heinrichs, R. J., & Baade, L. E. (2019). Research methods in performance validity testing studies: Criterion grouping approach impacts study outcomes. *The Clinical Neuropsychologist*, *33*(3), 466–477. https://doi.org/10.1080/13854046.2018.1484517

Sperling, S. A., Cimino, C. R., Stricker, N. H., Heffelfinger, A. K., Gess, J. L., Osborn, K. E., & Roper, B. L. (2017). *Taxonomy for Education and Training in Clinical Neuropsychology*: Past, present, and future. *The Clinical Neuropsychologist*, *31*(5), 817–828. https://doi.org/10.1080/13854046.2017.1314017

Sternberg, R. J. (2003). The job search. In M. J. Prinstein & M. D. Patterson (Eds.), *The portable mentor: Expert guide to a successful career in psychology* (pp. 297–308). Springer. https://doi.org/10.1007/978-1-4615-0099-5_23

Sweet, J. J., Klipfel, K. M., Nelson, N. W., & Moberg, P. J. (2021). Professional practices, beliefs, and incomes of U.S. neuropsychologists: The AACN, NAN, SCN 2020 practice and "salary survey." *The Clinical Neuropsychologist*, *35*(1), 7–80. https://doi.org/10.1080/13854046.2020.1849803

PART **II** FOUNDATIONAL COMPETENCIES IN NEUROPSYCHOLOGY

8 TRAINING, EDUCATION, AND COMPETENCIES IN NEUROPSYCHOLOGY

BRAD ROPER AND SCOTT SPERLING

How did we get the current roadmap of training in the practice of clinical neuropsychology for students, interns, and fellows? Groups of stakeholders came together, at different points over more than 40 years, and did the hard work of developing consensus. Each step forward has helped to develop clinical neuropsychology into what it is today. Although some early steps are primarily of historical interest, other initiatives produced documents such as the Houston Conference Guidelines (HCG) that are essential to understand as you progress through training. Whereas HCG have been in place for over 20 years and are well known, recent developments are less well known but still important in understanding training experiences and mapping out your path to independent practice. The taxonomy for clinical neuropsychology allows students and trainees to compare across multiple programs at the doctoral, internship, and postdoctoral levels, and determine the intensity and percentage of time spent in clinical neuropsychology. Additionally, three recent initiatives have addressed the need for competencies that define the knowledge and skills needed for practice.

In this chapter, we review the history of training and education guidelines, HCG and the current structure and process of training, the taxonomy that provides common descriptors for training programs, and recent competency

https://doi.org/10.1037/0000250-009
The Neuropsychologist's Roadmap: A Training and Career Guide, C. Block (Editor)

initiatives. Whereas the various documents are complementary, their purpose and best use are not always obvious. Our coverage of the documents is intended to help students and trainees in mapping their pathway to independent practice. Additionally, our review may be helpful in planning training programs or rotations for those who are training directors or supervisors, or have an interest in joining the training community.

HISTORY OF EDUCATION AND TRAINING GUIDELINES

The initial steps to developing training guidelines followed not long after the establishment of organizations promoting neuropsychology as a multidisciplinary research field and clinical neuropsychology as a specialized area of psychology practice. As many organizations were involved, whose abbreviations may seem like an alphabet soup of acronyms, Table 8.1 provides a quick reference to the organizations referenced in this chapter.

TABLE 8.1. Explanation of Acronyms

Acronym	Organization
AACN	American Academy of Clinical Neuropsychology
ABCN	American Board of Clinical Neuropsychology
ABPP	American Board of Professional Psychology
APA	American Psychological Association
APA Division 40	The APA Division representing clinical neuropsychology, now the Society for Clinical Neuropsychology (SCN40)
APPCN	Association of Postdoctoral Programs in Clinical Neuropsychology
CNS	Clinical Neuropsychology Synarchy, now called the Clinical Neuropsychology Specialty Council, it is the specialty council representing clinical neuropsychology to the Council of Specialties in Professional Psychology
CoA	APA Commission on Accreditation
CoSPP	Council of Specialties in Professional Psychology
CPA	Canadian Psychological Association
CRSSPP	Commission for the Recognition of Specialties and Subspecialties in Professional Psychology
HCG	Houston Conference Guidelines: common shorthand form to refer to the Policy Statement of the Houston Conference on Specialty Education and Training in Clinical Neuropsychology
INS	International Neuropsychological Society
NAN	National Academy of Neuropsychology
SoA	APA Standards of Accreditation
TFEAC	Task Force on Education, Accreditation, and Credentialing, initially formed by the INS and later an INS/Division 40 task force

INS/APA Division 40 Guidelines for Doctoral Training Programs in Clinical Neuropsychology

The International Neuropsychological Society (INS; https://www.the-ins.org) was formed in the mid-1960s, in part because clinical neuropsychology did not have a home within the American Psychological Association (APA) at that time. Although primarily comprised of psychologists, INS became an interdisciplinary and international organization focused on promoting and disseminating scientific research on brain–behavior relationships and related areas. Over time, growing recognition of the need to address professionalization of the specialty became apparent, and in the 1970s, the INS formed the Task Force on Education, Accreditation, and Credentialing (TFEAC). A steering committee originating from TFEAC began advocating for a new Division of Clinical Neuropsychology to be created within APA, which was ultimately established in 1980 (APA Division of Clinical Neuropsychology, APA Division 40; https://www.scn40.org). Division 40, now known as the Society for Clinical Neuropsychology, gradually assumed full responsibility for TFEAC, whose efforts culminated in publication of the first set of guidelines for doctoral, internship, and postdoctoral residency programs as well as continuing, education programs in clinical neuropsychology (Costa, 1998; INS/Division 40 Task Force, 1987; Meier, 1981), commonly referred to as the INS/Division 40 Guidelines.

The INS/Division 40 guidelines established doctoral training within a regionally accredited university as the standard for specialization in clinical neuropsychology. The guidelines also indicated that training should encompass generic psychology and clinical cores; specialized education in clinical neuropsychology, the neurosciences, and basic human and animal neuropsychology; practicum experience; and a doctoral internship. The latter was to include at least 50% of the overall time dedicated to training in clinical neuropsychology, including supervision by a board-certified neuropsychologist and didactic and clinical training, within a program accredited by the APA or listed in the Association of Psychology Postdoctoral and Internship Centers directory (INS/Division 40 Task Force, 1987).

At the time, completion of an internship in clinical neuropsychology and its prerequisites were deemed sufficient for competent independent practice in the specialty. That said, the guidelines also clearly outlined the value of fellowship training as a method of developing an advanced level of competence. Fellowship training was thus recommended, and suggested to occur within a program directed by a board-certified neuropsychologist, associated with a hospital or neurological/neurosurgical service, and over the course of a 2-year period. At least 50% of time was to be devoted to clinical services and at least 25% of time was to be spent engaged in research. With completion of postdoctoral training, individuals would be eligible for board certification in clinical neuropsychology by the American Board of Professional Psychology (ABPP). As such, the INS/Division 40 guidelines implicitly appeared to be describing two levels of competence achieved within formal training (i.e., advanced vs. minimally qualified), depending on whether or not a fellowship was completed.

Houston Conference on Specialty Education and Training in Clinical Neuropsychology

In the late 1980s and early 1990s, professional psychology as a whole saw a push to formalize doctoral, internship, and postdoctoral training experiences. Within clinical neuropsychology, the INS/Division 40 guidelines emphasized specialty training needs independently at the doctoral, internship, and post-doctoral levels, lacking in integration and reflecting typical training activities at the time. (Bieliauskas, 1998a). On the heels of other successful national professional psychology training conferences (Belar et al., 1989, 1993; Belar & Perry, 1992; Bickman & Ellis, 1990), in 1997, a conference planning committee comprised of members from the Clinical Neuropsychology Synarchy (CNS), a group comprised of representatives of the major national organizations in clinical neuropsychology, began preparations for a national clinical neuro-psychology conference, focused on the establishment of consensus education and training guidelines based on an overarching and integrative model of training within the specialty.

The Houston Conference on Specialty Education and Training in Clinical Neuropsychology convened from September 3 to 7, 1997. The conference planning committee selected 37 delegates from different cultural back-grounds and regions of the country and with diverse training interests, subspecializations, and levels of seniority to participate (Bieliauskas, 1998b; Bieliauskas & Hamsher, 1998). These delegates were joined by five delegates from neuropsychology organizations, which included the American Academy of Clinical Neuropsychology (AACN), the American Board of Clinical Neuro-psychology (ABCN), the Association of Postdoctoral Programs in Clinical Neuropsychology (APPCN), Division 40 of the APA, and the National Academy of Neuropsychology, all of which provided financial support for the confer-ence. Four overarching questions were addressed via small group discussions, subsequent larger plenary sessions, and ultimately a vote:

1. For what professional roles is it necessary to have education and training in the specialty of neuropsychology?

2. What knowledge base and skills are needed?

3. How can training and education in the specialty of clinical neuropsychology be accomplished?

   a. Can all training and education in neuropsychology be accomplished at a single level?

   b. How should the different levels of training and education be integrated?

   c. What is the role of continuing education for the specialty of neuro-psychology?

4. How should the outcome of the conference be implemented?

The consensus guidelines reached in each area are outlined in the Houston Conference on Specialty Education and Training in Clinical Neuropsychology Policy Statement (Bieliauskas, 1998b; Hannay et al., 1998). A link to the HCG policy statement is found on the website of the Council of Specialties in Professional Psychology (CoSPP; https://www.cospp.org/clinical-neuropsychology) and continues to define the process of education and training in clinical neuropsychology.

HCG specifies that training and education in clinical neuropsychology must be scientist–practitioner based and stipulate that specialization in clinical neuropsychology begins at the doctoral level at a regionally accredited institution. The percentage of time devoted to training in neuropsychology during the doctoral internship could vary depending on individual needs, but must occur in an APA- or Canadian Psychological Association–approved professional psychology training program. In a departure from the previous INS/Division 40 guidelines, HCG specified completion of a 2-year postdoctoral residency as required for independent practice in the specialty. To promote advanced training and subsequent board certification in clinical neuropsychology by the ABPP, HCG specified that postdoctoral programs provide the following assurances (Bieliauskas, 1998b, pp. 163–164):

- The faculty consists of a board-certified neuropsychologist and other professional psychologists.

- Training is provided at a fixed site or on formally affiliated and geographically proximate training sites, with primarily on-site supervision.

- There is access to clinical services and training programs in medical specialties and allied professions.

- There are interactions with other residents in medical specialties and allied professions, if not other fellows in neuropsychology.

- Each resident spends significant percentages of time in clinical service, and clinical research, and educational activities, appropriate to the individual resident's training needs.

HCG also provide a list of knowledge and skill domains and indicates that training is competency-based. Included among these competency domains are generic psychology and clinical cores, knowledge related to brain–behavior relationships, and knowledge related to the practice of clinical neuropsychology. Also listed among competency domains are skills in assessment, treatment and intervention, consultation, research, and teaching and supervision.

Importantly, HCG acknowledge differences in education and training pathways and allows for differences in when and how the knowledge and skills requisite to becoming a neuropsychologist are obtained. For example, whereas you may develop competency in functional neuroanatomy primarily via doctoral level coursework, other trainees may develop this knowledge in a more distributed time over the course of their training, and via specialized training programs, seminars, and imaging rounds. Although the pathways may be different, you should all be in a similar place as other trainees at the conclusion of a 2-year fellowship. Moreover, newly minted neuropsychologists will need training consistent with HCG to become board certified. In fact, if you earned your doctoral degree in 2005 or later, you cannot take the ABCN board exam without having HCG-consistent training, including a 2-year residency (ABCN, 2020).

How have HCG performed in the years following their establishment? A 2010 survey demonstrated that HCG have received widespread acceptance. Also, those receiving training consistent with the guidelines reported being well-prepared for practice (Sweet et al., 2012).

The Clinical Neuropsychology Taxonomy

As training in specialty practice areas has burgeoned, so too has the range of terms employed to describe the intensity or scope of specialty training experiences. For example, education departments and training programs have used a range of terms to describe training experiences, such as "neuropsychology area of study" or "neuropsychology concentration" at the doctoral program level, or "neuropsychology track" or "neuropsychology emphasis" at the internship level. As such, students encountering the range of terms had little guidance in discriminating and comparing training experiences across training sites and institutions. The lack of consistency also hinders students' and psychologists' ability to easily describe their education and training experiences when communicating to prospective employers and the public. Over the last two decades, considerable efforts have been put forth to promote greater "truth in advertising" and consistency in how departments, training programs, and professional organizations describe their specialty training opportunities. In 2005, the APA Task Force on Quality Assurance of

Education and Training for Recognized Proficiencies in Professional Psychology indicated a need for the development of a clear taxonomy of terminology to describe the structure of education and training in professional psychology (APA, 2020). Over the next several years, the Commission for the Recognition of Specialties and Proficiencies in Professional Psychology, now known as the Commission for the Recognition of Specialties and Subspecialties in Professional Psychology (CRSSPP), in collaboration with other stakeholder organizations, worked to develop such a taxonomy, which was ultimately adopted as APA policy in 2012 and revised in 2020 as *APA Guidelines: A Taxonomy for Education and Training in Professional Psychology Health Service Specialties and Subspecialties* (APA, 2020; https://www.apa.org/ed/graduate/specialize/taxonomy.pdf).

Following the adoption of these guidelines as APA policy, CRSSPP tasked each health service psychology specialty with developing their own specialty-specific taxonomy, using the same general framework and terminologies. Specifically, each specialty was tasked with defining the minimum breadth and depth of education and training experiences required for departments and training programs to describe their offerings as either a Major Area of Study, Emphasis, Experience, or Exposure. The development of a taxonomy for neuropsychology was spearheaded by CNS, thereby providing opportunities for input from each of the major organizations. The *Taxonomy for Education and Training in Clinical Neuropsychology* was formally adopted by the CNS in 2015 and may be found on via a link on the CoSPP website (http://www.cospp.org/clinical-neuropsychology). Importantly, Sperling et al. (2017) provided a detailed explication of the taxonomy, with examples on its application across the range of training settings.

The clinical neuropsychology taxonomy establishes hierarchical definitions of education and training opportunities within academic, clinical, and research domains at each of the four stages in the sequence of professional training: doctoral, internship, postdoctoral, and postlicensure. It also establishes guidelines regarding what constitutes a neuropsychology course and a practicum in neuropsychology with the aim of creating consistency across departments and programs. Specifically, a Major Area of Study at the doctoral level would require that programs provide students the opportunity to complete a minimum of (a) three neuropsychology courses with content that prominently addresses foundations for the study of brain–behavior relationships and the practice of clinical neuropsychology as outlined in HCG; (b) two clinical neuropsychology practica; (c) additional coursework, practica, or didactics in clinical neuropsychology; and (d) completion of a dissertation or research project in neuropsychology. Designation as an Emphasis requires that programs offer two neuropsychology courses and two neuropsychology practica, whereas designation as an Experience requires at least one neuropsychology course and one neuropsychology practicum. An Exposure requires only that programs offer a course or practicum in clinical neuropsychology.

Designation of internship programs as a Major Area of Study in neuropsychology requires that they offer at least 50% of training time devoted to clinical neuropsychology and didactic experiences consistent with the HCG for knowledge and skill. Programs that offer students supervised clinical neuropsychology training between 30% and 50% and between 10% and 30%, coupled with HGC-consistent didactic experiences, would define these training experiences as an Emphasis and Experience, respectively. Internship training that includes only 5% to 10% of supervised experience in clinical neuropsychology and/or didactic training would be defined as an Exposure. As the clinical neuropsychology taxonomy was intentionally constructed to be consistent with HCG, clinical neuropsychology residency programs must provide training opportunities consistent with those defined within the taxonomy as a Major Area of Study. To meet said criteria, programs must offer trainees 2 years of full-time (or equivalent) formal training in neuropsychology, with the inclusion of relevant didactic, clinical, and research activities. The training must encompass clinical assessment and interventions that incorporate neuropsychological theories, perspectives, or methods and exposure to related health care disciplines. Postlicensure, any continuing education or training experience, irrespective of its duration and intensity, would be considered at the level of an Exposure.

As departments and training programs increasingly adopt the taxonomy and its terminology to describe their training opportunities, prospective students and trainees will find it easier to accurately evaluate and compare graduate, internship, and postdoctoral training programs as they matriculate through their educational careers. In turn, this may allow students to feel more confident that choosing to apply to or attend a specific program will allow them to engage in specialty-specific training of an intensity best suited to their career aspirations, particularly if attainment of board certification in clinical neuropsychology is a goal. It should, however, be underscored that neither the quality of education or training programs nor the competency of students matriculating through such programs should be evaluated solely based upon the intensity of their neuropsychology training offerings. The clinical neuropsychology taxonomy is instead designed to be *descriptive* rather than *prescriptive* in providing a common language that programs may use to accurately define their training opportunities, and in this way, can be best used by students as one of many tools in their pursuit of training opportunities.

THE COMPETENCIES MOVEMENT

Up to this point, we have covered clinical neuropsychology's overarching training model (i.e., HCG) and the taxonomy used in describing training experiences (i.e., the CNS taxonomy), but neither of those documents address the details of what makes a clinical neuropsychologist *competent* to practice. *Competence* has been defined as "the habitual and judicious use of communication, knowledge, technical skills, clinical reasoning, emotions, values, and reflection in daily practice for the benefit of the individual and community being served" (Epstein & Hundert, 2002, p. 226). As reported by Hoge et al. (2005), the first Annapolis Coalition on Behavioral Health Workforce Education in 2001 noted the relative lack of progress in articulating competencies and how to measure competence within mental health professions as compared to general medicine, business, and industry. To put it bluntly, it was much easier to describe what every brain surgeon should do than what every psychologist should do. Furthermore, most developments in what is now called the competencies movement in professional psychology have taken place after the development and publication of HCG in 1998.

Competency Initiatives in Professional Psychology

Just 4 years after the publication of HCG, a major psychology conference, the 2002 Competencies Conference: Future Directions in Education and Credentialing (Kaslow et al., 2004) aimed to address the core competencies expected of all graduates of professional education and training programs in psychology. One article resulting from the conference introduced the "cube model" of competency development in professional psychology (Rodolfa et al., 2005). In the model, a three-dimensional matrix was defined, consisting of foundational competency domains, functional competency domains, and stages of professional development. Foundational competencies were described as the building blocks of what psychologists do, including domains such as reflective practice/self-assessment, scientific knowledge and methods, and interdisciplinary systems. Functional competencies describe the knowledge, skills, and values necessary to perform distinct activities as a psychologist, such as assessment, intervention, and consultation. Finally, the stages of professional development reflect the context of competency development. Several years later, professional psychology competencies were articulated in a highly detailed manner, with behavioral anchors describing the appropriate competency level for readiness for practicum training, readiness for internship, and readiness for entry-level practice (Fouad et al., 2009). The so-called competency benchmarks document has been revised and simplified, and may be found on the APA website (https://www.apa.org/ed/graduate/competency).

The competencies benchmarks document has served to provide guidance to doctoral and internship training programs on competencies in professional psychology as well as how they can be concretely measured among individual trainees, and the interested reader is encouraged to review the document to better understand how competencies can be effectively measured. Furthermore, the Standards of Accreditation (APA CoA, 2018) and associated regulations specify the *profession-wide competencies* that are required of doctoral and internship programs in health service psychology. If you are a student in an APA-accredited psychology doctoral or internship program, chances are very good that you have seen the profession-wide competencies covered in graduate coursework and on competency evaluation forms.

Competency Initiatives in Neuropsychology

Specifying what every clinical neuropsychologist should be competent to do is hard and time-consuming work. The first hurdle to jump pertains to the level of detail needed to describe competencies that are distinct and measurable, for example in the context of a training program. Moreover, the second hurdle is to develop consensus across individuals and stakeholder organizations. In the sections below, we cover some of the competency development efforts completed over the past several years.

Initial Entry-Level Competencies

By definition, the articulation of competencies and benchmarks pertaining to professional psychology did not address competencies in specialty practice areas, such as clinical neuropsychology, clinical health psychology, and rehabilitation psychology, recognized by APA and ABPP. Broadly conceived, competencies had long been recognized as important within clinical neuropsychology, as was reflected in reference to "essential knowledge and skill competencies" within HCG (Bieliauskas, 1998b, p. 161). However, the Houston Conference occurred prior to the emerging perspective of the competency movement, which values articulation of competencies in more detailed, declarative form and embeds them in a conceptually rigorous structure. Clinical health psychology provided an early example in the development of specialty practice competencies, as detailed by France et al. (2008). Several years later, Rey-Casserly et al. (2012) proposed the first framing of HCG through a modern competencies perspective, which focused on the development of entry-level competencies for independent practice following the completion of 2 years of formal postdoctoral training in clinical neuropsychology. Rey-Casserly et al. served as a catalyst for several subsequent developments that revised and elaborated on the original proposal, which are covered in the following section.

CNS Entry-Level Competencies

HCG focus primarily on the process of training. In contrast, entry-level competencies define the expected outcomes of that training (Smith, 2018). Accordingly, competencies can be viewed as putting "flesh on the bones" of the structure provided by HCG. After the initial proposal by Rey-Casserly et al. (2012), there was a need to broadly vet and revise the competencies, which was initiated by a task force formed in 2014 by CNS. A first revision of the competencies was developed and then forwarded to all CNS-member organizations, inviting comment at the CNS meeting in February 2015, and subsequently over the following year (Smith, 2018). After an additional round of revision and response in 2016, member organizations were asked to affirm the revision. The final version of entry-level competencies (CNS, 2016) was included within the specialty's petition for continued recognition by APA, posted via a link on the CoSPP website (https://www.cospp.org/education-and-training-guidelines), and included within the publication by Smith (2018).

The competencies and their elements are lengthy, publicly available within the source documents listed previously and not reproduced here. However, we include a section of the preamble to the competencies to emphasize their potential uses:

- Serve as a helpful resource for training programs, especially programs seeking accreditation at the postdoctoral level. Common materials could also be developed that greatly streamline the process of initiating and maintaining accreditation.

- Enhance the process of specialty credentialing of clinical neuropsychologists.

- Provide a framework for more senior clinical neuropsychologists to consider continuing education opportunities.

- Serve to identify the unique knowledge, skills, and abilities of clinical neuropsychologists that will enhance broad advocacy efforts in a changing health care environment.

The CNS competencies are structured as eight foundational competencies that are relevant to multiple aspects of clinical neuropsychology practice, and seven functional competencies regarding specific domains of practice. Each of the competencies are further broken down into a number of elements. For example, the Scientific Knowledge and Methods competency is a foundational competency and includes one element that states, "The clinical neuropsychologist demonstrates knowledge of the clinical and cognitive neurosciences, including neurology, neuroanatomy, neurobiology, neuropathology, brain development, and neurophysiology." Likewise, within the Assessment functional competency, one element states, "The clinical neuropsychologist will be able to interpret assessment results, with formation of an integrated conceptualization that draws from all relevant information sources (e.g., interview, test results, behavioral observations, records)" (Smith, 2018, pp. 6–7).

Competency-Based Practicum Guidelines in Clinical Neuropsychology. Whereas most efforts related to training have been developed with the involvement of the CNS, a substantial effort related to practicum training was undertaken by the AACN, a CNS-member organization that developed a task force to address the historical lack of emphasis or guidance related to practicum training in clinical neuropsychology (Nelson et al., 2015). The approach aimed to provide best-practice guidelines and was framed as aspirational as opposed to mandatory. The resulting practicum guidelines broadly characterize practica in clinical neuropsychology and detail the nature of supervision and the relationship between training sites and the doctoral program. Additionally, the approach is strongly competency-based and addresses benchmarks or milestones for each competency element, defined at two developmental levels, namely, "readiness for practicum" and "readiness for internship." Finally, in its Appendix, the practicum guidelines include a rating form that may be used by practicum sites as a way to provide detailed feedback on students' competency levels to their doctoral program.

Competency-Based Fellowship Guidelines in Clinical Neuropsychology. Following the January 1, 2017, implementation of the Standards of Accreditation (SoA; APA CoA, 2018), all accredited doctoral programs and doctoral internship programs are expected to adhere to a set of nine profession-wide competencies and their elements, as specified in the Implementing Regulations of the APA Commission on Accreditation (CoA), the accrediting body for psychology training programs (APA CoA, 2020). In contrast, only three profession-wide competencies are expected, irrespective of specialty, of all postdoctoral programs, including Integration of Science and Practice, Ethical and Legal Standards, and Individual and Cultural Diversity. For postdoctoral programs in a specialty practice area such as clinical neuropsychology, programs are required to use specialty-specific competencies (also called Level 3 competencies) that are consistent with the specialty's consensus training guidelines (APA CoA, 2018). In December 2016, the CoA sent a request to specialties via the CoSPP to provide Level 3 competencies to the CoA, and within clinical neuropsychology, the CNS formed a workgroup in response (Smith, 2018). In contrast to other efforts at competency development, Level 3 competencies are not aspirational and would be expected of all postdoctoral programs seeking or maintaining postdoctoral accreditation in clinical neuropsychology through APA. Likewise, postdoctoral residents in an APA-accredited postdoctoral program would be required to meet competency expectations in order to complete the program. As such, the CNS workgroup made efforts to ensure that all accredited programs could provide training in the Level 3 competencies, and the workgroup sought feedback from CNS-member organizations and accredited clinical neuropsychology postdoctoral programs. Level 3 postdoctoral competencies for clinical neuro-psychology were included in Smith (2018) and were also posted on the CoS website (https://www.cospp.org) under Postdoc Competencies.

Competencies were provided to the CoA in July 2017. In 2019 and 2020, two successive drafts by the CoA of Level 3 competencies were released for public comment, and extensive feedback was provided by the CNS work-group on each draft. At this writing, the CoA has not formally incorporated Level 3 competencies into its implementing regulations. When finalized, Level 3 competencies will be included as a revision of the CoA Implementing Regulation C-9 P, entitled Profession-Wide Competencies. Accredited post-doctoral programs will then be expected to incorporate those competencies into their training.

CONCLUSION AND FUTURE DIRECTIONS

The field has come a long way in a relatively short time in developing clin-ical neuropsychology as a vibrant practice area. HCG define the structure and process of training in clinical neuropsychology. More recently, advances in training, education, and competencies in clinical neuropsychology have complemented HCG and include a taxonomy of training offerings, overarching entry-level competencies, detailed practicum guidelines, and a draft of required competencies for accredited postdoctoral programs. Table 8.2 summarizes the resources reviewed here, including the purpose, primary target, and relevant audiences. More obvious examples of the uses of the documents include the importance of HCG to potential and current trainees planning each step of the training pathway. Trainees may also compare training offerings in clinical neuropsychology across sites by gaining familiarity with the taxonomy, and they can consult the entry-level competencies as a guide to what needs to be

TABLE 8.2. Training and Education Documents Based on Their Purpose, Target, and Relevant Constituencies

Document	What it does	What it does not	Target	Relevant constituencies
Houston Conference Guidelines[a]	Describes the structure and process for training in neuropsychology	Specify detailed competencies	Trainees	Those considering training, training programs, credentialing and accrediting bodies, and employers
Clinical Neuropsychology Taxonomy[b]	Provides a standardized terminology for differing intensities of training experiences	Define training standards or guidelines	Graduate, internship, and fellowship training programs	Trainees
CNS Entry-Level Competencies[c]	Provides a detailed description of entry-level competencies for neuropsychologists	Define the structure or process of training or specify benchmarks during training	Individual neuropsychologists	Training programs, credentialing and accrediting bodies
AACN Practicum Guidelines[d]	Promotes quality of training in neuropsychology at the practicum level, including specification of relevant competencies and benchmarks for the beginning and end of practicum	Address graduate training outside of the practicum experience	Practicum sites and associated graduate training programs	Students and practicum supervisors
CNS Draft Level 3 Postdoctoral Competencies[e]	Specifies the competencies that are required for all APA-accredited postdoctoral fellowship programs in neuropsychology	Define competencies for graduate schools or predoctoral internship programs	Fellowship programs	APA's Commission on Accreditation[f]

Note. CNS = Clinical Neuropsychology Synarchy; AACN = American Academy of Clinical Neuropsychology; APA = American Psychological Association.
[a] Bieliauskas (1998b). [b] CNS (2016), Smith and CNS (2018; Tables 3–10). [c] CNS (2015). Sperling et al. (2017). [d] Nelson et al. (2015). [e] CNS (2015), Smith and CNS (2018; Tables 11–12). [f] Fellowship competencies were provided to APA Commission on Accreditation in 2017, but at this writing have not been formally incorporated into APA Implementing Regulations.

in place at the end of formal training. They are also relevant to credentialing bodies (e.g., ABCN). Additionally, established practitioners may use the entry-level competencies to identify weak spots in their knowledge and skill to guide which continuing education they need. In addition to expecting that job applicants have training consistent with HCG, search committees could formulate interviews intended to reveal the extent to which applicants possess the full range of entry-level competencies. More broadly, from a health care systems standpoint, the entry-level competencies have relevance in workforce analysis when considering the breadth of application of the competencies.

This chapter captures a snapshot of the current state of the art in clinical neuropsychology training and education. Although recent efforts on HCG have greatly expanded, a number of potential enhancements remain, including (a) developing competency measurement tools that apply to the doctoral, internship, and postdoctoral training levels; (b) moving toward standardization of the relative roles of graduate school, internship, and postdoctoral training in competency attainment; (c) developing a broad curriculum of materials aimed at bolstering competencies; (d) more closely linking entry-level competencies to board certification; and (e) leveraging recent advances in training and education into advocacy efforts promoting the importance of clinical neuropsychology practice. Regarding (a), currently no consensus-based measurement tool has been developed to assess neuropsychology competencies, except at the practicum level, which appears as an appendix within Nelson et al. (2015). In contrast, professional geropsychology has had a consensus-based measurement tool available since 2008 (Karel et al., 2010). Development of measurement tools based on the entry-level competencies and rating levels with clear behavioral anchors would be a boon to training programs. Furthermore, a modern competency approach could contribute to greater consistency of training across training sites. Specifically, benchmarks that specify "readiness for internship" and "readiness for postdoctoral residency" for each competency would go far in achieving the integrated model of training conceived by HCG. At this writing, a workgroup within APPCN has been developing a competency-measurement tool for use by postdoctoral programs (Heffelfinger et al., 2020), which will become publicly available in the near future.

Regarding curriculum development, much work is needed in this area, with several encouraging examples. The APPCN maintains for its member programs a practice board-certification written exam, mock oral exam, fact-finding and ethics vignettes, and a growing library of video didactics. Additionally, a group of VA-based postdoctoral programs have engaged in shared didactics and discussion via teleconferencing. The COVID-19 pandemic, while leading to the cancellation of numerous in-person conferences and other training events, has also been accompanied by increasing availability of online training in clinical neuropsychology topics to a far-flung audience. Regarding the linkage between competencies and board certification, review of written and oral examination procedures based on entry-level competencies would reflect in the board certification process the competency advancements realized in the training and accreditation communities. Finally, the explication of entry-level competencies aid ongoing advocacy efforts. The knowledge and skills possessed by clinical neuropsychologists have broad application across settings, including general and specialty integrated health care settings (Festa, 2018; Kubu et al., 2016). All of the applications of the documents covered in the chapter are meant to promote consistently competent practice, and that is an excellent goal indeed.

REFERENCES

American Board of Clinical Neuropsychology. (2020, September 29). *Written examination frequently asked questions.* https://theabcn.org/written-examination-frequently-asked-questions

American Psychological Association. (2020). *Education and training guidelines: A taxonomy for education and training in professional psychology health service specialties and subspecialties.* http://www.apa.org/ed/graduate/specialize/taxonomy.pdf

APA Commission on Accreditation. (2018). Standards of accreditation for health service psychology and accreditation operating procedures. http://www.apa.org/ed/accreditation/about/policies/standards-of-accreditation.pdf

Belar, C. D., Bieliauskas, L. A., Klepac, R. K., Larsen, K. G., Stigall, T. T., & Zimet, C. N. (1993). National conference on postdoctoral training in professional psychology. *American Psychologist, 48*(12), 1284–1289. https://doi.org/10.1037/0003-066X.48.12.1284

Belar, C. D., Bieliauskas, L. A., Larsen, K. G., Mensh, I. N., Poey, K., & Roelke, H. J. (1989). The national conference on internship training in psychology. *American Psychologist, 44*(1), 60–65. https://doi.org/10.1037/0003-066X.44.1.60

Belar, C. D., & Perry, N. W. (1992). The national conference on scientist–practitioner education and training for the professional practice of psychology. *American Psychologist, 47*(1), 71–75. https://doi.org/10.1037/0003-066X.47.1.71

Bickman, L., & Ellis, H. (Eds.). (1990). *Preparing psychologists for the 21st century: Proceedings of the National Conference on Graduate Education in Psychology.* Routledge.

Bieliauskas, L. (1998a). History and background of the conference. *Archives of Clinical Neuropsychology, 13*(2), 167–168. https://doi.org/10.1093/arclin/13.2.167

Bieliauskas, L. (1998b). The Houston conference on specialty education and training in clinical neuropsychology. *Archives of Clinical Neuropsychology, 13*(2), 160–166.

Bieliauskas, L., & Hamsher, K. deS. (1998). Delegate selection. *Archives of Clinical Neuropsychology, 13*(2), 170–171. https://doi.org/10.1093/arclin/13.2.170

Clinical Neuropsychology Synarchy (CNS). (2015). *Taxonomy for clinical neuropsychology.* https://3de0bcf9-0846-41d0-af8e-e2968fb7707d.filesusr.com/ugd/146c2d_d55cec138dd343288e2549c97732f2be.pdf

Clinical Neuropsychology Synarchy. (2016). Entry-level competencies in clinical neuropsychology. https://3de0bcf9-0846-41d0-af8e-e2968fb7707d.filesusr.com/ugd/12cc9c_14c7e4ba69a2447e9b125a2d279346c8.pdf

Costa, L. (1998). Professionalization in neuropsychology: The early years. *The Clinical Neuropsychologist, 12*(1), 1–7. https://doi.org/10.1076/clin.12.1.1.1723

Epstein, R. M., & Hundert, E. M. (2002). Defining and assessing professional competence. *Journal of the American Medical Association, 287*(2), 226–235. https://doi.org/10.1001/jama.287.2.226

Festa, J. R. (2018). Introduction to the special issue on neuropsychology practices in integrated care teams. *Archives of Clinical Neuropsychology, 33*(3), 257–259. https://doi.org/10.1093/arclin/acy017

Fouad, N. A., Grus, C. L., Hatcher, R. L., Kaslow, N. J., Hutchings, P. S., Madson, M. B., Collins, F. L., & Crossman, R. E. (2009). Competency benchmarks: A model for understanding and measuring competence in professional psychology across training levels. *Training and Education in Professional Psychology, 3*(4, Suppl), S5–S26. https://doi.org/10.1037/a0015832

France, C. R., Masters, K. S., Belar, C. D., Kerns, R. D., Klonoff, E. A., Larkin, K. T., Smith, T. W., Suchday, S., & Thorn, B. E. (2008). Application of the competency model to clinical health psychology. *Professional Psychology, Research and Practice, 39*(6), 573–580. https://doi.org/10.1037/0735-7028.39.6.573

Hannay, H. J., Bieliauskas, L. A., Crosson, B. A., Harmneke, T. A., Hamsher, K. deS., & Koffler, S. P. (1998). Proceedings of the Houston conference on specialty education and training in clinical neuropsychology. *Archives of Clinical Neuropsychology, 13*(2), 157–250. https://doi.org/10.1093/arclin/13.2.160

Heffelfinger, A. K., Janecek, J. K., Johnson, A., Miller, L. E., Nelson, A., & Pulsipher, D. T. (2020). Competency-based assessment in clinical neuropsychology at the post-doctoral level: Stages, milestones, and benchmarks as proposed by an APPCN work group. *The Clinical Neuropsychologist.* https://doi.org/10.1080/13854046.2020.1829070

Hoge, M. A., Morris, J. A., Daniels, A. S., Huey, L. Y., Stuart, G. W., & Adams, N., Paris, M., Goplerud, E., Horgan, C. M., Kaplan, L., Storti, S. A., & Dodge, J. M. (2005). Report of recommendations: The Annapolis coalition conference on behavioral health work force competencies. *Administration and Policy in Mental Health and Mental Health Services Research, 32*, 651–663. https://doi.org/10.1007/s10488-005-3267-x

INS/Division 40 Task Force. (1987). Reports of the INS/Division 40 task force on education, accreditation, and credentialing. *The Clinical Neuropsychologist, 1*(1), 29–34. https://doi.org/10.1080/13854048708520033

Karel, M. J., Emery, E. E., & Molinari, V. (2010). Development of a tool to evaluate geropsychology knowledge and skill competencies. *International Psychogeriatrics, 22*(6), 886–896. https://doi.org/10.1017/S1041610209991736

Kaslow, N. J., Borden, K. A., Collins, F. L., Forrest, L., Illfelder-Kaye, J., & Nelson, P. D., Rallo, J. S., Vasquez, M. J. T., & Willmuth, M. E. (2004). Competencies conference: Future directions in education and credentialing in professional psychology. *Journal of Clinical Psychology, 60*(7), 699–712. https://doi.org/10.1002/jclp.20016

Kubu, C. S., Ready, R. E., Festa, J. R., Roper, B. L., & Pliskin, N. H. (2016). The times they are a changin': Neuropsychology and integrated care teams. *The Clinical Neuropsychologist, 30*(1), 51–65. https://doi.org/10.1080/13854046.2015.1134670

Meier, M. J. (1981). Report of the task force on education, accreditation and credentialing of the International Neuropsychological Society. *The INS Bulletin*, September. 5–10.

Nelson, A. P., Roper, B. L., Slomine, B. S., Morrison, C., Greher, M. R., Janusz, J., Larson, J. C., Meadows, M.-E., Ready, R. E., Rivera Mindt, M., Whiteside, D. M., Willment, K., & Wodushek, T. R. (2015). Official position of the American Academy of Clinical Neuropsychology (AACN): Guidelines for practicum training in clinical neuropsychology. *The Clinical Neuropsychologist*, *29*(7), 879–904. https://doi.org/10.1080/13854046.2015.1117658

Rey-Casserly, C., Roper, B. L., & Bauer, R. M. (2012). Application of a competency model to clinical neuropsychology. *Professional Psychology, Research and Practice*, *43*(5), 422–431. https://doi.org/10.1037/a0028721

Rodolfa, E., Bent, R., Eisman, E., Nelson, P., Rehm, L., & Ritchie, P. (2005). A cube model for competency development: Implications for psychology educators and regulators. *Professional Psychology, Research and Practice*, *36*(4), 347–354. https://doi.org/10.1037/0735-7028.36.4.347

Smith, G. (2018). Education and training in clinical neuropsychology: Recent developments and documents from the Clinical Neuropsychology Synarchy. *Archives of Clinical Neuropsychology*, *34*(3), 418–431. https://doi.org/10.1093/arclin/acy075

Sperling, S. A., Cimino, C. R., Stricker, N. H., Heffelfinger, A. K., Gess, J. L., Osborn, K. E., & Roper, B. L. (2017). *Taxonomy for Education and Training in Clinical Neuropsychology:* Past, present, and future. *The Clinical Neuropsychologist*, *31*(5), 817–828. https://doi.org/10.1080/13854046.2017.1314017

Sweet, J. J., Perry, W., Ruff, R. M., Shear, P. K., & Guidotti Breting, L. M. (2012). The Inter-Organizational Summit on Education and Training (ISET) 2010 survey on the influence of the Houston Conference training guidelines. *The Clinical Neuropsychologist*, *26*(7), 1055–1076. https://doi.org/10.1080/13854046.2012.705565

9 CLASSROOM TEACHING AND CLINICAL SUPERVISION COMPETENCIES

LESLIE GUIDOTTI BRETING AND DOUGLAS M. WHITESIDE

One of the truly exciting aspects of a career in neuropsychology is the multitude of options for teaching, including working in the classroom and in the clinic providing clinical supervision. Many neuropsychologists are involved in clinical teaching through supervision of practicum students, interns, and postdoctoral fellows, but others may want a career involving traditional classroom teaching. While in the minority of neuropsychologists (Sweet et al., 2015), a number of very successful neuropsychologists work in traditional academic departments, including current leaders in the field, such as Yana Suchy (University of Utah), Maureen Schmitter-Edgecombe (Washington State University), Julie Suhr (Ohio University), Steven Paul Woods (University of Houston), Maria Schultheis (Drexel University), Monica Rivera-Mindt (Fordham University), Rebecca Ready (University of Massachusetts Amherst), and many more.

There is also a need for neuropsychologists to be faculty members at the doctoral level of training, given that many doctoral graduate students have expressed a need for mentoring in neuropsychology (Whiteside et al., 2016). For neuropsychology students interested in this career path, there are several critical considerations, and there are various ways to achieve this career

https://doi.org/10.1037/0000250-010
The Neuropsychologist's Roadmap: A Training and Career Guide, C. Block (Editor)

objective. Because professional psychology is moving to a competency model of training, it is important to consider the competencies involved in teaching, as well.

This chapter focuses on the competencies involved in becoming a successful teacher, both in the classroom and in the clinic. We begin by discussing the various clinic/counseling psychology training models, followed by the skills and competencies involved in teaching in the classroom and clinic, and tips on how to achieve competence in training. It is important to understand that there are different models for clinical training programs.

TRAINING PROGRAMS

There are three primary models of clinical/counseling psychology doctoral training programs in the United States (Routh, 2015), based primarily on the balance between clinical and research training provided in the program. As Chapter 1 of this text noted, the three main types of training programs are as follows:

- *scientist–practitioner model:* This is the traditional "Boulder" model program (Routh, 2015), which originated after World War II and today remains the most common training program. The model emphasizes the integration of research and clinical training, typically with a required dissertation for graduation, and extensive clinical training. The classic Boulder model scientist–practitioner program would have approximately equal emphasis on both clinical and research training.

- *practitioner–scholar model:* In contrast, the training model for these programs was first developed at the Vail Conference on Professional Training in Psychology in Colorado, in 1973. These programs tend to emphasize clinical training, with less emphasis on research training. Some may not require dissertations, but often have alternative capstone projects with a more clinical focus. Many of these programs are found in free-standing professional schools and usually offer a doctor of psychology (PsyD) degree. However, several PsyD programs are also found in more traditional university settings (e.g., Rutgers University, Baylor University, and several others).

- *clinical scientist model:* Of the three main models, this is the newest (developed at the Bloomington Conference titled "Clinical Science in the 21st Century," held by the National Institute of Mental Health and the

Association for Psychological Science, Indiana, in 1994; Routh, 2015) and the one that emphasizes research most heavily. Most of the clinical scientist model programs have as their goal to train researchers in clinical psychology, and their training model is geared to achieve this end. Thus, clinical training, while not unimportant, is less of an emphasis.

Depending on interest and background, neuropsychologists are generally well positioned to be faculty in any of these training model programs depending upon their particular course of study. However, there are other options for classroom teaching besides a full-time job in a traditional liberal arts college or free-standing program. In particular, adjunct teaching is viable option for psychologists and neuropsychologists at almost any level of experience. Frequently, community colleges and smaller undergraduate liberal arts-based programs are looking for qualified psychologists to teach undergraduate level psychology courses (e.g., Introduction to Psychology, Abnormal Psychology, Developmental Psychology). One potential drawback is that this option is usually lower paying than having a full-time teaching/research position. However, adjunct teaching is a great way to gain experience and connections in classroom teaching.

For the scientist–practitioner and clinical scientist model programs, research training and experience is typically a major factor in obtaining and retaining positions in those programs. Being in traditional settings, positions in these programs are often tenure-track, with the idea that once one obtains tenure, there is increased job security to pursue academic interests. Thus, tenure is typically heavily weighted on research productivity, and the student interested in this is advised to carefully read and consider Chapter 7 on research careers. It should be noted that many of the free-standing (and at least some university-based) practitioner–scientist model programs do not have a tenure system but often rely on contracts lasting one or more years. It is also possible for neuropsychologists to become adjunct faculty in programs that allow them to teach an occasional course. However, regardless of training model, most programs also value and evaluate candidates for jobs and promotion based on their classroom teaching skills and mentoring. Unfortunately, while it is important to get high-quality didactic training and experience in classroom teaching, few programs have a formal program that teaches about teaching. Rather, most new neuropsychologists (and, frankly, most faculty across disciplines) received at most on-the-job training through teaching assistantships, where they assist faculty with large undergraduate lecture format classes.

TEACHING

This section focuses first on the competencies involved in becoming an effective classroom teacher, whether this is your primary position or something you do occasionally. After that, various tips for being an effective classroom teacher are discussed.

Teaching as a Competency

What are the ways to gain competence in teaching? There are several options. One option would be to volunteer to teach an undergraduate or lower level graduate course in your department. If you wish to do this, be sure you have a good faculty mentor/supervisor for that class. Usually these types of teaching opportunities are reserved for advanced graduate students with strong academic records. We recommend asking your primary mentor/faculty member in your department about who would be an excellent faculty member to make sure your classroom teaching experience is successful. If opportunities are not available in your home department, another option is to seek out opportunities at local community colleges. There are some drawbacks to this option, particularly limited assistance and mentoring by many community colleges. However, some of your faculty may be willing to advise and consult with you. Further, you may need special permission to teach a class outside of your home department, and faculty will consider your overall track record and standing in the program. We encourage interested students to seek out opportunities in classroom teaching and then solicit feedback on your performance (from faculty as well as the students). Finally, for those with a strong interest in classroom teaching, resources are available through Division 2 (Society for the Teaching of Psychology) of the American Psychological Association (APA) and their official journal, *Teaching of Psychology* (Sage Publishing). Table 9.1 provides examples of resources to assist with teaching.

Tips for Teaching

Tip 1: Reflect on your own past courses. One of the first suggestions is to simply think about courses you have taken and identify what you liked and did not like about various instructors' teaching methods, materials, exercises, examinations, and so on. Your peers may also have insights on what they find valuable in the classroom setting. Thus, you can use your own experiences to make the classroom an effective teaching environment.

Tip 2: Reflect on what you already know about psychology. Utilize your psychology background to be a better teacher. Neuropsychologists, with their

TABLE 9.1. Sample Resources for Psychology Teaching and Supervision

Organizations	URLs
APA Society for Teaching of Psychology	https://www.teachpsych.org
APA Society of Counseling Psychology	https://www.div17.org
Association for Psychological Science	https://www.bit.ly/3hinOqT
KnowNeuropsychology	https://www.knowneuropsych.org
TeachPsychScience	https://www.teachpsychscience.org
Electronic resources	
Preparing the new psychology professoriate	https://www.teachpsych.org/page-1862898
Society for the Teaching of Psychology e-books on: • advising • research on teaching • teaching topics and techniques • early career • theoretical	https://www.teachpsych.org/ebooks/index.php#Teaching
Print resources	
McKeachie's Teaching Tips	https://www.bit.ly/2UxlUfY
Teaching for Thinking	https://www.apa.org/pubs/books/4316790
Evidence-Based Teaching for Higher Education	https://www.apa.org/pubs/books/4317288
Teaching Ethically: Challenges and Opportunities	https://www.apa.org/pubs/books/4311035
Constructing Undergraduate Psychology Curricula	https://www.apa.org/pubs/books/4316116
Clinical Supervision: Competency Based Approach	https://www.apa.org/pubs/books/4317045
Casebook for Clinical Supervision	https://www.apa.org/pubs/books/4317154
Supervision Essentials for the Practice of Competency-Based Supervision	https://www.apa.org/pubs/books/4317427
Multiculturalism and Diversity in Clinical Supervision	https://www.apa.org/pubs/books/4317344
Essentials of Psychological Assessment Supervision	https://www.wiley.com/learn/psychologyessentials
Other resources	
This is How I Teach blog	https://teachpsych.org/page-1703896?
Graduate Student Teaching Association Blog	https://www.teachpsych.org/page-1784686
Supervisory Styles Inventory	https://www.bit.ly/3cQ74sp
Sample Supervision Contract	https://www.bit.ly/2KdppVU
Sample psychology lecture videos	https://www.bit.ly/1tLcSGs
Sample cognitive neuroscience lecture videos	https://www.bit.ly/2AVWEue
Sample psychology classroom data set	https://www.osf.io/te54b

Note. APA = American Psychological Association.

particularly strong understanding of cognition, are in an excellent position to develop and implement teaching strategies that improve retention of material and critical thinking skills.

Tip 3: Seek mentorship and use it effectively. Of course, having an experienced mentor to help guide you through your early classroom teaching experience is critical for success. Try to identify faculty you feel are particularly strong teachers. They do not have to be neuropsychologists or even in the clinical psychology program. One particularly influential graduate school faculty member for one of us (Whiteside) was a quantitative psychologist who taught the statistics sequence. His teaching style made abstract and difficult statistical concepts understandable to first-year graduate students.

Tip 4: Take the time to prepare and plan, and do so thoughtfully. It takes considerable time to "prep" a class. Be prepared to spend extensive time getting ready for the first time you teach a class. Preparing coherent and engaging classroom lectures is time consuming and challenging. It's not just about relating a bunch of facts to students. You should plan in advance about how you will promote class discussion and critical thinking. The course evaluations/ assignments should be carefully considered and match the topic. For example, fact-based classes are often more amenable to short-answer type exams (e.g., biopsychology), whereas theoretical and experiential classes are more amenable to papers/essays (e.g., cognitive behavioral theory and therapy).

Tip 5: Be patient—mastery takes time. Classroom teaching may be a satisfying part of a professional career. Strong teachers make it look effortless, but the reality is that the skills needed to be an effective teacher take time to master, just like clinical skills.

Tip 6: Stay current with the field. After teaching the same course several times, make sure to update with new material and peer-reviewed articles. Use of technology can also be a terrific addition to engage students more actively and hold their attention. For example, many professors are now using interactive polls and quizzes or incorporating videos, animation, or graphics into their lectures.

Up to now, this section has focused primarily on traditional classroom teaching. However, many times neuropsychologists have the opportunity to use these didactic skills in other settings. For example, opportunities for one-time didactic presentations in academic medical centers or Veterans Affairs medical centers with internships or postdoctoral fellowships are common (e.g., grand rounds, didactics for interns and postdoctoral fellows). Further, neuropsychologists are often asked to provide educational programs to community groups, such as the Brain Injury Alliance or the Alzheimer's

Association. Being able to present complex and abstract neuropsychological concepts in a compelling and accessible manner will be very beneficial to the community members. Additionally, if you are in private practice, providing high quality education as a community outreach service (e.g., presenting to your local Alzheimer's disease support group) is an excellent way to increase your visibility and referral base.

Finally, teaching skills will serve you well in future job interviews, since interviews in academic settings almost always include some sort of "job talk," where you will be expected to provide a formal presentation, typically about a topic related to the position. These talks are meant to provide the faculty a chance to evaluate your formal teaching skills; doing well with these presentations will give you a competitive advantage. The topic of a job talk should be tailored to the setting where you are applying. For example, for a position with a significant research component, you should present on a research project you have completed (your dissertation is typically a good topic). Taking advantage of formal teaching opportunities and resources will help you prepare for all types of classroom-type teaching.

CLINICAL SUPERVISION

This section covers the various competencies that are important to be a successful clinical supervisor. Various tips are provided to help you become an effective supervisor.

Clinical Supervision as a Competency

While classroom teaching is sought out by a relatively small number of neuropsychologists, clinical supervision by neuropsychologists is more common and is a fundamental piece of the training of future clinical psychologists and neuropsychologists; however, there is limited literature regarding how to get training in supervision specifically for the neuropsychologist. A 2014 survey showed that only 27% of clinical neuropsychologists reported having training specific to neuropsychology supervision (Shultz et al., 2014). This is surprising, given that APA considers clinical supervision a professional competency. There is, however, a consensus statement related to the defining competencies in psychology supervision to provide guidance to aspiring clinical supervisors (Falender et al., 2004). Stucky et al. (2010) provided a framework for the development of suggested competency standards for training of neuropsychology supervisors, which is similar to the one proposed by Falender and Shafranske (2008) for clinical psychology. Stucky et al. suggested that a competency-based approach advocates for "a science-informed, formalized, and objective process that clearly delineates the competencies required for good supervisory practice" (p. 738). Kaufman and Kaufman (2006) reviewed the many models of supervision in professional psychology, and Stucky et al. (2010) built off of those models to propose a supervision model for neuropsychology that is an individually tailored, process-based, developmental approach. What this means is that a supervisor should be able to provide foundational experiences while assuming multiple roles (e.g., teacher, consultant, administrator, assessor) that are flexible to meet the trainee at their experience level, change as the trainee develops additional skills, and utilize the trainee's strengths. Six goals of supervision were outlined: "(a) the development of neuropsychological knowledge and skills, (b) critical thinking and decision making, (c) high-quality clinical care, (d) investment in career-long learning, (e) meaningful patient outcomes, and (f) development and fostering of essential attitudes for ethical practice" (Stucky et al., p. 740).

Many theories and models of supervision in clinical psychology have been proposed; while a thorough discussion of these models is outside of the scope of this chapter, readers are encouraged to consult Kaufman and Kaufman (2006) for a more detailed discussion of these supervision models. Kaufman and Kaufman described several examples of supervision models including psychotherapy-based, developmental, process-based, discrimination, systems, parallel process, interactional, interpersonal, supervisee-as-patient, comprehensive/integrative, one-size-fits-all, and no-model.

Three factors that the majority of the more general supervision models tend to focus on are administrative issues, clinical issues, and the supervisee's developing skills in psychotherapy. The model outlined above (Stucky et al., 2010) is the first one of which we are aware that is specifically for clinical neuropsychology supervision. Within this model, supervisors should encourage trainees to discuss ethical issues. Per Stucky et al. (2010), the applied competencies of a neuropsychology supervisor include

- providing effective training in the foundations of assessment, psychometric theory, and the administration/scoring of neuropsychological measures;

- providing effective training in developing and asserting one's professional identity and role as a clinical neuropsychologist;

- providing effective training in neuropsychological interviewing, test interpretation, case conceptualization, report writing, and the development of tailored recommendations;

- providing effective training in the treatment planning following an evaluation and how to effectively deliver feedback; and

- demonstrating sensitivity to individual and cultural differences in supervisory contexts.

TRAINING TO BECOME A COMPETENT AND EFFECTIVE SUPERVISOR

One of the best ways to learn how to supervise is to observe your clinical and/or research supervisors and then ask questions. Similar to teaching Tip 1 above, it is also important to reflect on your prior supervision experiences to incorporate what you found effective in your own experiences as a supervisee into your role as a supervisor. One valuable way to gain experience and training in supervision is to utilize vertical supervision, which is when a more advanced trainee, such as an intern or postdoctoral fellow supervises trainees at a lower level (e.g., externs). Vertical supervision does not replace the role of direct supervision; in your role as a supervisor, you must supervise both the trainee providing supervision and the trainee receiving the supervision. This is a nice opportunity for trainees to learn aspects of supervision and receive direct feedback. For additional information on vertical supervision, see Nelson et al. (2015).

Additionally, if your program offers supervision courses, take them seriously. For example, at Adler University Dr. Marla Vannucci teaches a required course titled Supervision and Management in Clinical Psychology that provides advanced graduate student didactic and experiential training in clinical supervision through role playing with live and videotaped sessions. However, the majority of training in supervision happens during the internship and postdoctoral fellowship; one continues to refine their supervisory skills throughout their professional career. It would be quite rare for a student to receive supervision training during a neuropsychology externship placement; however, this is still a great time for observation of your supervisors. Additionally, if interested in teaching/supervising let your faculty know so that if opportunities arise, they think of you. We encourage prospective interns and postdoctoral fellows to inquire about training opportunities in supervision during the application and interview process.

Medical schools are placing increasing importance on the quality of the training experience that their students obtain. Being a supervisor for many doctoral students in the Chicago metropolitan area, one of the authors (Guidotti Breting) was invited by Rosalind Franklin University of Medicine and Science to participate in the Preceptor Enhancement Program (PEP), an online continuing education (CE) module aimed at enhancing one's ability to instruct, mentor, and assess students in training. This type of online CE course aimed at supervision is being offered more frequently. If you would like additional training in supervising trainees, reach out to local medical school programs to see if they offer similar CE courses. (To learn more about the program at Rosalind Franklin University, visit https://www.rosalindfranklin.edu/about/strategic-initiatives/clinical-partnerships/clinical-preceptor-enhancement).

Tips for Supervision

Tip 1: Define your role. A common pitfall of being a new supervisor in neuropsychology includes failing to recognize the role differences between trainee and supervisor, such as the inherent power differential in these respective roles. On the other hand, some supervisors emphasize this role difference too much. As with most things in life, the supervisory role requires a fine balance between the roles and a clear understanding of appropriate professional boundaries (e.g., not "friending" supervisees on Facebook).

Tip 2: Allocate ample time for supervision. The time required to be an effective supervisor is often significant, particularly during the early career phase when the neuropsychologist is less experienced at clinical supervision. Time allotment for supervision can also be a significant challenge for some clinical neuropsychologists, and careful time management is an important skill for clinical supervisors (and neuropsychologists in general). For example, there are times when competing demands limit time in the day for proper supervision and training. Conversely, it is a temptation to spend too much time on supervision and training, which interferes with a healthy work–life balance. In spite of these issues, there are specific time requirements related to supervision that must be met (e.g., for internships, for doctoral programs, licensure, board certification).

Tip 3: Have self-confidence. New supervisors may struggle when one of their trainees is their own age or older. However, having the training and experience to supervise is not a direct function of age. When working with postdoctoral fellows in this situation, we encourage supervisors to have confidence in their competencies and ability to train anyone.

Tip 4: Provide constructive feedback. One of the more challenging aspects of supervision is providing the clinical neuropsychology trainee with appropriate and constructive feedback and assessment for their graduate program. When providing summative feedback for trainees, it is important to include both strengths and weaknesses, as well as goals. Try to frame weaknesses in the context of the level of training and encourage the trainees to remember that everyone has areas where they are more and less proficient. Aside from the more formal quarterly or biannual evaluation forms that a program may require you to complete for a trainee, it is also important, as a supervisor, you provide regular formative feedback and offer additional information related to neuropsychology competencies that a supervisee needs to acquire. It is also helpful to have trainees evaluate your own supervision skills, effectiveness, and availability.

Tip 5: Meet a trainee at their level. It can be challenging to provide the appropriate level of supervision for trainees at different stages. To assist with this, Nelson et al. (2015) published a comprehensive guideline for practicum in clinical neuropsychology, which delineates competency expectations at various stages of training (i.e., novice, basic, intermediate, advanced, proficient, expert). For example, at the advanced level of training, one would only require supervision for unusual or complex situations; whereas, at the basic level of training one would require intensive supervision requiring a significant time commitment.

Tip 6: Acknowledge and manage "impostor syndrome." As a final note, many early career professionals and advanced trainees experience imposter syndrome, which commonly manifests as doubts about your competence to effectively complete important professional responsibilities (e.g., neuropsychological evaluations) and the sense that you "fooled" your supervisors throughout training. Based on many conversation with other neuropsychologists, this is a very common feeling among early career professionals in many fields (including the authors of this chapter). It should be noted that imposter syndrome can occur not only when you work to complete your first neuropsychological evaluation report independently under your license, but also in the context of supervision. Importantly, if you do not feel comfortable in the supervisory role, then seek additional training and consultation from peers or senior faculty who have demonstrated themselves as effective supervisors.

Tip 7: Continually evaluate principles of diversity and ethics. As a supervisor, one must intentionally examine and integrate diversity/inclusion considerations and ethical standards into all aspects of practice. The field of neuropsychology is actively working to be more responsive to diversity issues and be more inclusive, and supervisors who can help facilitate development of these issues in trainees will be highly valuable. At the same time, the supervisor should evaluate the trainee on these dimensions to protect the public and further the field of neuropsychology. Despite these common challenges, being a valued clinical and/or research supervisor can be a rewarding and valuable experience that helps to shape the future of neuropsychologists in training.

CONCLUSION AND FUTURE DIRECTIONS

Based on the discussion and limited literature outlined in this chapter that is specific to teaching and training/supervision within the field of neuropsychology, it is evident that in the future additional research on effective clinical supervision in neuropsychology would be valuable, as well as specific teaching and supervision methods or standards. It will be imperative for future clinical neuropsychologists who are interested in teaching and supervising trainees to receive mentorship, coursework, and CEs related to this topic. Teaching and supervising future clinical neuropsychologists can be a very valuable experience in one's career; we encourage you to seek out these tremendous opportunities throughout your career.

REFERENCES

Falender, C. A., Cornish, J. A. E., Goodyear, R., Hatcher, R., Kaslow, N. J., Leventhal, G., Shafranske, E., Sigmon, S. T., Stoltenberg, C., & Grus, C. (2004). Defining competencies in psychology supervision: A consensus statement. *Journal of Clinical Psychology*, *60*(7), 771–785. https://doi.org/10.1002/jclp.20013

Falender, C. A., & Shafranske, E. P. (2008). *Casebook for clinical supervision: A competency-based approach*. American Psychological Association. https://doi.org/10.1037/11792-000

Kaufman, A. S., & Kaufman, N. L. (2006). *Essentials of clinical supervision*. Wiley.

Nelson, A. P., Roper, B. L., Slomine, B. S., Morrison, C., Greher, M. R., Janusz, J., Larson, J. C., Meadows, M.-E., Ready, R. E., Mindt, M. R., Whiteside, D. M., Willment, K., & Wodushek, T. R. (2015). Official position of the American Academy of Clinical Neuropsychology (AACN): Guidelines for practicum training in clinical neuropsychology. *The Clinical Neuropsychologist*, *29*(7), 879–904. https://doi.org/10.1080/13854046.2015.1117658

Routh, D. K. (2015). Training models in clinical psychology. In R. L. Cautin & S. O. Lilienfeld (Eds.), *The encyclopedia of clinical psychology*. Wiley. https://doi.org/10.1002/9781118625392.wbecp061

Shultz, L. A., Pedersen, H. A., Roper, B. L., & Rey-Casserly, C. (2014). Supervision in neuropsychological assessment: A survey of training, practices, and perspectives of supervisors. *The Clinical Neuropsychologist*, *28*(6), 907–925. https://doi.org/10.1080/13854046.2014.942373

Stucky, K. J., Bush, S., & Donders, J. (2010). Providing effective supervision in clinical neuropsychology. *The Clinical Neuropsychologist*, *24*(5), 737–758. https://doi.org/10.1080/13854046.2010.490788

Sweet, J. J., Benson, L. M., Nelson, N. W., & Moberg, P. J. (2015). The American Academy of Clinical Neuropsychology, National Academy of Neuropsychology, and Society for Clinical Neuropsychology (APA Division 40) 2015 TCN Professional Practice and 'Salary Survey': Professional practices, beliefs, and incomes of U.S. neuropsychologists. *The Clinical Neuropsychologist, 29*(8), 1069–1162. https://doi.org/10.1080/13854046.2016.1140228

Whiteside, D. M., Guidotti Breting, L. M., Butts, A. M., Hahn-Ketter, A. E., Osborn, K., Towns, S. J., Barisa, M., Santos, O. A., & Smith, D. (2016). 2015 American Academy of Clinical Neuropsychology (AACN) student affairs committee survey of neuropsychology trainees. *The Clinical Neuropsychologist, 30*(5), 664–694. https://doi.org/10.1080/13854046.2016.1196731

10

CONSULTATION, ASSESSMENT, AND INTERVENTION COMPETENCIES IN NEUROPSYCHOLOGY

AMY HEFFELFINGER AND JULIE JANECEK

If you have gotten this far into this book, then you must be intrigued by the science of neuropsychology. You are considering a career studying how the brain's genetic, developmental, and aging processes, its neurons and glial cells, and its neural networks and systems influence our thinking, learning, feeling, and behavior. In this chapter, we discuss what you will be learning in school, and what you will be doing in your career, if you choose the clinical practice of neuropsychology. We delineate the steps for training as well as the expected clinical practice competencies necessary for neuropsychological assessment, consultation, and intervention, in a way that we hope will help you decide whether you would like a clinical career in neuropsychology.

First, it is important for you to understand what it means to be evidence based. Neuropsychology as a field is built on its science, and our clinical practice demonstrates this in all aspects of what we do. What does this mean? Our process of assessing our patients' neuropsychological functioning and deciding whether it is impaired or not, and the interventions and treatments that are recommended are driven by scientific evidence. Some clinical neuropsychologists use their data to conduct clinical research to allow for a better understanding of patients and their unique and diverse backgrounds, common and rare disease states, and brain development throughout the

https://doi.org/10.1037/0000250-011
The Neuropsychologist's Roadmap: A Training and Career Guide, C. Block (Editor)

lifespan. Driven by science and furthering science: This is what it means to be an evidence-based field.

The practice of clinical neuropsychology involves strong knowledge of how brain functions and brain systems develop and operate, and how they can be damaged with injury or disorder. With this knowledge, the clinical neuropsychologist conducts a comprehensive clinical interview and uses neuropsychological tests that measure neuropsychological functions and standardized normative data to determine whether that function has declined. Each component of this process has been carefully designed through empirical research and study. The clinical neuropsychology competencies describe each of the areas of knowledge and skill that are necessary to function independently in practice. The Houston Conference Guidelines were established to determine requirements for training in clinical neuropsychology (Hannay et al., 1998). This chapter uses the competencies for clinical neuropsychology as described in Smith (2019) and Heffelfinger et al. (2020), which are based on those originally proposed by Rey-Casserly et al. (2012). The competencies include

- integration of science and practice
- ethical and legal standards and policy
- individual and cultural diversity
- professional identity and relationships/self-reflective practice
- interdisciplinary systems and consultation
- assessment
- intervention
- research
- teaching, supervision and mentoring
- management and administration

At the conclusion of a full-time, 2-year, postdoctoral fellowship in clinical neuropsychology, trainees should be prepared for independent practice, having developed a strong knowledge base and well-developed skills in each of the competencies This chapter describes what you will be able to do in clinical practice after you graduate from your 2-year fellowship.

EXPECTATIONS FOR PROGRESSION THROUGH TRAINING

As you have read earlier in this book, the path to becoming a clinical neuropsychologist starts in graduate school and continues through your predoctoral internship and postdoctoral fellowship. The core of each step in the training process is the development of the knowledge and skills essential for neuropsychological assessment, consultation, and intervention. Cognitive assessment is the primary role of most clinical neuropsychologists with consultation to other areas of medicine, schools, and industry typically playing a lesser role. The intervention component of practice for most clinical neuropsychologists involves providing feedback on the assessment results and empirically supported treatment recommendations specific to the patient.

It is important to understand the expectations for training. The major professional and training organizations in neuropsychology in the United States established a taxonomy for clinical neuropsychology to outline the recommended sequence of education and training (Sperling et al., 2017). This taxonomy identifies the types of coursework and quantity of practical experiences necessary for training in doctoral, internship, and postdoctoral programs to spend on neuropsychology training, but not the specific knowledge and skills that should be acquired at each step of the training process. The primary requirement for each aspect of training is learning how to administer, score, interpret, integrate and report the results of the neuropsychological assessment. A workgroup was formed to generate guidelines for specific competencies to be achieved at the graduate student or practicum levels (Nelson et al., 2015), and recently specific competencies and a procedure for competency-based evaluation have been proposed at the postdoctoral fellowship level (Heffelfinger et al., 2020; Smith, 2019). The remainder of this section describes the trajectory of knowledge and skill development at each stage of training in clinical neuropsychology.

Graduate School Level

The initial training in clinical neuropsychological assessment, consultation, and intervention occur during graduate school, and typically a graduate student will complete 2 to 3 years of supervised clinical training experiences called practicum placements. Over the course of the practicum, students are exposed to aspects of clinical neuropsychology and require intensive supervision. The main areas of training include test administration, interpretation of tests, and report writing. At this stage, it is expected that you will observe your supervisor performing aspects of the neuropsychological evaluation such as conducting an interview, administering neuropsychological tests, and giving feedback, as well as being directly supervised as you develop your own assessment skills (see Table 10.1).

Internship Level

In order for an internship program to offer a Major Area of Study in neuropsychology, at least 50% of the training time must be devoted to clinical

TABLE 10.1. Practicum Level

Domain	Expectation
Test administration	A core feature of your neuropsychology practicum will be learning to administer commonly used neuropsychological tests. You will learn to give standardized instructions, record responses, and document behavioral observations—these are things that the patient does during the testing process that are clinically meaningful, such as making word substitutions or interacting with the test materials in a repetitive or unusual manner.
	You will learn to score the tests by comparing how the patient performed to how a group of healthy people who are demographically similar to them did on the same tests.
Interpretation	During your neuropsychology practicum, you will talk about interpretation of tests and integration of test data with the information that was learned in the clinical interview, record review, and behavioral observations with your supervising neuropsychologist.
	You will start to learn about patterns of cognitive performance that are commonly seen in certain cognitive disorders, such as learning disabilities and memory disorders.
	You will begin to understand the relationships between brain structure and function, you repeatedly see language and verbal memory deficits associated with strokes or seizures in the left temporal lobe or neglect associated with a brain tumor or brain injury that affects the right parietal lobe.
Report writing	After developing test administration skills, you may be asked to write some or all the neuropsychological report. Typically, this consists of several sections including background information, behavioral observations, summary and conclusions, and recommendations.
	At this stage of training, it can be difficult to know what information is important and the best way to pull it all together. Your supervisor will provide extensive feedback at this stage about the content and structure of your reports.
Consultation	At the practicum level of training, you will be exposed to different referral sources and you may be working with other clinical services (e.g., rehabilitation, neurology, psychiatry) under the direct supervision of a clinical neuropsychologist.
	You will observe how your supervisor communicates with patients, referral sources, and colleagues.
Intervention	You will learn about evidenced-based interventions for different cognitive and behavioral populations. You will likely observe your supervisor providing feedback to individuals and families and recommending scientifically validated interventions to treat particular cognitive conditions.

neuropsychology and some of the didactic experiences must address aspects of knowledge and skill that are relevant to clinical neuropsychology. At this level of training, the student is expected to administer, score, and interpret neuropsychological tests, provide verbal and written feedback of the results integrated with the broader clinical picture, and provide recommendations for what the patient should do regarding their results. You will learn to consult to referral sources in the medical setting and community, and establish a base for your knowledge of empirically based interventions for the types of patients you are seeing. All of this occurs with ongoing direct supervision, and significant growth occurs in your knowledge and skills during your internship year (see Table 10.2).

Fellowship Level

At the postdoctoral fellowship level, you should have advanced knowledge and skills in clinical neuropsychology. While you still require ongoing supervision, the focus starts to shift to more apprentice-based training. The supervisor guides the thinking and decision making, but the postdoctoral fellow determines the reason for referral, the possible differential diagnoses and neurobehavioral syndromes, how to assess for these, how to integrate them into the clinical history, and what is needed to treat them. You gain independence in all the basic aspects of clinical neuropsychology and rely on your supervisor more for complex or atypical situations as you progress through the program. By the end of your 2-year fellowship, you are able to function independently as a clinical neuropsychologist, with the expectation that you will seek continuing education and consultation as needed (see Table 10.3).

COMPETENCY-BASED ASSESSMENT OF NEUROPSYCHOLOGICAL ASSESSMENT, CONSULTATION, AND INTERVENTION

As you progress through the stages of training in clinical neuropsychology, the development of your knowledge and skills will be supervised and evaluated at each step along the way. The competency-based approach to supervision and evaluation was established by the American Psychological Association (APA) as a systematic way to articulate training goals and learning objectives, identify specific knowledge, skills, and attitudes that form each competency, and provide a behaviorally anchored basis for feedback and evaluation (Falender & Shafranske, 2012). In 2015, the APA Commission on Accreditation (APA CoA) published the *Standards of Accreditation for Health Service Psychology and Accreditation Operating Procedures,* which provides guidelines

TABLE 10.2. Internship Level

Domain	Expectation
Test administration	By the time you start internship, you will likely have completed at least one practicum in clinical neuropsychology.
	You will be proficient in the basics of test administration and scoring for commonly used neuropsychological tests. You may be exposed to a few new tests or some less commonly used tests.
	The main developmental goal for test administration during internship is to increase accuracy and efficiency, and to increase attention to clinically relevant behavioral observations.
Interpretation	This is a significant area of growth during internship, when you start to put all the pieces of the clinical interview, medical records, test data, and behavioral observations together.
	More time in supervision will likely be dedicated to case conceptualization and integration.
	You will discuss patterns of performance that are consistent with various cognitive disorders.
	The link between neuroanatomical structure and cognitive function will be strengthened as you see more clinical cases and participate in higher-level didactic experiences (e.g., case conferences, brain cutting, radiology rounds).
Report writing	During internship, you may be exposed to different report writing styles, such as very brief reports for consultation services or longer reports to legal or educational assessments. Over the course of your internship year, you should become proficient in writing background and behavioral observation sections of the report and demonstrate growth in your ability to integrate information in the summary/conceptualization section and provide appropriate recommendations.
Consultation	You may have the opportunity to participate in more consultation work during internship. This may involve working side by side with another provider such as a neurologist or a psychiatrist.
	Along with your supervisor, you may be asked to conduct inpatient consultations or work as part of a rehabilitation team.
Intervention	At this level of training, you will likely be providing feedback to patients and families under the direct observation of your supervisor. You will become more knowledgeable about different evidenced-based treatments and recommendations. In some settings, you may provide cognitive rehabilitation services or participate in support groups for individuals with neurological (e.g., epilepsy, stroke, multiple sclerosis, dementia) or psychiatric (e.g., psychogenic neurological disorders) problems.

TABLE 10.3. Fellowship Level

Domain	Expectation
Test administration	At the postdoctoral level, you will likely already be proficient in test administration and scoring. You may continue to test patients yourself or you may supervise students at the practicum or internship level, or psychometrists who administer and score the tests.
	You will be expected to understand the tests, their normative samples, and how to consider individual differences in age, race, ethnicity, and other aspects influencing individual performance.
Interpretation	During your postdoctoral fellowship, you will be responsible for gathering data from multiple sources (conducting a clinical interview, reviewing records, behavioral observations, test data) and generating a summary of the patient's clinical presentation.
	These activities will be observed by and discussed with your supervisor, though over the course of your postdoctoral program you will do this with increasing independence.
Report writing	You will be writing reports from start to finish and submitting them to your supervisor for review.
	You will learn to tailor your reports for different consumers (e.g., schools, physicians, courts).
	During the course of your postdoctoral program you should notice that you become increasingly efficient and concise, and that your reports need less editing than when you started.
Consultation	In some postdoctoral programs, you will be leading consultation activities (with oversight from your supervisor), such as inpatient consultations, multidisciplinary clinics, or team conferences.
	You can expect to independently provide these services, initially with direct observation from your supervisor, in order to help you prepare for independent practice.
Intervention	You will be providing feedback to patients and discussing that rationale for the recommendations you provide. You may be asked to implement interventions at the postdoctoral level as well. Your supervisors will likely expect you to independently research evidence-based recommendations that may be implemented for the patients that you see and discuss this in supervision.

for evaluation at the doctoral, internship, and postdoctoral levels. All APA-accredited training programs are required to define a developmentally appropriate minimum level of achievement that is needed to demonstrate each competency. These competency-based minimum levels of achievement provide the basis for evaluation that takes place at multiple time points during the training program. At the postdoctoral level, the expectation for the student is that they are increasing in their independence in neuropsychological assessment, consultation and intervention, and the supervisory process for this is essential to developing, honing, and refining these skills.

This competency-based model of training and supervision has been applied to the specialty of clinical neuropsychology. Entry-level competencies for clinical neuropsychology practice were developed (Rey-Casserly et al., 2012) and revised for broad use across training centers (see Smith, 2019, for a summary). These competencies are based on the Houston Conference policy statement, which delineated broad educational and training guidelines that provide the foundation for many clinical neuropsychology training programs (Hannay et al., 1998). To address evaluation at the first level of training, the American Academy of Clinical Neuropsychology published guidelines for competency-based practicum training that takes place at the doctoral level, as well as an evaluation form for practicum supervisors that is competency-based (Nelson et al., 2015). The Association of Postdoctoral Programs in Clinical Neuropsychology also published a paper proposing a process for evaluation of competencies as well as an assessment tool for the postdoctoral level (Heffelfinger et al., 2020).

Supervision of clinical neuropsychology trainees should follow a competency-based approach that is evidence based, formalized, objective, process based, and considers developmental level and individual differences (Stucky et al., 2010). Goals and expectations for progress should be addressed at the beginning of the training experience and are sometimes formalized in a supervision contract or individualized training plan. The structure of weekly supervision and feedback in clinical neuropsychology often differs from that of therapy-based clinical psychology training experiences. In clinical neuropsychology, patients are typically being evaluated over the course of 1 day to address a specific clinical question. This often requires an open-door or "elbow-to-elbow" model of supervision that occurs over the course of the entire day rather than a 1-hour weekly supervision time as is common in areas of psychology primarily conducting therapy. Thus, feedback related to the assessment portion of the evaluation process often occurs in real time in addition to the subsequent supervision and feedback regarding case conceptualization and report writing (Schwent-Shultz et al., 2014).

In addition to real-time supervision and feedback, both formative evaluations (i.e., those that occur during the process of training) and summative evaluations (i.e., those that occur at the completion of a training program) should be completed. Specific evaluation forms and procedures differ between programs. However, it has been recommended that multiple tools are employed to assess progress as well as program exit criteria (Stucky et al., 2010). Examples of formative evaluation procedures include the use of behavior checklists, skills rating forms, evaluation of case presentations or lectures, patient satisfaction ratings, oral or written examinations, measurement of patient outcomes, or ratings of written vignettes or simulated patients. Summative evaluations may include rating forms that specify benchmarks for a specific level of training (e.g., readiness for internship, readiness for postdoctoral training, readiness for entry to practice), completion of a project, completion of a state licensing examination, or completion of a mock oral examination. Thus, trainees should be able to monitor their progress toward goals and/or minimum levels of achievement that were identified at the beginning of their training program by participating in competency-based self-evaluations and reviewing formative evaluations with their supervisors during the course of their training.

DEVELOPMENT OF COMPETENCY IN ASSESSMENT

If you become a clinical neuropsychologist, you will spend most of your time conducting neuropsychological assessment with patients, as this is the core defining role of the profession. Most assessments determine current intellectual functioning; suspected functioning before the injury or disease onset or "premorbid functioning"; and specific neuropsychological functions in areas such as attention, executive functioning, language, visual spatial construction and memory. The results of assessments are used to help patients, their families, and their treating medical teams understand what has happened to the brain systems of the patient and what interventions or treatments may help brain system recovery in some situations, slow the rate of decline in others, and in some, change expectations and provide necessary accommodations for permanently injured neuropsychological functions.

Defining the Question

The first goal of the assessment is to determine the goal of your assessment, because this is your guide for the entire evaluation process. What is the referring provider asking? Who is the consumer for your work product? How will the results be used? Much of the time the question is whether patients are having cognitive problems that are abnormal for their age and what level of skills and abilities the patient has in various neuropsychological domains. Sometimes the question can be broad, such as "Assess the cognitive functioning of this patient to help them get the appropriate help in school or work," but at other times it can be very specific, such as "Has this patient had a decline in their memory since their previous evaluation 2 years ago?" The consumer of the assessment results also varies. Many times, the results are used by the patient and their family to understand the impact of a disease or neurological disorder. Other times, the referring doctor needs the results to know how to treat the problem, or a school may need the results to design an appropriate special education plan. At times, the results may be for a research protocol to help understand a disease, an attorney in consideration of cause and damages in legal cases, or a county disability officer helping the individual get disability resources. Once you have defined the question, the consumer, and how the results will be used to care for the patient, you can conduct the evaluation.

Gathering Supporting Clinical Information to Address the Assessment Questions

The clinical neuropsychologist begins the clinical assessment by conducting a clinical interview, typically with the patient and their family, and reviewing available medical, educational, or work records with the goals of generating a list of possible problems for consideration, which are called differential diagnoses or neuropsychological syndromes. The clinical interview is usually with the patient and possibly corroborating family members, such as spouse/ significant other, parents, or children. If the patient is a child (usually defined as under 18) or an adult who is not able to provide their own history, then the parent or legal guardian will complete the interview with or without the patient present. Once the clinical neuropsychologist has conducted the interview and the record review, considered possible limitations and concerns for the specific patient, and defined the possible differential diagnoses, they then list appropriate tests to be administered to conduct the assessment.

The clinical neuropsychologist always needs to be mindful of the potential considerations and limitations in the process when conducting neuropsychological evaluations with individuals from diverse backgrounds. Clinical neuropsychologists must continuously evaluate their own biases or "blind spots," as well as their values and beliefs and their level of cultural competence, which can impact the results of an evaluation. At the current time, the majority of clinical neuropsychologists continue to be from middle to upper socioeconomic status, White, English speaking, American backgrounds. Similar to other health care disciplines in American society, the field of clinical neuropsychology has historically defined processes and expectations that naturally apply to individuals from similar backgrounds. This can make it difficult for Black, Brown, and Native individuals, or individuals who are not monolingual English-speakers, to have access to care or to understand and trust the care of clinical neuropsychologists. Additionally, when assessments are being conducted with individuals from diverse backgrounds, the clinical neuropsychologist may not understand the patient's background or history. Moreover, most neuropsychological tests were developed based on the cultural expectations of predominantly White, English-speaking individuals, and the normative data almost always includes a majority of White individuals and rarely includes an oversampling of individuals from non-White, non-English speaking backgrounds. Therefore, all clinical neuropsychologists need to endeavor to evaluate their own biases, understand how the system they work for may limit or restrict care for certain individuals, know which tests are most inclusive in their development, and integrate and apply their knowledge to truly understand their patient.

Corroborating records are reviewed at several stages of the evaluation. Most clinical neuropsychologists can review medical records in an electronic medical record system or will receive relevant records from the referral source. In some cases, the patient needs to sign a release of information so that you can look at records from doctors in other medical systems or school, employment, or treatment records. It is important to identify in the records if previous cognitive or neuropsychologist testing has been completed. Previous neuropsychological testing can be used as a comparison or baseline for change in skills and abilities at the current evaluation. Neuropsychologists can use a variety of methods to determine change over time, including statistical approaches like reliable change analyses, which help determine whether clinically meaningful change has occurred (Duff, 2012). Please see Table 10.4, which outlines information and essential considerations in the clinical interview. After the interview and record review, you will establish a set of differential diagnoses of neuropsychological syndromes that will guide your assessment. Depending on the referral question, some examples of differentials may include dementia versus normal aging, nonfluent aphasia versus global cognitive impairment, anxiety versus autism. You then select the tests that you want to administer to evaluate your patient's cognitive functioning, which is essentially selecting tools to fill in the gaps in your knowledge needed to complete the puzzle. Neuropsychological tests have been developed to measure specific neuropsychological functions (e.g., attention, language,

TABLE 10.4. Information and Essential Considerations in the Clinical Interview

Information that the neuropsychologist can address or treat

Patient's neuropsychological abilities	Now and in the past
	Whether these abilities have regressed or improved:
	• attention language abilities
	• processing speed memory abilities
	• executive functioning visuospatial abilities
Functional markers of cognition	Day-to-day living skills in the home and community
	Academic achievement
Other aspects	Emotional well-being
	Behavioral functioning
	Social functioning

Necessary supporting information

Medical concerns (course, treatment, and current)	Neurological, medical, psychiatric, or genetic illness/disorder(s) that may have caused or influenced neuropsychological problems
	Medical treatments, such as surgical interventions or medications that may have caused or influenced neuropsychological problems
Patient's story	With whom do they live? Where do they live?
	How do they define their race, ethnicity, language(s), and gender?
	What are their significant relationships (spouse, family, friends)?
	What is their educational history? How did they perform in school?
	What is their occupation? If a child, what do they like to play?
Other aspects	Family history of neurological, medical, psychiatric, and/or genetic illness/disorder(s)

Essential considerations

Patient's neuropsychological abilities	Does anything prevent the patient from being able to show their true cognitive skills on our tests?
	Do they have any sensory disorders (blindness, deafness)?
	Do they have any motor disorders (hemiparesis, movement disorder)?
Cultural or ethnic factors affecting assessment	Level of acculturation
	Trust in the medical profession
	Cultural views of disease and medicine
	Access to quality education and medical care
Other aspects	Handedness, both original and current
	Language development and primary language at time of assessment (you may need an interpreter if you do not speak the patient's primary language)

memory) and have been standardized. Standardization requires that the test is always given in the same manner. The results are then compared with the normative sample, which ranges from dozens to hundreds of individuals who have been grouped based on demographic factors typically determined by the U.S. Census results (e.g., by age, education level, sex). Comparison of your patient's performance with the normative sample allows you to estimate whether their performance is normal or abnormal, and to what degree. The best practice is to use a normative database that includes other individuals like your patient in terms of age, gender, race/ethnicity, and geographical region. When this is not available, it is important to explicitly address the limitations of the data. As a clinical neuropsychologist, you will be trained to carefully consider individual differences in experiences, education, and other living and psychosocial factors. Conducting culturally competent neuropsychological evaluations requires training and self-reflection. It is critically important to consider the impact of age, gender, gender identity, race, ethnicity, culture, national origin, religion, sexual orientation, disability, language, and socioeconomic status, both for yourself and for your patient (Fujii, 2017). Misinterpreting data can have dire consequences for a patient, and we always strive to help each patient and to do no harm. For more information related to individual and cultural diversity in neuropsychological evaluation please see Chapter 15 of this text.

Test Interpretation and Case Conceptualization

The goal after testing is to put the pieces together to solve the puzzle and answer the referral question. Test interpretation includes defining and describing how the individual performed on each test by comparing the patient's performance with the normative database, with consideration for age, gender, race, ethnicity, and language. Once you understand how the individual did on each test, you then combine all your data to date to identify the following:

- Is the test data a valid estimate of the patient's functioning? If not, why?

- General intellectual functioning, both currently and before any changes may have occurred (premorbid functioning).

- Neuropsychological strengths and weaknesses defined as having significantly better or worse performance consistently on specific domain areas compared to intellectual functioning.

Case conceptualization should be the most important and careful step of your evaluation. What do the areas of weakness mean? Are they consistent with normal individual variability, or do they represent a neuropsychological disorder? If they are abnormal, what happened to cause them? It could be that these neuropsychological impairments or problems are related to a disease process, injury, medical treatment, or diagnostic procedure, and they may be familial or genetic, or idiopathic (i.e., of unknown cause). We use our empirical knowledge of the disease, disorder, or injury process to help the patient understand the likely course of recovery, development, and disease state, the best interventions or treatments, and how the patient can get support or accommodations to function maximally in the home, school, or workplace. The most common types of recommendations that are provided to patients and families include those related to supervision and independence, driving, educational resources, mental health and substance use, health and rehabilitation referrals, health, employment, education, and compensatory strategies (Meth et al., 2019). We give verbal feedback about test results to the patient or family in most situations and provide a copy of test results in a written report that is given to the patient and the referral source.

DEVELOPMENT OF COMPETENCE IN INTERDISCIPLINARY SYSTEMS/CONSULTATION

Communication is always key, right? Being a great clinical neuropsychologist requires excellent communication skills. First, you have to be a savvy and attentive listener. Patients are referred for a neuropsychological evaluation by other professionals and the clinical neuropsychologist must discern what is needed. A neurologist may be concerned that their patient with epilepsy is having problems with memory. A family practice physician might ask you to evaluate whether a 45-year-old woman has early onset dementia, because she is becoming forgetful, and her mother died from dementia when she was 55. A critical care neurologist who treated a man who was having a stroke may want you to evaluate whether he now has aphasia, because he is no longer able to answer questions. A hospitalist might ask you to evaluate the cognitive consequences for a 12-year-old recovering from meningitis. You may be asked to determine if a child has attention-deficit/hyperactivity disorder or autism. Sometimes the referral question is clear, as in the previous examples, and other times it may be more complex. For example, you may be asked whether a 12-year-old who is having problems in school and was crying every night had experienced a concussion when he fell on the playground playing kickball, which requires consideration of both a possible brain injury and long-standing learning problems. Clinical neuropsychologists often have strong collaborations with many disciplines, and it is important to be able to communicate with each of them. To care for our patients, we often work with neurologists who evaluate and treat individuals with brain-based disorders like epilepsy, stroke, and movement disorders. Psychiatrists assess and treat psychiatric disorders like schizoaffective disorder, depression, and anxiety, which are often co-occurring with neuropsychological syndromes. Psychiatrists also help differentiate causes of complex presentations of psychosis that can present in specific neurological disorders such as frontotemporal dementia and antiNMDA receptor encephalitis versus schizophrenia. Although many clinical neuropsychologists have a basic understanding of neuroimaging, we need neuroradiologists to read brain imaging to help us understand and define structural or functional brain abnormalities. We often work closely with rehabilitation physicians who assess and treat the acute motor and cognitive deficits from brain injuries or strokes. Each of these disciplines views the patient through a different lens, and the clinical neuropsychologist often integrates each of these views into our conclusions to holistically help the patient achieve optimal recovery, treatment, accommodations, or care. For more information on integrated care approaches, see Chapter 18 of this text.

Clinical neuropsychologists also often communicate in consulting roles in nonclinical settings. Because of our unique expertise in the cognitive consequences of injury, we are often called on to be expert witnesses in legal cases in which an injury to the brain may have occurred. The clinical neuropsychologist may be hired by the plaintiff who is claiming the injury or the defense attorney who is defending the individual or entity allegedly responsible for the injury. Clinical neuropsychologists may be asked to explain the injury and impact on brain functions and are typically asked to provide an opinion about whether the injury caused permanent cognitive impairment. Some fictional examples of these legal cases could include

- a 3-year-old who cannot walk or talk and was given an erroneous medication as a newborn

- a 10-year-old who was struck by a truck when riding her bike and now is not able to pay attention in school

- a 25-year-old who fell off a ladder at work and now has headaches, constant fatigue, and cannot work

- a 45-year-old who was struck by a box that fell off the shelf at a store and continues to have word-finding problems

- a 70-year-old who was in a car accident and now cannot remember much of his childhood

Clinical neuropsychologists also are important for public policy and lobbying efforts that involve our profession and the patient populations that we work with regularly. For example, it is important for us to work to get insurance companies to pay for our services, which sometimes requires local, state, or federal lobbying. We may lobby for changes in the law to help protect patients, such as legislation on seat belt use or special education. We may need to help agencies that pay for special education to understand the treatment needs associated with hemiplegia or a learning disability. For more information on neuropsychology and advocacy, please see Chapter 20 of this volume.

As is discussed at greater lengths elsewhere in this book, clinical neuropsychologists often are principal investigators, coinvestigators, or collaborators in research. We often design research to study neuropsychological domains or systems, such as the development of language or the degradation of memory. Or we might work to help define the actual brain systems involved in a specific cognitive function, like word repetition. We often study the course of diseases of interest, like spina bifida or multiple sclerosis. Sometimes, we also are called on to consult about a topic of someone else's research. For example, one might need an expert in how to define specific diseases or how to best assess attention in a 4-year-old.

This is not an exhaustive list of the ways that clinical neuropsychologists work with other disciplines or consult with others, but as you can see, communication about what we do and how we do it is an essential competency to promote and protect our profession, science, and our patients.

DEVELOPMENT OF COMPETENCE IN INTERVENTION

Your job is not over when the assessment is completed. Giving feedback about assessment results is one of the most important parts of a neuropsychological evaluation, and the explanations of the assessment conclusions can be influential in improving a patient's quality of life, emotional experience, and social adjustment (Rosado et al., 2018). Some clinical neuropsychologists may also provide treatment such as cognitive behavioral therapy or cognitive rehabilitation. Others use the results of their assessments to guide evidence-based recommendations and interventions. Discussing assessment results can be a powerful intervention in and of itself. Sometimes your role is to provide education and reassurance. Simply providing education about the typical course of recovery can improve outcomes. For example, you may tell a parent that their child will not have permanent brain damage following a mild concussion, which can promote faster recovery, as the child will be encouraged to be more active in thinking and learning. You may be able to reassure an older adult that they have no signs of memory loss, thereby providing an intervention for anxiety and improving day-to-day functioning. In other situations, you can empower individuals and families to access and benefit from services or accommodations. Diagnosing a learning disability can be used to support the provision of special education services or employment accommodations. Understanding the nature of impairments in attention and language after brain injury or stroke can be used to tailor cognitive rehabilitation strategies.

Because clinical neuropsychologists are trained in clinical psychology and research methods, we are uniquely suited to help patients navigate the wide array of treatment options that are available. While many have scientific support, others are not evidence-based and result in wasted time and financial resources. For example, you may refer someone for speech therapy after they have a stroke that affects language areas of the brain, because there is research that supports this speech therapy as an intervention. On the other hand, there are currently no evidence-based curative treatments for dementia, yet thousands of dollars are spent on services such as hyperbaric oxygen therapy, neurofeedback, and nutritional supplements despite no evidence to support that these interventions improve memory or day-to-day functioning. Part of your job is to educate patients about the scientific support that exists for various interventions to help them be informed consumers.

It is also important to know what works for whom. Interventions are not one-size-fits-all. Some individuals and families might have the resources to make lifestyle changes related to eating a healthy diet, improving their physical health, accessing psychotherapy or cognitive rehabilitation services, and attending support groups. For others, barriers exist, such as lack of financial resources, unreliable transportation, lack of family support, or availability of providers. Moreover, there are some conditions that can affect the applicability of interventions. For example, someone with aphasia and depression would likely not be a good candidate for traditional psychotherapy but could benefit from cognitive rehabilitation and behavioral therapy. Someone without insight or awareness of their condition, such as some individuals with dementia, may need social support to facilitate interventions or benefit from an intervention as simple as sending a supplemental letter after the appointment to enhance recall and follow-through with your recommendations (Meth et al., 2016). Additional strategies and real-world examples of how to deliver meaningful feedback and recommendations to individuals and their families has been collected from practicing clinical neuropsychologists and compiled in an excellent book entitled *Feedback That Sticks: The Art of Effectively Communicating Neuropsychological Assessment Results* (Postal & Armstrong, 2013).

CONCLUSION AND FUTURE DIRECTIONS

In summary, the education and training process to become a clinical neuropsychologist includes a well-defined set of competencies with curriculum for building knowledge about brain functions, how they develop, and what can harm them, as well as several years of supervised clinical experiences that increase in responsibility, complexity, and independence. If you are interested in becoming a clinical neuropsychologist, apply for each level of training (graduate, internship, and postdoctoral) to programs that provide training experiences consistent with the APA *Taxonomy for Education and Training in Clinical Neuropsychology* (Sperling et al., 2017). Hopefully, you have mentors around you who can help you take your next steps in training in clinical neuropsychology. If you do not, please reach out to the mentoring groups within all the various neuropsychology organizations to help you find a mentor. There are mentors who want to help you, so reach out!

REFERENCES

American Psychological Association Commission on Accreditation. (2015). *Standards of accreditation for health service psychology and accreditation operating procedures.* http://www.apa.org/ed/accreditation/about/policies/standards-of-accreditation.pdf

Duff, K. (2012). Evidence-based indicators of neuropsychological change in the individual patient: Relevant concepts and methods. *Archives of Clinical Neuropsychology, 27*(3), 248–261. https://doi.org/10.1093/arclin/acr120

Falender, C. A., & Shafranske, E. P. (2012). The importance of competency-based clinical supervision and training in the twenty-first century: Why bother? *Journal of Contemporary Psychotherapy, 42*(3), 129–137. https://doi.org/10.1007/s10879-011-9198-9

Fujii, D. (2017). *Conducting a culturally informed neuropsychological evaluation.* American Psychological Association. https://doi.org/10.1037/15958-000

Hannay, H. J., Bieliauskas, L. A., Crosson, B., Hammeke, T., Hamsher, K. D., & Koffler, S. P. (1998). The Houston conference on specialty education and training in clinical neuropsychology. *Archives of Clinical Neuropsychology, 13*(2), 160–166. https://doi.org/10.1093/arclin/13.2.160

Heffelfinger, A. K., Janecek, J. K., Johnson, A., Miller, L. E., Nelson, A., & Pulsipher, D. T. (2020). Competency-based assessment in clinical neuropsychology at the post-doctoral level: Stages, milestones, and benchmarks as proposed by an APPCN work group. *The Clinical Neuropsychologist.* https://doi.org/10.1080/13854046.2020.1829070

Meth, M., Calamia, M., & Tranel, D. (2016). Does a simple intervention enhance memory and adherence for neuropsychological recommendations? *Applied Neuropsychology: Adult, 23*(1), 21–28. https://doi.org/10.1080/23279095.2014.996881

Meth, M. Z., Bernstein, J. P. K., Calamia, M., & Tranel, D. (2019). What types of recommendations are we giving patients? A survey of clinical neuropsychologists. *The Clinical Neuropsychologist, 33*(1), 57–74. https://doi.org/10.1080/13854046.2018.1456564

Nelson, A. P., Roper, B. L., Slomine, B. S., Morrison, C., Greher, M. R., Janusz, J., Larson, J. C., Meadows, M.-E., Ready, R. E., Rivera Mindt, M., Whiteside, D. M., Willment, K., & Wodushek, T. (2015). Official position of the American Academy of Clinical Neuropsychology (AACN): Guidelines for practicum training in clinical neuropsychology. *The Clinical Neuropsychologist, 29*(7), 879–904. https://doi.org/10.1080/13854046.2015.1117658

Postal, K., & Armstrong, K. (2013). *Feedback that sticks: The art of effectively communicating neuropsychological assessment results.* Oxford University Press.

Rey-Casserly, C., Roper, B. L., & Bauer, R. M. (2012). Application of a competency model to clinical neuropsychology. *The Clinical Neuropsychologist, 43*(5), 422–431. https://doi.org/10.1037/a0028721

Rosado, D. L., Buehler, S., Botbol-Berman, E., Feigon, M., León, A., Luu, H., Carrión, C., Gonzalez, M., Rao, J., Greif, T., Seidenberg, M., & Pliskin, N. H. (2018). Neuropsychological feedback services improve quality of life and social adjustment. *The Clinical Neuropsychologist, 32*(3), 422–435. https://doi.org/10.1080/13854046.2017.1400105

Schwent-Shultz, L. A., Pedersen, H. A., Roper, B. L., & Rey-Casserly, C. (2014). Supervision in neuropsychological assessment: A survey of training, practices, and perspectives of supervisors. *The Clinical Neuropsychologist, 28*(6), 907–925. https://doi.org/10.1080/13854046.2014.942373

Smith, G. (2019). Education and training in clinical neuropsychology: Recent developments and documents from the clinical neuropsychology synarchy. *Archives of Clinical Neuropsychology, 34*(3), 418–431. https://doi.org/10.1093/arclin/acy075

Sperling, S. A., Cimino, C. R., Stricker, N. H., Heffelfinger, A. K., Gess, J. L., Osborn, K. E., & Roper, B. L. (2017). *Taxonomy for Education and Training in Clinical Neuropsychology*: Past, present, and future. *The Clinical Neuropsychologist, 31*(5), 817–828. https://doi.org/10.1080/13854046.2017.1314017

Stucky, K. J., Bush, S., & Donders, J. (2010). Providing effective supervision in clinical neuropsychology. *The Clinical Neuropsychologist, 24*(5), 737–758. https://doi.org/10.1080/13854046.2010.490788

11 NEUROANATOMY TRAINING AND COMPETENCIES

MICHAEL PARSONS AND CADY BLOCK

In this chapter, we attempt to delineate an approach to learning and maintaining a competent knowledge of functional neuroanatomy. It is impossible to provide all the necessary information a neuropsychologist might want or need in a single chapter. Thus, the goal here is to provide some foundational knowledge about neuroanatomy—and, more important, some suggestions and guidance on training activities that can help facilitate the iterative development of your knowledge base.

Put more specifically, in this chapter we provide historical background and some context for the importance of neuroanatomical knowledge to neuropsychologists, outline important principles and concepts central to the understanding of functional neuroanatomy, and suggest a sequence of training in an attempt to address the following four questions:

1. Why is this information critical to the field of neuropsychology, and why is it critical for you as a neuropsychologist to have a working understanding of this information?

2. What functional neuroanatomy material should you master as a neuropsychologist?

https://doi.org/10.1037/0000250-012
The Neuropsychologist's Roadmap: A Training and Career Guide, C. Block (Editor)

3. When during the course of neuropsychological training should you under-take the study of functional neuroanatomy?

4. How should you approach the initial acquisition and lifelong learning of neuroanatomical principles?

NEUROANATOMY: A BRIEF HISTORY

Humans have long sought an understanding of the structure and function of the human body—including the brain. A review of this topic is enriched by some historical context, so let's take a quick trip back in time. Some of the earliest hypotheses regarding brain structure and function date back to antiquity. You probably recognize the name Aristotle (384–322 BC), and indeed it was he who posited that the brain was a "radiator" of sorts, important for cooling the heart and blood. A little later on, Herophilus (335–280 BC) added to our understanding by being the first—through careful (but often very public) dissections—to distinguish cerebrum from cerebellum and motor from sensory nerves. Several centuries later, Galen (129–199 AD) attempted to tie together brain structure and function (though he erroneously posited that intellect came from the fluid-filled ventricles). During the years of the Reformation, Andreus Vesalius (1514–1564 AD) continued dissections—against the rule of papal law—and produced stunningly detailed depictions of the human body and brain in his widely known text *De Humani Corporis Fabrica*. History also contains pseudoscientific endeavors, namely the phrenology movement propagated by Franz Gall (1758–1828 AD) and his protégé Johann Spurzheim (1776–1832 AD). Regardless of scientific cred-ibility, all of these people contributed to the evolution in our understanding of brain structure and function, laying the eventual foundation for neuro-psychology as methods of assessment became increasingly codified and standardized.

Before the development of neuroimaging, neuropsychology was the primary tool for localizing a lesion within the brain—and it served a purely diagnostic role. During the 20th century, the struggle to understand brain function vacillated between opposing theories of brain organization. On one hand were the localizationists, such as Paul Broca and Carl Wernicke, who firmly believed that neurocognitive and behavioral functions arose from specific, dedicated regions within the brain. On the other hand were indi-viduals like Pierre Flourens and Karl Lashley, who believed that all brain matter was *equipotential* in nature, meaning that the brain operated in a more holistic manner (rather than as discrete faculties). In this case, the extent of an injury—not its location—was a greater determinant in the effects of brain injury or disease.

In an attempt to balance the two theories, Russian neuropsychologist Alexander Luria developed a model in which the brain consists of discrete units (responsible for tasks as basic as wakefulness to higher level information processing and behavior). These units comprise three larger functional systems operating in a successively more complex and integrative manner. Because all behavior requires the interaction of all three units across all three functional systems, all behavior thus reflects activity of the entire brain. As Luria (1980) noted, "The higher mental functions may be disturbed by a lesion of one of the many different links of a functional system; nevertheless, they will be disturbed differently by lesion of different links" (p. 79).

This principle of *pluripotentiality* continues to represent a basic premise of current neuropsychology, pointing out the importance of understanding multiple operating and interacting layers of functional neuroanatomy. Our understanding of the brain has since evolved substantially over the past century, influenced by studies of the neurobehavioral effects of circumscribed lesions (see Table 11.1). Although a comprehensive review of historically significant case studies is beyond the scope of this chapter, see the Classic Cases in Neuropsychology series by Code et al. (2003, 1996). More recently, our understanding of the brain has been derived from the study of brain activity during performance of neurocognitive and behavioral tasks.

THE WHY: EXPLAINING THE IMPORTANCE OF FOUNDATIONAL KNOWLEDGE

Why is a foundation in functional neuroanatomy important for neuropsychology and for you as a developing neuropsychologist? For neuropsychologists practicing in the current era of neuroimaging, the primary goal of neuropsychological investigation continues to be to identify behavioral correlates of neuropathology in the service of differential diagnosis, prognosis, and treatment of a huge range of conditions that effect cognition. As Muriel Lezak and colleagues noted (Lezak et al., 2012): "Even when the site and extent of a brain lesion have been shown on imaging, *the image will not identify the nature of residual behavioral strengths and the accompanying deficits: for this neuropsychological assessment is needed*" (p. 5, italics added for emphasis). So, although a computed tomography or magnetic resonance image (MRI) may itself be an elegant depiction of brain structure, it speaks little to brain function—and the implications of brain injury or disease for

TABLE 11.1. Famous Case Studies

Case	Description
Tan	At just 30 years old, Frenchman Louis Leborgne lost the ability to speak. He could utter only the singular syllable *"Tan"* (though often this was twice in succession, i.e., *"Tan Tan"*). He was admitted to Bicêtre, a Parisian hospital.
	In 1861, Tan was admitted for surgery under physician Paul Broca. Broca noted that all of Tan's mental faculties except speech were intact; he dubbed this *aphémie*, the loss of articulated speech—what we now call *aphasia*.
	Tan passed away at age 51, and a posthumous biopsy revealed a large lesion in the posterior inferior frontal gyrus. This area became recognized for its involvement in the brain's language network and was named *Broca's area*.
Phineas Gage	Gage was an American foreman with the Rutland & Burlington Railroad company. Railroad was laid down by using gunpowder to create deep holes in which tamping rods could be placed. In 1848, an errant explosion caused a nearly 4-foot rod to strike Gage in the head, entering through below his left cheekbone and exiting at the top of his skull, resulting in severe brain injury.
	Gage survived, though his physician, John Harlow, noted a profound change in his personality that has since been attributed to frontal lobe damage. Once kind and even tempered, Gage was now impatient, unreliable, and often foul. With an odd sense of pride, he later made public appearances and posed for photographs with the tamping rod.
H. M.	American Henry Molaison (H. M.) had suffered from minor seizures since childhood, but at age 16 these erupted into severe tonic-clonic seizures. Medications did not help, so he was referred to neurosurgeon William Beecher Scoville, who believed that they stemmed from his left and right temporal lobes.
	To control his seizures, in 1953 H. M. underwent removal of both medial temporal lobes, where a structure called the *hippocampus* lies. His seizures disappeared, but with them went the ability to form new memories.
	Neuropsychologist Brenda Milner worked closely with H. M. for many years. Through careful study, she discovered that H. M. did retain motor skills learning and spatial memory. Her work and his case helped to revolutionize our understanding of memory.
Chuck Close	Chuck Close is an American artist who suffers from a neurological condition called *prosopagnosia*, also known as *face blindness*. This condition stems from dysfunction in an area of cortex called the fusiform face area. Interestingly, his specialty is human portraits.
	Close completes his paintings by working in a series of grids, filling in each grid and ultimately constructing an entire human face. The end result is an incredibly photorealistic portrait. His story has been told in a documentary called *Chuck Close: A Portrait in Progress* (Cajori, 1998).

each individual, or what may be helpful in terms of recommendations or treatment. Thus, the practice of neuropsychology depends on an understanding of basic principles of brain organization as a starting point—and embarks on an understanding of the individual patient's expression of brain pathology through the lens of cognition and behavior.

Indeed, the structural anatomy of the brain is incredibly complex, and so developing a mature understanding of neuroanatomy and the pathologies that affect the brain may seem overwhelming. As a neuropsychologist, your job is even more complicated because the goal of each evaluation is to integrate an understanding of brain structure and neuropathology with the neurocognitive and behavioral functioning of the patient in front of you. To make these abstract principles more concrete, consider the following example:

A 47-year-old right-handed man with no known history of neurologic injury or illness presents to you for neuropsychological evaluation; he was referred by his primary care physician because of concerns about memory loss. During the interview, you discover that the patient has developed problems with word-finding in his spontaneous speech over the past several weeks to months. He can communicate clearly but has frequent circumlocution, and when you test him with an object naming task you find that he performs in the severely impaired range. As you evaluate him, you note some minor reading errors and difficulty finding visual objects in right upper portion of his visual field. To investigate, you perform simple visual field testing and find a clearly demarcated right upper quadrant field cut (right upper quadrantanopsia).

In this case, a patient was referred with a vague concern about "memory loss," and the evaluation revealed a visual field defect. Because this rarely occurs outside the context of a structural brain lesion, you as the neuropsychologist have just identified some very important information relating to the visual pathway within the brain, specifically, at the point in which this pathway courses through the left temporal lobe. You also know that left temporal lobe lesions commonly produce naming difficulty. A solid foundational knowledge of functional neuroanatomy—in this case, the visual and language pathways—helps you localize a potential issue in the left temporal region. You consider the fact that this patient's symptom onset was relatively recent, which is worrisome because it indicates a rapidly progressing etiology. You request that his physician place a referral for a brain MRI, which indeed indicates a high-grade tumor in the left temporal lobe. Of course, such discoveries are rare in the neuropsychology clinic, and many patients referred for memory loss concerns may turn out not to have any such localizing or focal signs. Nonetheless, it is the responsibility of the competent neuropsychologist to be able to identify these patterns if and when they arise, and that recognition depends on a solid understanding of functional neuroanatomy and neuropathology. Alternatively, you may be called on to understand the relevance of an already-identified focal brain lesion in relation to a patient's neurocognitive symptoms. Consider the following example:

A 70-year-old woman has been referred to you by her neurologist because of memory decline over the past year. The neurologist has already ordered and reviewed a brain MRI, which showed a right frontal lobe mass measuring about 1 cm in diameter, with no surrounding edema. They have been following the mass with scans over the past 5 years; it has not grown and is presumed to be a benign tumor called a *meningioma*. During your evaluation, the patient denies any neurocognitive symptoms, but her family reports gradual memory decline in the past 2 years. Your evaluation demonstrates moderate to severe impairment in memory as well as milder deficits in executive function and object naming.

In this situation, it is difficult to ascribe the patient's diffuse and fairly severe neurocognitive issues to what is essentially a stable lesion. The nature and course of her neurocognitive symptoms more strongly suggest a neuro-degenerative disorder such as a form of dementia. Again, your ability to integrate neuropsychological data and patient history with your understanding of the brain is critical to an accurate diagnosis. It also has significant implications for prognosis as well as treatment recommendations. All of these rest on an understanding of the principles of functional neuroanatomy and neuropathology.

THE WHAT: IDENTIFYING FOUNDATIONAL KNOWLEDGE

What do neuropsychology trainees need to learn about neuroanatomy and neuropathology? As we noted previously, a list of functional neuroanatomical details really cannot be adequately covered in a single book chapter. In fact, we don't even venture to propose that it is necessary to memorize and retain everything there is to know about neuroanatomy and neuropathology to be a competent neuropsychologist. We instead suggest that training in neuro-psychology should include core concepts and principles of neuroanatomy and specific patterns of neuropathology, providing a basis for further investigation. In other words, once you have a clear understanding of the brain then you are able to generate and reason through clinical hypotheses about the root cause.

Guiding Principles

We have attempted to identify several guidelines that we feel serve as useful principles for neuropsychology students and trainees in organizing functional neuroanatomical knowledge. We frequently teach these principles to our own students and trainees, including applied examples, and hope that you, the reader, find them equally useful. An abbreviated list of these principles is presented in Table 11.2.

Principle 1: Brain structure and function are reciprocally interrelated. As we discussed, there is a meaningful relationship between brain structure and function. Although there is some level of variability between and within individual brains, there are certain hard-wired neurologic functions that provide anchor points for functional neurogeography. Two areas of the highly specialized intra-lobar cortex, the primary motor strip and primary somatosensory strip, are a prime example of this principle. Consider that one main function of the central nervous system is to create internalized representations, or "maps," of different aspects of the individual and the world around them. This occurs as information flows into our various sensory organs and then is mapped onto the brain's primary sensory cortices. For example, the *primary somatosensory cortex* (also known as the *somatosensory homunculus*; see Figure 11.1) resides in the post-central gyrus of the parietal lobe contralateral to the body side represented. Similarly, the primary motor system depends on the brain's representation of the body musculature and motor planning of actions—both of which are externalized via projections from a map residing in the *primary motor cortex* (also known as the *motor homunculus*). The structure of these systems has developed over the course of evolutionary history, and their organization is highly reliable from one person to another. The functional neuroanatomy of numerous cortical and subcortical systems are even preserved across species, including complex systems like those that support recent memory (Squire, 1992).

TABLE 11.2. Guiding Principles in Neuroanatomy

Number	Principle
1	Brain structure and function are reciprocally interrelated.
2	The brain operates in the context of life span development.
3	A spatial map of the brain in three dimensions is important to develop.
4	The brain operates on the basis of a division of labor between hemispheres.
5	The brain operates locally as well as in networks.
6	The brain operates in a series of systems that surround and support its function.

FIGURE 11.1. Somatosensory and Motor Homunculus

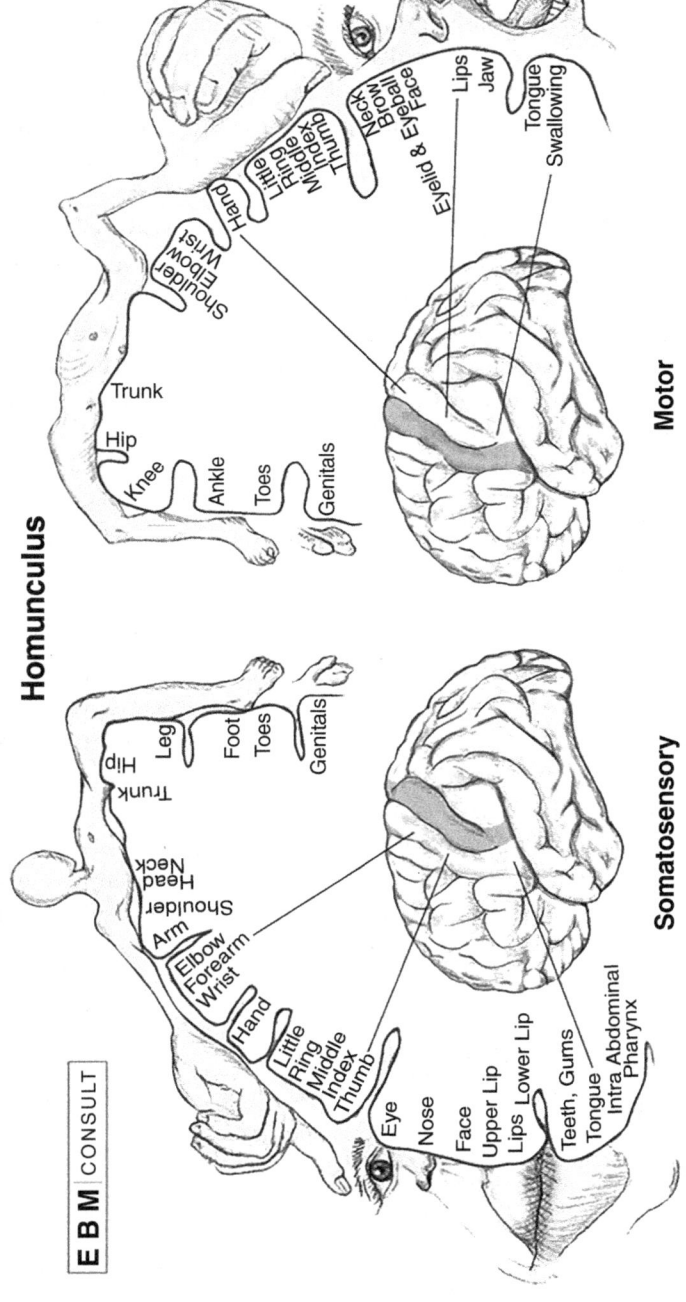

Note. From *Homunculus: Somatosensory and Somatomotor Cortex*, by A. J. Busti and D. Kellogg (Eds.), 2015, Evidence-Based Medicine Consult (https://www.ebmconsult.com/articles/homunculus-sensory-motor-cortex). Copyright 2015 by EBM Consult, LLC. Reprinted with permission.

Because of the accessibility and reliability across individuals and species, these pathways have been studied for centuries and are well described in countless texts. These hard-wired systems can be used to anchor our efforts at localization of function in the evaluation of patients. For this reason, examination of simple motor functions, body sensation and perception, and visual fields has a high degree of localizing value.

These systems are composed of multiple overlapping layers, including peripheral input and output neural processes; spinal cord or cranial nerve pathways; subcortical synapses; and cortical representations at the primary, secondary and tertiary levels. Thus, you as the neuropsychologist must carefully consider all of these factors while observing, measuring, and characterizing a patient's functional performance (i.e., during a neurobehavioral examination and/or across neurocognitive measures) in order to localize the focus of a potential disruption. A thorough understanding of these hard-wired systems is of great benefit, and examination of these functions is often an important component of the evaluation.

Principle 2: The brain operates in the context of lifespan development. In hearing the term *neurodevelopment* you might be inclined to think of the process of brain development early in life. But neurodevelopment is not static; instead, it is an ongoing process over the course of one's life. True, there is a hustle and bustle of activity within the first several years of life, beginning with the creation and proliferation of neuronal and glial cells in the first trimester of pregnancy. Throughout the rest of pregnancy, neurons in the fetus begin to migrate to various regions within the brain. In the 2 years that follow birth, neurons develop the synapses and axons necessary for intracellular communication; this is followed by a massive pruning process whereby redundant or unnecessary cellular connections are trimmed in the name of neurologic efficiency. As this exciting cellular process is unfolding, the embryonic precursor to the structures that make up our central nervous system—known as the *neural tube*—begins to coalesce and then differentiate into the spinal cord, cerebellum, and cerebrum. The latter includes the telencephalon, which eventually forms the two cerebral hemispheres. Rapid expansion of this telencephalon bestows a distinct *C* shape to many internal structures, such as the lateral ventricles, corpus callosum, cingulate gyrus, caudate nucleus, and fornix.

However, the neuropsychologist is aware that the brain continually operates within the context of time, meaning that changes are happening throughout and even in the later part of life. Up through the second decade of life, axons undergo myelination to support and enhance information transfer across the brain. The concept of *neuroplasticity*—the innate ability of the brain to respond and adapt to change—both positive (e.g., cognitively challenging tasks such as learning a new language or musical instrument) and negative (e.g., normal and abnormal effects of aging)—is an important one. You as the neuropsychologist will understand how these factors interact and manifest functionally.

Principle 3: A spatial map of the brain in three dimensions is important to develop. Much of neuroanatomy and neuropathology education and training comes from reviewing visual depictions of the brain and its many constituent parts. Many of these depictions are clearly drawn, nicely organized, labeled, and even color coded; however, in actuality the brain is none of these things. As such, we encourage students of neuropsychology to learn the brain as it exists in the third dimension; that is to say, learn the brain so that no matter where you are looking within the brain—whether in the left parietal lobe, down in the fourth ventricle, in the anterior limb of the internal capsule, somewhere along the arcuate fasciculus, or down the tail of the caudate nucleus—you can readily orient yourself by using familiar, nearby markers. A clear understanding of the dimensional brain is particularly helpful when reviewing neuroimaging. The savvy neuropsychologist is well aware of radiologic convention, or the fact that left and right orientations are reversed in any neuroimaging such as computed tomography, MRI, positron emission tomography, or other types of image. They are also aware of the three major anatomical planes (see Figure 11.2) that allow one to explore the brain across superior–inferior (up–down), anterior–posterior (front–back), and lateral–medial (outermost–innermost) directional gradients.

A three-dimensional understanding of the brain offers two major benefits: (a) no matter where you are within the brain, you can easily and quickly orient yourself to nearby structures, pathways, and vasculature, and (b) by recognizing the geographic location of a suspected lesion or area of dysfunction, you understand where it falls within a larger pathway or network and thus better able to predict accompanying neurocognitive, behavioral, and/or psychiatric deficits.

Principle 4: The brain operates on the basis of a division of labor between hemispheres. Pop science dictates that one is relatively more left brained or right brained; however, we hope that by now you know that people use both hemispheres of the brain at all times. That being said, there are divisions of labor between the two cerebral hemispheres; this is known as *lateralization of function*. An excellent example to illustrate the concept of lateralization of function involves the visual system. Functional neuroanatomy of visual fields is an exercise in lateralization, crossing, and localization of function. The optic nerves, optic chiasm, lateral geniculate, and

FIGURE 11.2. The Three Major Radiologic Planes

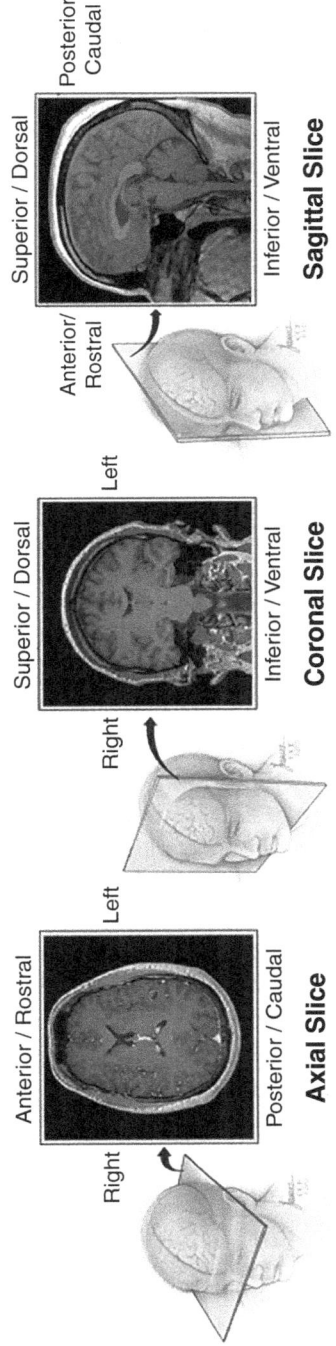

Note. Adapted from "Structural and Functional Brain Imaging for the Neuropsychologist," by M. W. Parsons, S. E. Jones, and T. Krewson, in M. W. Parsons and T. A. Hammeke (Eds.), *Clinical Neuropsychology: A Pocket Handbook for Assessment* (3rd ed., p. 77), 2014, American Psychological Association (https://doi.org/10.1037/1433-005). Copyright 2014 by the American Psychological Association.

optic pathways provide a useful set of anchor points that are a special instance of the hard-wired networks we discussed earlier. As we noted in our earlier example of a patient with a visual field defect, a thorough knowledge of these pathways can be combined with other aspects of functional neuroanatomy to provide localizing information regarding brain lesions. By developing the ability to conduct a gross visual field examination the neuropsychologist can quickly localize focal lesions when visual field defects are present.

As an educational tool, an excellent learning exercise is to track the visual pathways from retinal projection through optic chiasm, around the various projections of optic radiations, and ultimately to the receptive fields in the occipital lobe. This complex anatomy allows the student to integrate a clear behavioral sign of a lesion with a specific focal lesion. That lesion can then be identified on brain imaging studies (which because of radiological convention induce another left–right flip). The mental rotation required to work through this process can be intimidating, in particular early on in the study of functional neuroanatomy, and a clear understanding of this system can greatly enhance one's self-confidence when studying neuroanatomy.

Principle 5: The brain operates locally as well as in networks. Neuropsychological functions are often *localized*, meaning that small networks of neighboring brain regions work together to accomplish specific functions. A basic understanding of the functional neuroanatomy of language systems and the disorders of language—also known as *aphasiology*—is perhaps the most well-known example of localization of function and is a critical cornerstone in the knowledge base of a neuropsychologist. The study of aphasia dates back to Paul Broca's description of an individual with severe language output difficulty. As noted in Table 11.1, this patient, known simply as "Tan," lost the ability to articulate but remained able to comprehend language. In the localizationist tradition, Broca ascribed Tan's language difficulty to a single lesion in the left frontal lobe (Broca, 1865). Not long afterward, Carl Wernicke described a language disorder characterized by impaired comprehension but spared speech production, which he ascribed to a single lesion in the posterior part of the superior left temporal gyrus (Wernicke, 1874). Both Broca's and Wernicke's areas are connected by a thick bundle of white matter fibers called the *arcuate fasciculus*. Now recognized as *Broca's* (language production) and *Wernicke's* (language recognition and comprehension) *aphasias*, these disorders were used to found a theoretical understanding of the functional neuroanatomy of language.

The evolution of neuroscience, however, has significantly changed our historical view of aphasia and the functional neuroanatomy of language.

It remains true that there are critical cortical regions related to language comprehension and production, but modern neuropsychology and neuroscience have demonstrated that many other brain regions in the dominant and nondominant hemispheres play an important role in language (Mayeux & Kandel, 1985; Sabsevitz & Hammeke, 2014). This modernization of the classical model integrates network and localizationist perspectives and guides our understanding of neuropathology in patients with aphasia.

Principle 6: The brain operates in a series of systems that surround and support its function. Many neuropathological issues arise from, or include damage to, the cerebrovascular system, skull, ventricular system, and even the meningeal structures. An understanding of the organization of these systems can greatly aid neuropsychologists when attempting to make sense of the relationship between neuropathology and neuropsychology.

The importance of this relationship is perhaps most obvious in the instance of cerebrovascular disease. The layout of the arterial supply of the brain has very specific implications for the combination of symptoms that might be induced by a cerebrovascular accident in a specified distribution. A basic understanding of brain regions supplied by anterior, middle, and posterior cerebral arteries is a critical starting point, and further knowledge of the hemodynamics of these systems can provide helpful information when trying to understand neurobehavioral phenomena. For instance, a *watershed distribution infarct*, which refers to a loss of blood flow to the tiny arterioles at the ends of large vessel distributions, can produce stereotypical patterns of cognitive impairment, depending on the severity of infarction and the hemisphere affected. Similarly, a sudden loss of blood pressure, or *hypoperfusion*, to areas supplied by the posterior arteries can lead to a classic syndrome of amnesia due to the way these arteries supply the hippocampus.

Similarly, a basic understanding of the layout of the ventricular system, the direction of flow of cerebrospinal fluid through these compartments, and general familiarity with the expected size and shape of the main components of the ventricular system can be extremely informative. For example, an appreciation of the size of the temporal horn of the lateral ventricle is relevant to interpretation of cognitive findings and differential diagnosis in the context of temporal lobe epilepsy and dementia (e.g., Macdonald et al., 2013).

Familiarity with the relative shape and positions of the bony and meningeal structures surrounding the brain is also useful. In the context of intracerebral hemorrhage, for example, a basic recognition of the differences among epidural, subdural, and subarachnoid hemorrhages carries important implications for the expected neurocognitive sequelae and clinical course of the injury. Similarly, it is important to have a basic understanding of the location of major aspects of the meningeal linings when considering factors such as mass effect related to tumors or other space-occupying lesions. For instance, the *falx cerebri*, the firm interhemispheric lining, may limit mass effect to one hemisphere if there is no midline shift.

Other Core Concepts

It is critical that you also gain an understanding of the relationship between different types of neuropathology and neurocognitive symptoms. The process of neuropsychological evaluation is an exercise in hypothesis testing. As we have discussed in some detail, a thorough understanding of functional neuroanatomy can provide a great deal of guidance to that hypothesis-testing exercise. Similarly, a few key concepts can provide critical information during the process of differential diagnosis when dealing with neuropathology.

Onset

Characterizing the onset of a neuropsychological problem has important implications for categories of neuropathology. An acute onset, with symptoms developing over seconds or minutes, typically occurs in the context of stroke, epilepsy, and traumatic brain injury. A subacute onset, with symptoms occurring over days to weeks, may be seen in the context of brain tumor, subdural hematoma, or infection. At the other end of the scale, a gradual or insidious onset may herald a neurodegenerative etiology (e.g., Alzheimer's disease, Parkinson's disease) or may even end up indicating typical neurocognitive problems related to normal aging.

Course

Like neuropsychological conditions, the course of a cognitive disorder carries important information about the likely etiology and potentially even the prognosis. Cognitive symptoms that wax and wane, or have an episodic course with intervals of normal function, may be observed in the context of epilepsy, metabolic disorders, and autoimmune conditions such as multiple sclerosis. The time course of these fluctuations is typically relevant to the underlying condition as well. A progressive course is typically observed in neurodegenerative conditions, though the rate of deterioration may be very gradual. Neurocognitive problems that are caused by a single instance of neural injury, such as traumatic brain injury or stroke, will often initially have an improving course followed by stabilization. The extent of cognitive impairment and rate of improvement during the early phase of recovery may carry prognostic information about the overall expectations for outcome (Pedersen et al., 1995).

Lesion Type

It is important to recognize that different types of lesions may have different effects on neural function, even when they occur in the same location. For example, as noted earlier, a stroke in the left frontal operculum (e.g., Broca's area) will produce a devastating aphasia syndrome, whereas a low-grade brain tumor (e.g., diffuse infiltrative low-grade glioma) in the same region may not produce any observable deficits. Similarly, a developmental venous anomaly in that same location may be present throughout a person's life span without ever inducing any dysfunction. This variability in how different types of neuropathology affect the surrounding neural tissue is complex and may be related to many factors, including the extent to which there is neuronal destruction induced by the lesion, the time course over which the pathology develops, the potential for neuroplasticity (both of the specific region involved and within the individual), and history of prior neurologic injury.

THE WHEN AND HOW: GAINING FOUNDATIONAL KNOWLEDGE

When, exactly, should the process of learning about functional neuroanatomy and neuropathology take place? The answer to this is relatively simple: It is an ongoing, lifelong process. We all must consistently refresh and update our knowledge base, or risk information decay. This has been empirically studied: A group of senior medical students was tested on neuroanatomy knowledge acquired during their first year of school—scores dropped more than 45% at retesting, indicating a decline in factual knowledge over time (D'Eon, 2006). If at any point you feel that your knowledge and understanding of functional neuroanatomy and neuropathology are inadequate, rest assured that you are not alone. Integrating the study and practice of considering neuroanatomy in your everyday practice is challenging but essential, starting early in the training process and continuing well throughout the rest of your career.

Because the "when" and the "how" questions we have discussed go hand in hand, we address both in this section. It is important to note that it is always important to seek balance in your training: To be a good neuropsychologist, you must first be a good clinical psychologist—meaning, do not seek neuroanatomy or neuropsychology experiences to the exclusion of foundational clinical psychological knowledge and skills. With that precaution in mind, how should you approach the initial acquisition and lifelong learning of neuroanatomical principles?

As an undergraduate, seek out relevant formal coursework. Because there are no recognized undergraduate programs in neuropsychology, this coursework will likely relate to neuroscience, sensation and perception, and/or physiological psychology/biopsychology. If no opportunities exist but there is a local doctoral program in clinical psychology or neuroscience at your institution, you might see whether it is possible to audit a course. Supplement your coursework by volunteering in a research laboratory—preferably with a faculty mentor whose line of research relates to neuroimaging, neuroscience, or neurocognition specifically—though at this level of training any exposure to conducting and/or disseminating research (e.g., publications and presentations) is helpful.

When searching for potential American Psychological Association–accredited PhD or PsyD graduate programs, do so with a careful consideration of what neuropsychology educational, clinical, and research opportunities exist as part of the program. The same would apply if you are a graduate student matriculated in a doctoral clinical psychology program. Are there any faculty who conduct research in (or related to) neuropsychology, neurocognition, and/or neuroscience? Are there formal courses in neuropsychological assessment, structural and functional neuroanatomy, cognitive and/or behavioral neuroscience, or neuroimaging? Is there a diversity of clinical experiences available in which you can receive supervised training in traumatic brain injury; stroke; epilepsy; dementia; and other pediatric, adult, and geriatric neurological populations? Are these experiences offered across a variety of settings, such as inpatient or outpatient training in an academic medical center, VA medical center, community hospital, or private practice? Would any of your supervisors be board certified in neuropsychology?

At the internship and postdoctoral fellowship levels, you should be seeking programs that are in accordance with the Houston Guidelines Criteria and the more recent Commission for the Recognition of Specialties and Subspecialties in Professional Psychology Taxonomy (Hannay et al., 1998; Sperling et al., 2017; Smith, 2018). At this level, you should be seeking routine exposure to neuroimaging in your clinical work and supervision sessions. As much as possible, you should attend any available medical center didactics (e.g., neurology grand rounds, neurosurgery grand rounds, and/or neuropathology/brain-cutting conference). These offer excellent opportunities to learn about the specific anatomy and pathologies of neurological disease and injury—and any potential neuroanatomical implications of other medical, psychiatric, and/or developmental conditions (e.g., cancer, autoimmune conditions, genetic disorders, pain) as well as treatments (e.g., chemotherapy, radiation, transplant surgery). There may also be specific surgical conferences that permit trainees to attend (e.g., epilepsy presurgical case conferences, deep brain stimulation presurgical case conferences, neuro-oncology surgical case conferences).

Specific to the fellowship level, attending a program that involves a neuroanatomy and neuropathology educational component is ideal. Many programs require that their Fellows take a medical school neuroanatomy and neuropathology course—for a grade. In addition to consolidating any previous learning, this has the added benefit of preparing outgoing Fellows for their upcoming board certification examination. Of course, at all levels of training, including continuing education throughout your career, there are very helpful ancillary resources that we can recommend; see Table 11.3.

TABLE 11.3. Ancillary Neuroanatomy and Neuropathology Resources

Type	Resource
Courses	Clinical Neuroanatomy online course, National Academy of Neuropsychology: https://www.bit.ly/2mmfEer
	Neuroanatomical Dissection Course: Human Brain and Spinal Cord, Marquette University College of Health Science: https://www.bit.ly/2nPvUF3
	Neuroimaging training programs, Harvard Massachusetts General Hospital Center for Biomedical Imaging: https://www.bit.ly/2nXUIAO
Web	Neuroanatomy series, University of British Columbia: https://www.neuroanatomy.ca
	Atlas of Functional Neuroanatomy, University of Ottawa: https://www.atlasbrain.com
	Whole Brain Atlas, Harvard University: http://www.med.harvard.edu/AANLIB/
	Digital Anatomist Project, University of Washington: http://www.da.si.washington.edu/da.html
	Salamon's Neuroanatomy and Neurovasculature Web-Atlas Resource, University of California, Los Angeles: http://www.radnet.ucla.edu/sections/DINR/index.htm
	MRI Atlas, University of Chicago: https://hpmribrainatlas.rcc.uchicago.edu
	Neuropathology: An Illustrated Interactive Course for Medical Students and Residents: https://www.neuropathology-web.org
	Neuroanatomy Open Access Lab Exercises, University of Texas Health System: https://med.uth.edu/nba/resources/neuroanatomy-online/
	Neuroanatomy Quizzes, University of Utah: https://www.library.med.utah.edu/kw/hyperbrain/quiz/

(continues)

TABLE 11.3. Ancillary Neuroanatomy and Neuropathology Resources (*Continued*)

Type	Resource
Textbooks	Blumenfeld, H. (2002). *Neuroanatomy through clinical cases.* Oxford University Press.
	Mendoza, J., & Foundas, A. (2007). *Clinical neuroanatomy: A neurobehavioral approach.* Springer Science+Business Media.
	Arciniegas, D. B., Anderson, C. A., & Filley, C. M. (Eds.). (2013). *Behavioral neurology and neuropsychiatry.* Cambridge University Press.
	Berkowitz, A. (2016). *Lange clinical neurology and neuroanatomy: A localization-based approach.* McGraw-Hill Education.
	Ho, M. L., & Eisenberg, R. L. (2014). *Neuroradiology signs.* McGraw-Hill.
	Diamond, M. C., & Scheibel, A. B. (1985). *Human brain coloring book.* HarperCollins.

Note. MRI = magnetic resonance imaging.

CONCLUSION AND FUTURE DIRECTIONS

A competent neuropsychologist must be able to describe the behavioral correlates of neural structures, systems, and networks as well as anticipate the potential cognitive and behavioral ramifications of damage to those systems. The development of this knowledge base is no small feat, and maintenance of competency in this arena requires constant study. Of course, it must be acknowledged that the scientific study of functional neuroanatomy is an ongoing process, and it is very likely that in the decades and centuries to come our current understanding of these principles will seem simplistic and juvenile. Nonetheless, to develop competency in neuropsychology, each student, trainee, and professional must commit to learning and maintaining the core concepts of functional neuroanatomy and neuropathology.

REFERENCES

Broca, P. (1865). Sur la siège de la faculté du langage articulé [On the seat of the faculty of articulated language]. *Bulletins et Mémoires de la Société d'Anthropologie de Paris, 6,* 377–393.

Cajori, M. (Director). (1998). *Chuck Close: A portrait in progress* [Film]. Art Kaleidoscope Foundation.

Code, C., Joanette, Y., Lecours, A. R., & Wallesch, C. W. (Eds.). (2003). *Classic cases in neuropsychology* (Vol. II). Psychology Press.

Code, C., Wallesch, C. W., Joanette, Y., & Lecours, A. R. (Eds.). (1996). *Classic cases in neuropsychology.* Psychology Press.

D'Eon, M. F. (2006). Knowledge loss of medical students on first year basic science courses at the University of Saskatchewan. *BMC Medical Education, 6*(1), 5.

Hannay, J., Bieliauskas, L., Crosson, B. A., Hammeke, T. A., Hamsher, K., & Koffler, S. (1998). Proceedings of The Houston Conference on Specialty Education and Training in Clinical Neuropsychology. *Archives of Clinical Neuropsychology, 13*, 157–250. https://doi.org/10.1186/1472-6920-6-5

Lezak, M., Howieson, D., Bigler, E., & Tranel, D. (2012). *Neuropsychological assessment* (5th ed.). Oxford University Press.

Luria, A. (1980). *Higher cortical functions in man* (2nd ed., rev.). Basic Books.

Macdonald, K. E., Bartlett, J. W., Leung, K. K., Ourselin, S., Barnes, J., & The ADNI Investigators. (2013). The value of hippocampal and temporal horn volumes and rates of change in predicting future conversion to AD. *Alzheimer Disease and Associated Disorders, 27*(2), 168–173. https://doi.org/10.1097/WAD.0b013e318260a79a

Mayeux, R., & Kandel, E. (1985). *Principles of neural science*. Elsevier.

Pedersen, P. M., Jørgensen, H. S., Nakayama, H., Raaschou, H. O., & Olsen, T. S. (1995). Aphasia in acute stroke: Incidence, determinants, and recovery. *Annals of Neurology, 38*(4), 659–666. https://doi.org/10.1002/ana.410380416

Sabsevitz, D. H., & Hammeke, T. (2014). The aphasias. In M. Parsons & T. Hammeke (Ed.), *Clinical neuropsychology: A pocket handbook* (pp. 411–435). American Psychological Association. https://doi.org/10.1037/14339-019

Smith, G. (2018). Education and training in clinical neuropsychology: Recent developments and documents from the Clinical Neuropsychology Synarchy. *Archives of Clinical Neuropsychology, 34*(3), 418–431. https://doi.org/10.1093/arclin/acy075

Sperling, S. A., Cimino, C. R., Stricker, N. H., Heffelfinger, A. K., Gess, J. L., Osborn, K. E., & Roper, B. L. (2017). *Taxonomy for Education and Training in Clinical Neuropsychology*: Past, present, and future. *The Clinical Neuropsychologist, 31*(5), 817–828. https://doi.org/10.1080/13854046.2017.1314017

Squire, L. R. (1992). Memory and the hippocampus: A synthesis from findings with rats, monkeys, and humans. *Psychological Review, 99*(2), 195–231. https://doi.org/10.1037/0033-295X.99.2.195

Wernicke, C. (1874). *Der ahasische symptomenkomplex* [The aphasic symptom complex]. Cohn and Weigart.

12

RESEARCH DEVELOPMENT AND DISSEMINATION COMPETENCIES

DERIN COBIA, DALIN PULSIPHER, AND CADY BLOCK

Beginning your career as a scientist can seem daunting, but with the right preparation and focus, a lifelong journey in the research world can turn into an exciting and fulfilling experience. The first seeds of a research-minded career are often planted in graduate school, when your activities are generally restricted to the interests of your mentor; however, your own unique ideas and research questions will begin to emerge as you gain independence and experience over the course of your training path. There are many components to the development of your professional research career, and at the forefront will be the acquisition of essential skills for conducting neuropsychological research informed by Houston Conference Guidelines and the more recent *Taxonomy for Education and Training in Clinical Neuropsychology* (Hannay et al., 1998; Sperling et al., 2017). In this chapter, we outline detailed topic areas with which you should be familiar, to help you be successful in cultivating a research career as a neuropsychologist.

https://doi.org/10.1037/0000250-013
The Neuropsychologist's Roadmap: A Training and Career Guide, C. Block (Editor)

DEVELOPING AND CONDUCTING RESEARCH

The topics and strategies in this section are aimed at helping you make smart choices for decisions you will face early in your research career. Becoming familiar with and establishing best practices in selecting the right setting for your research, cultivating meaningful research ideas, and creating valuable research partnerships will put you on a strong trajectory for making a difference in the scientific community.

Selecting a Setting

Your early development as a junior scientist may be heavily influenced by the setting in which you choose to work (or it may be the reason you chose that setting). Selecting the right setting can be a tough decision that is influenced not only by geographic and financial factors but also by the balance of your other activities (e.g., clinical work or teaching), the type of institution, or that institution's research infrastructure, to name a few. If you are contemplating a career that includes a significant focus on research, then two potential scenarios are worth consideration: (a) an established setting and (b) a new or developing setting. Although admittedly an oversimplification, these are outlined in Table 12.1.

Your plans to pursue a research-driven career generally should be solidified by the time you begin your postdoctoral fellowship; however, it is not entirely uncommon to transition during or afterward. This is mainly a function of how postdoctoral training is structured in neuropsychology, with the availability of both clinical or research-focused positions and the rare blended ones. Going the research route in neuropsychology usually entails employment at a university and/or academic medical center, which are the most ideal institutions to help you succeed with this goal. Although it is possible to begin your career as a dedicated clinician and then switch to a research-focused career, this is more often the exception than rule given the unique challenges such a shift poses.

Regardless of when you start your career in research, selecting the right laboratory in which to begin your training will be critical to your success. Carefully evaluate your available options, and do not make prized attributes, such as abundant funding or a solid publishing record in high-impact journals, your only criteria. Choose a place where you also feel motivated, excited, and fascinated by the work being done there. Furthermore, look to the well-being and advice of current lab members on the relationship with the primary investigator: Does everyone appear happy and engaged?

TABLE 12.1. Selecting a Research Setting

Established setting	New or developing setting
This is a setting where the infrastructure and expectation for high-level research exist, for example, departments with faculty that have funded projects, institutional offices that govern sponsored research contracts, and dedicated centers and programs that support the logistics of research for faculty (e.g., center cores, clinical trial groups, faculty research development and mentorship institutes).	In this setting there is little or no established infrastructure to support independent research because the institution may have other priorities (e.g., teaching or clinical work).
Examples here include Research 1 universities or academic medical centers.	Examples here include non–Research 1 universities, community hospitals, or independent/private practices.
Benefits	*Benefits*
✓ More institutional resources for funding research, accessing valuable patient populations, and supporting conference travel to present research	✓ The opportunities may be exciting and in an area of direct interest to the trainee.
✓ Equipment to help collect, analyze, and store data	✓ There is a higher degree of perceived control over research.
✓ Means to connect to people with expertise in related fields	✓ Expectations for publishing frequency and journal impact may be less rigorous.
Drawbacks	*Drawbacks*
✗ Typically high expectations and pressure for obtaining external funding and publishing in higher impact journals	✗ There might be fewer or less developed institutional resources and/or mentorship available to the trainee.
✗ There may be expectations about the amount of time dedicated to primary research efforts versus other commitments.	✗ There may be a lack of research infrastructure related to laboratory environments and available work space or resources.
	✗ Clinical or teaching demands may limit the time available for research activities.

Are trainees able to have dedicated, regular access to research mentorship? Where do trainees end up after their time in the lab? As a general rule, choose a mentor whose mindset is oriented to developing the careers of trainees and is not just interested in cheap labor for their own projects. The ideal research mentor is one who will support your ideas and model positive mentoring behaviors; adopting these mentoring attitudes can be just as valuable as the specific research knowledge and skills you learn along the way.

It is not uncommon after postdoctoral training for young scientists to remain with their mentor in some capacity. Although this arrangement may have some degree of security, it can also create some challenges with long-term independence. In this situation it is often difficult to step out from under the shadow of your mentor (especially when they are prolific). If this is the case, others may begin to view your work as synonymous with the mentor's—or it may contribute more to their prestige than to your own. When it comes time for promotion, your review committee may be left wondering how independent you really are as a scientist. Knowing when to step out or away from that comfort zone can be a difficult decision, so consult friends and colleagues about the right timing for such a move. If you do it too early, you may not be ready; if you do it too late, it may be too inconvenient to leave. The path to independence in these situations usually involves transferring to a different institution to create a "fresh start." By and large, mentors want to see their trainees gain independence and move on, so do not hesitate (unless you have strong reasons otherwise) to counsel with them on selecting positions, preparing for interviews, and navigating the new-hire process. The experience ideally will be a meaningful one that you can pass on as you repeat the cycle of research mentorship.

Outside of the research setting examples described in Table 12.1, there are a variety of research opportunities that fluctuate across and even within a setting or job. Take time to learn how different institutions function in regard to research and what that may mean for your own career and research goals. In addition, although you may not be exposed to many behind-the-scenes administrative politics and activities, it is helpful to pay attention to how organizations work and ask mentors questions about the institutional infrastructures and hierarchies where you train. Learning how to conceptualize how the culture and operations of places you work will come in handy at many points in your career. A great resource for learning about different institutional research infrastructures is the Howard Hughes Medical Institute, which offers free electronic resources, including *Making the Right Moves: A Practical Guide to Scientific Management for Postdocs and New Faculty* (Burroughs Wellcome Fund & Howard Hughes Medical Institute, 2006), which contains more detail about different research settings, and offers helpful guidelines for plotting out a career trajectory. (For more information on research settings and careers in neuropsychology, see Chapter 7, this volume). There are four general settings for both training and employment in neuropsychology, each of which has a different perspective on the importance of research and how it should be done:

- *University/college (i.e., a setting where your primary responsibilities are to teach, mentor students, and conduct research).* The expectation here is that as a faculty member you will establish a lab with a focused line of research that will advance you through the promotion and tenure process as you involve both undergraduate and graduate students. A thorough understanding of the expectations (documented and unspoken) and balance of teaching, mentoring, and research as they relate to academic advancement, salary funding, and publications is key if launching a career on this path. As a trainee you are likely a member of these labs, directly contributing to projects and developing research skills from the lab director.

- *Academic medical center (i.e., hospital or health care system often associated with a medical school that offers full-time research effort or a mixture of clinical work and research; this may include Veterans Affairs [VA] settings).* There is likely to be administrative overlap with a university, and an academic medical center may offer different university-affiliated tracks defined by clinical or research-oriented positions. This setting typically offers collaborative opportunities (often with physicians) and access to medical resources (e.g., clinical and/or research scanners, electronic medical records). If primarily research oriented, these places expect you start your own lab and research program, but they also offer opportunities to join other grant-funded work to cover a portion of your time. It is common for the division of your effort to fluctuate from year to year. For example, you may find that one year your clinical/research/administrative percent effort is divided 50/40/10, but the following year this changes to 20/70/10 if you secure grant funding as a principal investigator (PI) or coinvestigator.

- *Nonacademic medical center (i.e., independent hospital or health care system that emphasizes clinical work with more limited research opportunities).* This setting may have academic affiliations but provide a completely different environment for research that may align more with a new or developing setting (see Table 12.1), although collaborative opportunities with other professionals and access to medical resources will resemble that of an academic medical center. Research infrastructure is generally limited, and research time may be capped to meet clinical demands.

- *Private practice (i.e., independent clinic driven by clinical or forensic work).* There are many well-respected researchers whose employment exclusively comprises private practice. The stakes may be higher because time not spent on billable activities comes at a higher personal cost, although research can be conducted during nonbusiness hours. Access to an institutional review board and compliance with laws and regulations pertaining to data collection must still be followed.

Cultivating Research Ideas

Now that you've spent all this time thinking about where you're going to conduct research, the content of that research should be the next top priority (although many people pick a setting on the basis of the type of research they conduct, it can go either way). Have you ever felt stumped about how to come up with a research idea? Know that you are not alone! This is perhaps a skill best gained by experience, and many students (who are by definition earlier on in their neuropsychology training) often feel intimidated when trying to develop a research topic of interest. Asking meaningful and relevant questions is a central component to the success and longevity of any research career; nothing is more frustrating that spending time headed in the wrong direction. In *The Psychology Research Handbook*, Leong and Muccio (2006) covered a variety of strategies aimed at addressing this problem. At the most basic level are individual strategies—you can brainstorm and generate interesting ideas simply from your own background! Many individuals take inspiration from the most personal of experiences. As psychologist Robert Sternberg (2017) once wrote

> Almost all my research has come out of my life experiences. I studied intelligence because I did poorly on IQ tests as a child. I studied creativity because I ran out of ideas at one point. I studied wisdom because I remembered a time when I gave a student really bad advice. I studied love because I was in a failing relationship. Well, you get the idea. (p. 77)

What in your life has made a real impression on you—and is there something there to study? More often than not, your finely crafted ideas will come about because of a systematic approach to discovery and not in some single spontaneous "Aha!" event. There are many ways this might happen. In one example, Russell and Morrison (2012) described a six-step process to generating ideas that includes (a) defining a niche area you want to develop, (b) collecting and critically analyzing the literature in this area, (c) generating and evaluating the ideas you develop, (d) assessing your idea's potential for success, (e) seeking constructive criticism from colleagues, and (f) continually refining ideas on the basis of feedback.

Although individual strategies can and should always be a point of influence in one's research, students and trainees also can rely on interpersonal strategies. These involve speaking with other students, attending talks and poster sessions at scientific meetings, or trying your hand at a research assistantship. Furthermore, as students and trainees advance in their scientific knowledge and sophistication, their appreciation for print and electronic resources increases as they read the latest literature via discipline-specific publications, or on preprint websites (e.g., bioRχiv [https://www.biorxiv.org/] or the SSRN [formerly the Social Science Research Network; https://www.ssrn.com/index.cfm/en/]).

What about social media? Social media provides an excellent way to follow colleagues, authors, or research groups on online platforms (e.g., ResearchGate, Social Science Research Network, or Twitter) to keep up with current thought leaders and become part of the daily flow of contemporaneous scientific dialogue. Beyond these individual and interpersonal strategies, we include some additional tips you may find useful.

Tip 1: Write, write, and write some more. A cross-cutting strategy not included in Leong and Muccio's (2006) original list is keeping a running record of your own ideas. Purchase a small notebook to jot down these ideas, and carry it with you at all times. Prefer a digital notebook? There are a number of great note-taking apps and even apps specifically designed for plotting new ideas and making connections between them. Record unique observations and research ideas—no matter how big or small, novel or mundane. Record anything and everything that comes to mind. The goal here is to build an actionable and consistent habit of reflective, creative thinking. Make a daily ritual of sitting down and reading what you have written that day, and then continue to write some more. *Nulla dies sine linea*, ("No day without a line," or simply "Write each day"), as the Romans said. When it comes to producing formalized manuscripts, establishing a routine for focused writing is essential (Gray, 2015; McDonnell, 2016). Experts agree that dedicating a regular protected time slot each day to scientific writing greatly enhances your scholarly productivity; some recommend 1-hour increments (McDonnell, 2016), whereas others suggest that even 15 to 30 minutes daily is enough (Gray, 2015; Silvia, 2007).

Tip 2: Manage time effectively. Time is perhaps one of your most valuable resources as a young researcher. Particularly in the realms of academia and academic medicine, your time must be accounted for through research dollars and/or clinical productivity (measured in relative value units that represent the amount of billable time and services), and it is not uncommon for research time to be the first thing to suffer in clinical settings. No matter what setting you are in, protecting this research time is critical. One of your best indicators for long-term success and satisfaction involves developing healthy research habits. Although much has been written on the topic (see, e.g., Bourne, 2005), most recommendations tend to be broken down into either practical applications or attitudes (Erren et al., 2007). For example, you will be amazed at how much writing you can accomplish by keeping to a routine, but this involves setting boundaries. This may mean physically going to another location to work on research-related activities if your primary location is prone to frequent interruptions. Protecting your time from other obligations also includes knowing how to effectively supervise students and trainees in research if you are at that stage in your career. Whether an early-, mid-, or late-stage career scientist, you have to strike a balance between meeting your professional needs and holding trainees accountable without micromanaging. Furthermore, recognize that collaborators and coauthors may not work according to your timetable (or any timetable at all!), so be prepared for unexpected delays even in the face of looming deadlines, whether others meet them or not. Finally, setting realistic goals and sticking to your schedule is just as important as making sure you use your protected time wisely.

Tip 3: Utilize resources effectively. Although the first two strategies are helpful for just about everyone, know that your research topic may also in part be guided by your level of training. Many graduate programs accept students on the basis of potential fit with available mentors who have an established line of research. Entry into such programs means that your research topic will necessarily align with your prospective mentor's work. This is certainly the case for your master's thesis and doctoral dissertation, which are two of the most important (if not the most important) research projects you will complete during your education. Publishing your dissertation (and even your thesis) is a great way to begin a line of research and establish your name in a particular discipline; many great researchers started their career by publishing and expanding off of their dissertation projects. As a former mentor of one of the authors once wisely advised, "Make every project work twice." You could consider publishing your thesis and/or dissertation as a two-part document: one publication represents your literature review of the topic, the second comprises your actual study and results.

For more advanced trainees, such as predoctoral interns and postdoctoral fellows, research topics may be contingent on available research resources, such as patient populations, analytic approaches, and previously collected archival data. The limited timeline for these training experiences (1 or 2 years at the site) often means that an original research idea cannot be developed and carried out within that short window of time. In these instances, research is more feasible if it pulls from existing resources (e.g., an institutional review board–approved data set/repository at your training program, or a smaller side project representing an offshoot of your mentor's current line of research). Although it is not impossible to obtain funding and conduct a small project during the 2 years that you are on fellowship, remember that your 2 years also likely will be steeped in clinical obligations, coursework, studying, and taking the Examination for Professional Practice in Psychology or state licensure examination, and finding/procuring your first real job.

An efficient method of collecting data if you are working in a clinical setting is the creation of an original clinical database. This typically involves archiving demographic, clinical, cognitive, and other data from patient populations seen in the clinic. Several specialty organizations have made recommendations for partial or full test batteries in clinical populations (e.g., multiple sclerosis, congenital heart defects) that would facilitate efficient organization of the archived data. Adherence to these test guidelines can help with quality improvement and provide cross-site research opportunities given the uniform nature of the data. Finally, it is critical to consider compliance with institutional requirements regarding data collection; informed consent; and database access, storage, and backup. Private practice or other settings do not preclude adherence to the same safeguards and standards.

Tip 4: Read, read, and read some more. As your research program begins to develop and grow, sustaining that program is just as important as starting it in the first place. Staying informed of trends in your particular field ensures that the work you do is relevant and timely. Like many good practices, balancing between time spent producing and consuming research is a skillful habit that can be cultivated. Some simple activities include regularly browsing through table of contents alerts from the most recent editions of various journals or reading (and participating in) the latest science-related discussions on social media. In addition to neuropsychology, branch out into related disciplines such as neuroscience, cognitive/developmental psychology, rehabilitation, medicine, and beyond to glean themes and trends within and beyond the field; some of the most interesting ideas come from rather unexpected places. In addition to keeping current with published literature, you also can monitor the progress and output of relevant large-scale, multisite studies (e.g., the National Institutes of Health–funded Adolescent Brain Cognitive Development and Human Connectome Projects), which may even offer open-access data. Although these activities can be stimulating and thought provoking, they can easily monopolize your time, so don't be afraid to schedule specific "keeping up-to-date" times each week for reviewing journals and other relevant material. In sum, establishing strong habits for cultivating research ideas will not only improve your personal research agenda but also prepare you for important collaborative relationships with others.

Creating and Maintaining Meaningful Research Partnerships

Developing and building relationships with colleagues will be a vital part of your training and career as a research scientist and can reap many benefits.

In fact, the literature on conducting collaborative or team research across many fields indicates that teams tend to dominate individual efforts because they produce more innovative and highly cited research (Wuchty et al., 2007). Indeed, Fortunato and colleagues (2018) suggested that research in general is shifting toward team efforts, which have a greater overall impact and are more beneficial to science in terms of innovation and exposure. They also found that small teams are more likely than large teams to disrupt science and technology with new ideas that persist over time, so when you begin to build collaborative relationships, carefully think about the nature and composition of your team in terms of diversity in training, expertise, and size.

Relationships can be developed and built in many ways. For example, interdisciplinary teams are often found at major medical centers and academic institutions (for more about interdisciplinary science and practice, see Chapter 18, this volume). One of the simplest ways is by reaching out to friends and colleagues in your home department to start projects. Common interests usually will bring like-minded people together, but there is also value in interacting with those from different disciplines because it can increase your appreciation for thinking about questions differently. You can make these connections at seminars or meetings at your institution as well as at conferences. Take the time to attend presentations and poster sessions on various topics, or informally meet people at the conference socials or in the hallways. Developing relationships with colleagues at other institutions can be some of the most exciting because of the shared intellectual inspiration, tools and methods, or access to unique patient populations. Although making these new collaborations initially may come easily and naturally, maintaining them from a productivity standpoint is sometimes challenging; however, this can easily be managed with some simple planning. Casual interactions are helpful in that they build camaraderie but are usually infrequent given busy schedules and sporadic conference travel. Taking a planned approach to discussing ideas or monitoring progress on mutual projects (in particular if it is yours) tends to be the most effective, especially when they are regular, directed, and brief. Some creativity here may be helpful, but a few examples include monthly lunch meetings, weekly research updates, or short communications via phone/video conferencing (you'd be surprised how many people would prefer to Skype from their desk than go across the street for a meeting). Don't be afraid of ruining friendships by being the "stickler" and keeping to a schedule; most people will welcome it and are often at their best with this kind of structure.

As you continue to grow in your research, so will the range of possible research roles, such as PI, co-primary investigator (co-PI), coinvestigator, and eventually mentor. Knowing how and when to step into each one will help you successfully juggle all of your competing demands as well as your lab's efficiency. To some extent, if you have your own research project, you are technically the PI; however, functioning as a PI of a funded grant or project comes with many obligations depending on the amount of the award and scope of its responsibilities. Project PIs are responsible for leading a team through the completion of a funded award, which will require all of your organizational and logistical skills to be successful. Serving as the PI for just one grant can be stressful, so be careful if you want to do this for multiple projects, and know your limits. Acting as a co-PI or coinvestigator for a grant is less intensive because the role tends to be more circumscribed. In fact, one of the advantages of being a neuropsychologist is that many of your skills in clinical psychology, neuropsychological assessment, behavioral neuroscience, and beyond can make you a valuable team member on any project or grant, in particular in allied disciplines that study overlapping problems or populations (e.g., neurosurgery, neurology, psychiatry, nursing). As a coinvestigator, it will be important for you to accurately describe your roles and responsibilities on a project, develop a timeline for deliverables, and provide updates as needed. It is in your best interest to make PIs happy with your performance given that this can lead to future opportunities on funded projects, high-impact papers, and collaborations on your own work. Many people find themselves as both PIs and coinvestigators of multiple projects, which often can provide the right balance of effort, funding, and publishing. It is also quite common for neuropsychologists to serve only as co-PIs or coinvestigators, in particular, if they have a strong clinical obligation. If carefully constructed, this kind of arrangement can allow you to have that highly sought-after balance between research and clinical effort.

PROMOTING YOURSELF AND YOUR WORK

We have focused on developing your research, identifying the right setting, and understanding the more mundane (but hugely important!) aspects of research, but none of it means a thing if you aren't promoting yourself and your ideas. This means not just publications but also posters and presentations at local, regional, national, and international meetings and/or "data blitzes" (i.e., typically a series of very brief, fast-paced research talks that address the most critical elements). Nowadays, sharing your research with the world also means taking advantage of technologies at your disposal. This can include online repositories, blogs, and social media outlets such as

Facebook and Twitter. Equally important to the dissemination of your work product is cultivating and disseminating you as a researcher (yes, you).

Research Metrics

Your success as a researcher will frequently be evaluated against standard metrics that estimate the influence of your work. Understanding the metric nomenclature will help you make decisions on publication outlets, how to spread your ideas, and your level of preparedness for advancing in rank and tenure. We describe the most frequent journal- and author-level metrics in Table 12.2.

Although strong performance on the metrics listed in Table 12.2 is not necessarily required when applying for training positions (e.g., internship or fellowship), they can still be helpful as indices of productivity and will become more influential when applying for faculty positions, going up for promotion/tenure, and applying for research funding. Both journal- and author-level metrics vary across specialties, with lower index values expected for social and behavioral sciences versus the biomedical sciences; they also (on average) vary as a function of academic rank. For example, one may be considered a competitive candidate as a prospective assistant professor with an h-index between 3 and 5, for associate professors between 5 and 10, and 10+ for newly tenured professors in the field. However, there are no current hard-and-fast guidelines for what constitutes acceptable researcher metrics. Hirsch's individual m was developed in an attempt to balance number of citations against a scholar's active research time; it is calculated by dividing one's h-index by the number of years that have passed since the author's first publication. Here, a score of 1 is desirable, 2 is considered outstanding, and 3 truly exceptional.

TABLE 12.2. Research Metrics

Journal-level metrics	Author-level metrics
✓ *Impact factor*: Calculated as the number of citations in the current to previous two years divided by total number of citable articles from the past two years.	✓ *Hirsch index (h-index)*: Calculated by noting the highest number of publications (*h*) that receive a citation number greater than or equal to *h*.
✓ *5-year impact factor*: Similar to journal impact factor, except it encompasses the past five years.	✓ *i10-index*: A Google Scholar metric that represents the numbers of publications of an author that have at least 10 citations.
✓ *Eigenfactor*: Similar to 5-year impact factor, but instead selects out journal self-citations.	✓ *Average citations per item*: The average citation rate for any given author's publication.

Conference Presentations

Presenting your research in the form of a poster or talk at a conference is probably the most common method of sharing one's findings. First, choosing the "right" conference or conferences is important because that effectively determines your audience. Presenting at conferences geared toward neuropsychologists (e.g., the International Neuropsychological Society) is perfectly acceptable and often the best fit, but consider also stepping outside of neuropsychology and participating at specialty conferences or events (e.g., the American Epilepsy Society) to make interprofessional connections, establish collaborative opportunities, and solicit feedback from professionals in other disciplines. At a conference, your submission will be assigned to a session on the basis of thematic content and will be just one part of a broader session involving multiple poster or paper presentations related to a particular topic.

The question of "poster or paper?" often arises for trainees when submitting their research, which is understandable given that there are many similarities between the two, in particular with regard to content. Both include the following major sections: title, introduction, aims/hypotheses, methods (i.e., participants, measures/materials, and procedures), results, conclusions, implications/future directions, and your full name and academic institution with contact information. Both will also involve the presence of an interested audience, which encourages having either printed or electronic handouts ready for them. From there, a series of differences emerge (see Table 12.3).

For the unfamiliar, a conference poster is a large wall-mounted print product (either paper or fabric) typically designed using presentation software that briefly summarizes the findings of your research project. These can be printed by your local or online print store, and sometimes by your academic institution. With the advent of virtual conferences, posters are submitted as an electronic file and hosted on the conference website to be browsed by online attendees. Sometimes presenters are also asked to provide a brief audio file for viewers that describes the main points of the work. Poster sessions can involve as many as several hundred (or more) posters with attendees mingling throughout and interacting one on one with presenters, or virtually via an online portal.

When most effective, posters are well organized and rely on graphical representations of data rather than dense verbiage (see Hess et al., 2013). Posters are, in effect, an advertisement—of your research prowess, of you as the researcher, and of your institution. Making your research visible in conference venues can attract interested individuals for a number of reasons, including those looking for graduate schools, labs to work in, fellowships in which to train, and even other early career professionals like yourself.

TABLE 12.3. Academic Posters Versus Presentations

Academic poster	Academic presentation
✓ Your poster may be one of 100+ in a single 1- to 2-hour poster session.	✓ Your talk may be one of three to four 15-minute presentations as part of an hour-long symposium.
✓ Emphasis is on *conversing* rather than *presenting*. The contemporaneous nature of poster sessions allows for deviation and return to various points in the discussion, as well as for questions to be interjected.	✓ Emphasis is on *presenting* rather than *conversing*. Time is more constrained in a presentation, and the focus is on you as the speaker who guides the audience through your study.
✓ Impact and interaction are of greater *breadth* but lower *depth*. Large sessions can have many attendees who may spend less than a minute or 2 per poster.	✓ Impact is of greater *depth* but lower *breadth*. Sessions will likely have fewer attendees, but most are driven to attend by a shared interest in the topic at hand and will attend the entire session.
✓ Great way to share *preliminary* research ideas and findings with others, with the goal of getting informal thoughts and feedback.	✓ Great way to share more *polished* or fully developed research. This is an excellent means to practice for teaching and professional presenting in general.
	✓ Usually viewed as a stronger mark of research on your curriculum vitae relative to a poster.

Taking a creative angle to poster presenting can set you apart from the "sea of signs" that engulfs every poster session. Some newer trends advocate for a billboard-style poster that breaks up the monotony of text and figures by summarizing key points and facilitating more personal conversation during the poster-going experience (e.g., see Morrison, 2019). Adopting a creative poster style could, in fact, increase attendance and interest in your work just by being better at advertising. For example, creating a QR code that links to a copy of your poster is a creative way to easily and efficiently spread your work at conferences; however, know that some institutions may require you to work with public relations and information systems staff in order to do this.

In contrast to a poster, a conference presentation, sometimes referred to as an "oral" or "paper" presentation, is a time-limited thematic talk of your work made to a room filled with attendees. This involves briefly presenting a short series of slides detailing your study (background, methods, results, discussion of findings and implications for future research) and then fielding questions at the end. Your talk will be grouped with other presentations that are typically of the same general theme and each allotted approximately

10 to 15 minutes from start to finish. It is also good practice to encourage interested attendees to find you afterwards to talk should time run out. In the era of virtual conferences, these paper sessions are typically organized like an online webinar, with the speakers presenting and answering questions "live" one after the other. Often this content is recorded and archived by the society hosting the conference.

The importance of proper preparation for poster and paper presentation experiences cannot be stressed enough. Even within fields and subdisciplines, not all colleagues will be familiar with your ideas or work, so learn how to convey them using language that is clear, concise, and approachable for both student and seasoned academic alike. The key to success is practice, practice, practice. One way to prepare (after you have completed your poster or slides) is to first rehearse once or twice alone, to become accustomed with the words you will use. Next, find every opportunity to present your material to whomever will listen, which could include during lab meetings, at lunch brown bags, or at other department seminars. Some institutions have informal interdisciplinary seminars just for this purpose; they are organized as a space for trainees or faculty to practice presenting their work in a nonthreatening venue that encourages feedback. After each presentation, solicit and incorporate meaningful feedback from participants. You will find that as you spend more time crafting your message, you not only will become more comfortable describing your work, but you also will develop greater familiarity with it. A happy by-product of your preparation is that you also will be better prepared for describing your work to lay audiences or giving an impromptu "elevator pitch" should you find yourself in a promising situation for potential collaboration or funding. For more advice on helping scientists communicate their work to lay audiences and handling the media, see the excellent text *Am I Making Myself Clear?* (Dean, 2012).

Publishing

An added benefit of conference posters and paper presentations is that each provides a strong foundation for manuscripts—let no endeavor end at the presentation alone! Although an overview of all aspects of producing a manuscript is outside the scope of this chapter, there is an array of resources available, such as *Write It Up: Practical Strategies for Writing and Publishing Journal Articles* (Silvia, 2015).

When it comes time to write those manuscripts, there are several decisions to make beforehand that will save you time and stress in the long run. One of the first is how to decide authorship. Traditionally, the first author does the bulk of work with regard to the written manuscript and the scientific development of the study itself. All authors after that represent various degrees of contribution, with the second author contributing more than the third, and third more than fourth, and so on. The senior author (or last author) is traditionally reserved for your mentor or the one who is responsible for supplying the resources of the project (usually the PI of the grant or project from where the data came). Once author order has been decided, the question then becomes where to submit.

One of the more recent and easiest ways to solicit feedback before submitting your manuscript to a journal is through a process known as *preprint peer review*. Websites such as arXiv (https://arxiv.org/) and bioRχiv (https://www.biorxiv.org/) allow people to post early drafts of their manuscripts to encourage discussion and feedback from other scientists on the ideas, design, and interpretation of their work. Although this can be a great way to get much-needed commentary and improve your chance of having the manuscript eventually accepted in a traditional journal, some publishers explicitly state that they will not accept manuscripts that have gone through this process—so always be sure to check beforehand! These journals typically want to present the latest and greatest research, and if you already have shared the manuscript online (even if it later undergoes significant revisions), you have precluded yourself from those journals. So, if you decide to go through the preprint review process, be sure and check whether the journal(s) to which you plan on submitting does not restrict the practice.

When deciding where to submit a manuscript, it can be helpful for the author team to peruse various journal websites, because each will detail the journal aims and scope to help you know whether it will be a good home for your work. Alternatively, one can review recently published articles within a given journal to better understand current trends and topics of interest. There are now also reference management software packages that analyze your citations and their frequency, producing specific journal recommendations in which to publish. That being said, for better or worse, impact factors (see Table 12.2) remain the predominant deciding factor in choosing where to submit for publication. Again, keep in mind who you want your audience to be, whether your study meets the journal criteria with regard to content and methods, whether you want the manuscript to be open access, and whether you want (and are able) to share your study data. There are a number of open-access journals that are freely available for public consumption, with many other subscription-based journals beginning to offer the option of publishing your article in open-access format; however, those journals may charge a hefty fee in order to make the article accessible. Certain funding organizations (e.g., the National Institutes of Health) now require that any manuscript produced as a result of their support must be made publicly available after an embargo period (usually 1 year). Some official online repositories, such as PubMed Central (https://www.ncbi.nlm.nih.gov/pmc/), simplify this process for free. The debate over for-profit journal publishers' fees for single articles and institutional subscriptions is brewing, and more and more scientists are pushing for open access. Many even view it as an ethical responsibility, so be aware of these contemporary issues as you make publishing decisions.

Although some authors may take the approach of producing a manuscript first and then deciding on a journal, it can be to the advantage of the author team to produce a manuscript tailored to a specific journal. This way, you get to know all the ins and outs of a specific journal's expectations before you even begin outlining and writing. You then can prepare your submission in a manner consistent with the journal (e.g., length and word count, formatting of headings and statistics, allowable number of tables and figures), which is sometimes a more efficient approach. Although this may seem like a minor detail, failure to comply with manuscript preparation requests can result in unnecessary delays and even prompt rejection, something that is easily avoidable. The same goes for basic grammar, syntax, and punctuation: Accurate proofreading is essential to a quality article—do not shift that responsibility to the reviewers and editor! This is a quick ticket to rejection, or at the very least earns you the annoyance of those deciding on your submission. As neuropsychology grows around the globe, journals in the field will continue to experience an increase in submissions from individuals for whom English is not their first language, which may result in some difficulty with written communication. Support in the form of English language consultants are available in these situations to facilitate making quality research more suitable for publication and promote accessibility. The International Neuropsychological Society offers such a service through their Research and Editing Consultant Program (see https://www.the-ins.org/about-ins/ins-committees/international-resources).

If you decide you want to submit to a journal with a high impact factor, great! But understand that such journals generally accept a very low percentage of submissions. Sometimes this means putting a lot of work into a manuscript only to have it swiftly rejected. But that's okay! That is not a reflection of the quality of your work or who you are. Start out with realistic expectations and, if rejected by one journal, be prepared to move on. Once you submit to a journal, there are several potential outcomes. If your manuscript is accepted, congratulations; if revisions and resubmission are recommended, you're one step closer. The most important thing to remember is to follow the journal editor's instructions. Regardless of the extent of revisions required, always meet your deadlines, follow directions, and explicitly address each comment. Not only is this the professional thing to do, but also not following directions could result in rejection.

Finally, we offer some cautionary words about predatory publishers and journals. In brief, predatory publishers are organizations that often use spamming techniques to solicit work from researchers in the guise of a legitimate open-access operation. They charge exorbitant fees and often engage in unethical practices while failing to follow accepted standards for scholarly publishing (see https://predatoryjournals.com/about). Requests typically come as a seemingly legitimate email with company or journal titles that closely resemble authentic institutions. One of the easiest ways to tell whether a particular journal is legitimate or not is to check Beall's List (https://beallslist.net/), a listing of publishers considered potentially predatory; also, seek advice from mentors or colleagues when navigating this landscape. Despite the publish-or-perish pressures researchers face, submitting to these journals can deprive you of hard-earned funds and damage your reputation.

The Next Wave of Disseminating Research

There are also several ways to share your research that are not widely used in neuropsychology. In addition to social media, resources such as ResearchGate (https://www.researchgate.net/), OpenNeuro (https://openneuro.org/), and GitHub (https://github.com/) link work to projects, make data publicly accessible and allow the creation and sharing of programming and statistical code with networks of like-minded individuals. One new approach to address the replication crisis in the scientific community (see Tackett et al., 2019, for a review) is to publish in journals that use the registered-reports mechanism through the Center for Open Science (https://osf.io/). This is a process whereby the aims, hypotheses, and design of a project are submitted to a journal for peer review and accepted on the basis of the merits of these criteria. Once data collection, analysis, and interpretation have occurred and the manuscript is written, it is then published regardless of the results. This practice makes it different from the traditional peer-review process because it adds transparency and reflects the quality of scientific rigor instead of whether or not the findings are statistically significant.

CONCLUSION AND FUTURE DIRECTIONS

As you progress through your journey of becoming a scientist in neuropsychology, keep in mind it is not uncommon for your research interests to change over the course of your career. Those interests may take many unexpected turns, so be flexible and open to where they lead, in particular if they ignite your passions and motivate you to do your best work. These experiences can lead you to think more creatively, which is just as important as analytical and critical thinking. After many days on the battlefield of science you may find yourself dealing with the typical pressures and anxieties that plague all researchers, including (but not limited to) funding constraints, shifting interests, changes in staff, petty reviewers, and institutional demands that seemingly frustrate the research process. Have complete confidence in your research and the ideas behind it, because the simple belief that the work you do matters can sometimes be enough to sustain you during difficult times. In spite of discouragement, never lose sight of the thing that got you into the exciting world of scientific discovery. Remember what inspires you to be creative, thoughtful, and focused in your pursuit of advancing knowledge and discovering something new in the field of brain and behavior!

REFERENCES

Bourne, P. E. (2005). Ten simple rules for getting published. *PLOS Computational Biology*, *1*(5), e57. https://doi.org/10.1371/journal.pcbi.0010057

Burroughs Wellcome Fund & Howard Hughes Medical Institute. (2006). *Making the right moves: A practical guide to scientific management for postdocs and new faculty.* https://www.hhmi.org/science-education/programs/making-right-moves

Dean, C. (2012). *Am I making myself clear?* Harvard University Press.

Erren, T. C., Cullen, P., Erren, M., & Bourne, P. E. (2007). Ten simple rules for doing your best research, according to Hamming. *PLOS Computational Biology*, *3*(10), e213. https://doi.org/10.1371/journal.pcbi.0030213

Fortunato, S., Bergstrom, C. T., Börner, K., Evans, J. A., Helbing, D., Milojević, S., Petersen, A. M., Radicchi, F., Sinatra, R., Uzzi, B., Vespignani, A., Waltman, L., Wang, D., & Barabási, A. L. (2018, March 2). Science of science. *Science*, *359*(6379), eaao0185. https://doi.org/10.1126/science.aao0185

Gray, T. (2015). *Publish and flourish* (2nd ed.). Starline.

Hannay, H. J., Bieliauskas, L. A., Crosson, B., Hammeke, T. A., Hamsher, K. D., & Koffler, S. P. (1998). The Houston Conference on Specialty Education and Training in Clinical Neuropsychology. *Archives of Clinical Neuropsychology*, *13*(2), 160–166. https://doi.org/10.1093/arclin/13.2.160

Hess, G., Tosney, K., & Liegel, L. (2013). *Creating effective poster presentations: An effective poster.* https://projects.ncsu.edu/project/posters/

Leong, F. T. L., & Muccio, D. J. (2006). Finding a research topic. In F. T. L. Leong & J. T. Austin (Eds.), *The psychology research handbook: A guide for graduate students and research assistants* (2nd ed., pp. 23–40). Sage. https://www.doi.org/10.4135/9781412976626.n2

McDonnell, J. J. (2016). The 1-hour workday. *Science*, *353*(6300), 718. https://doi.org/10.1126/science.353.6300.718

Morrison, M. (2019, March 25). *How to create a better research poster in less time* [Video]. YouTube. https://www.youtube.com/watch?v=1RwJbhkCA58

Russell, S. W., & Morrison, D. C. (2012). *The grant application writer's workbook.* Springer.

Silvia, P. J. (2007). *How to write a lot: A practical guide to productive academic writing.* American Psychological Association.

Silvia, P. J. (2015). *Write it up: Practical strategies for writing and publishing journal articles.* American Psychological Association.

Sperling, S. A., Cimino, C. R., Stricker, N. H., Heffelfinger, A. K., Gess, J. L., Osborn, K. E., & Roper, B. L. (2017). *Taxonomy for Education and Training in Clinical Neuropsychology*: Past, present, and future. *The Clinical Neuropsychologist, 31*(5), 817–828. https://doi.org/10.1080/13854046.2017.1314017

Sternberg, R. J. (2017). *Starting your career in academic psychology.* American Psychological Association.

Tackett, J. L., Brandes, C. M., King, K. M., & Markon, K. E. (2019). Psychology's replication crisis and clinical psychological science. *Annual Review of Clinical Psychology, 15*(1), 579–604. https://doi.org/10.1146/annurev-clinpsy-050718-095710

Wuchty, S., Jones, B. F., & Uzzi, B. (2007). The increasing dominance of teams in production of knowledge. *Science, 316*(5827), 1036–1039. https://doi.org/10.1126/science.1136099

13 RESEARCH AWARDS AND GRANTSMANSHIP COMPETENCIES

STEPHANIE KIELB AND CADY BLOCK

Now that you've developed some of the foundational skills necessary to become a junior scientist (see Chapter 12), you are ready to begin thinking about ways to obtain financial support and recognition for your research work. Identifying and pursuing such opportunities can seem daunting, especially as a trainee. Indeed, this process can demand a lot of time and effort. It may seem high risk, but it can also be of high reward. Just like anything else, learning how to navigate and apply for research awards and grants comes through observation, practice, and learned experience.

First and foremost, you should understand the difference between a research grant and a research award. These can be fuzzy concepts, at times used interchangeably as nouns or even verbs (e.g., "Professor Jones was awarded a grant" or "Professor Jones was granted an award"), which can be very confusing. For the purposes of this chapter, a *grant* refers to monetary support given on the basis of an application for an intended research project. In contrast, a research *award* primarily recognizes a completed project or cumulative achievement. The basic difference is that a grant goes toward your specific research activities, whereas an award applies to you as a researcher and your scientific accomplishments.

https://doi.org/10.1037/0000250-014
The Neuropsychologist's Roadmap: A Training and Career Guide, C. Block (Editor)
Copyright © 2021 by the American Psychological Association. All rights reserved.

In this chapter, we describe some different types of research awards and grants and discuss how trainees can benefit from pursuing these opportunities. We also provide some resources and tips to help you locate, apply for, and obtain a research grant or award.

RESEARCH AWARDS

As we mentioned, research awards serve to recognize and honor an individual's scientific achievements. A multitude of award opportunities are available through academic institutions and professional organizations at local, state, national, and international levels. They can vary widely in terms of size, scope, and selection criteria. Not all awards involve a monetary component, but in some cases award recipients receive a monetary prize or funding for a specific activity or cause (e.g., the cost of tuition or textbooks).

Benefits of Research Awards

Pursuing a research award can have a number of immediate and longer term benefits for trainees. Those that come with a financial reward can obviously be helpful, in particular for graduate students operating on a tight budget. Awards also draw attention to your achievements, so they can signal to others that you are not just a trainee but also a competent and skilled researcher. Definitely list any award you receive on your curriculum vitae!

Receiving an award can also foster growth and professional advancement. First of all, it feels good to be recognized for your hard work and accomplishment(s). Having a documented history of awards will increase your visibility within the scientific community and could potentially open up opportunities for future collaboration and leadership/service positions (e.g., on an organization's science committee). Winning an award also highlights your scientific skills, which can make you look more competitive for other opportunities down the line.

Even if you don't necessarily win the award, submitting the application alone is a useful exercise that can be counted as a personal victory. Preparing an application encourages you to engage in personal and professional self-assessment. Applications often ask you to think about your accomplishments from a broader level: How have you developed as an individual? What do you see yourself doing in the future, should you win this award? Graduate school, internship, and postdoctoral fellowship training can be quite granular at times, so it can be challenging but helpful to step back and reflect on these big picture questions. In retrospect, applicants often find that they learn much about themselves and their professional interests as they go through the application process.

Pursuing awards can also help you craft your professional goals and future endeavors. More often than not, award-granting entities provide descriptions of previous winners on their website. You can use this information to gauge your competitiveness for the award right now and figure out how you can become a more competitive applicant in the future. Reviewing the award criteria and past winners may give you a sense of the skills and experiences you need to achieve your own professional goals.

Types of Awards

The term "award" is a broad one that can encompass many different kinds of honors and accolades. In this section, we highlight a few types of research awards that can be relevant for trainees. Many research awards are merit based, meaning that they reward someone for making a significant contribution to their field. Typically, the recipients of these awards have demonstrated outstanding achievements in terms of academic, scientific, and/or leadership performance. Merit awards give members of the scientific community an opportunity to recognize these achievements. They are often not accompanied by a monetary prize, although these awards can vary from organization to organization. You can apply directly to most merit awards, but some require you to be nominated by a mentor or peer. A number of professional organizations have awards that honor graduate students for exceptional master's theses and dissertations in the fields of neuropsychology and neuroscience.

Other types of awards provide financial support for trainees who wish to attend a professional or scientific conference. As anyone who has attended one of these meetings will know, conference registration, travel, and lodging expenses can add up quickly. Many academic institutions and professional organizations have awards designed to offset these costs. A lot of travel awards are restricted to trainees who have a poster or talk accepted for presentation at an upcoming conference; however, travel assistance programs, such as the one offered by the Association for Psychological Science (https://www.psychologicalscience.org/members/apssc/travel), offer financial opportunities to any trainee interested in attending a conference, regardless of whether or not they will be part of the scientific program at said conference.

Additional travel funds may be available for trainees who are willing to volunteer their services at a scientific conference. Some organizations have a student volunteer program associated with their annual meeting. Someone in a volunteer position might enjoy a waived registration fee and a small stipend to cover housing and travel costs in exchange for spending a few hours manning the registration booth or overseeing session attendance. Most of these programs have a formal application process, and selection can be competitive. Trainees serving in a volunteer capacity not only get to attend the conference but also may have unique opportunities to engage with presenters and attendees at the meeting. For students in the first few years of their training, this can be a great way to engage with the scientific community and begin to build a professional network.

How to Locate Relevant Awards

Although a multitude of research awards are available to students and trainees, locating these opportunities can be challenging, especially if you are not sure where to start your search. As a first step, ask about opportunities within your own academic institution; some departments, colleges, and graduate student organizations give small merit and/or travel awards to students. A number of professional and scientific organizations have awards that specifically recognize trainee accomplishments in neuropsychological or neuroscientific research. Some of these organizations are listed in Table 13.1. This is by no means meant to be a comprehensive list of organizations that offer research awards, because that is outside of the scope of this chapter. You may be able to locate relevant awards by browsing the websites of broad scientific societies in psychology and neuroscience as well as professional

TABLE 13.1. Sample Organizations Offering Research Awards

Category	Examples
National and international	American Academy of Clinical Neuropsychology (https://theaacn.org) American Board of Clinical Neuropsychology (https://theabcn.org) American Psychological Association (https://www.apa.org) Association for Psychological Science (https://www.psychologicalscience.org) International Neuropsychological Society (https://www.the-ins.org) National Academy of Neuropsychology (https://www.nanonline.org) Society for Clinical Neuropsychology (https://www.scn40.org) Society for Neuroscience (https://www.sfn.org)
Regional, state, and local	Ohio Psychological Association (https://ohpsych.org) Association for Women in Science, Chicago area chapter (https://www.awis-chicago.org) Pacific Northwest Neuropsychology Society (https://pnns.org/)
Honor societies	Psi Chi (https://www.psichi.org) Sigma Xi (https://www.sigmaxi.org)

organizations specific to neuropsychology. You might consider reaching out to regional-, state-, or city-based scientific organizations to see if they have research award mechanisms. Some academic honor societies can also sponsor relevant programs, such as the Sigma Xi's Young Investigator Award and an award from Psi Chi that covers travel to any psychology-related conference.

The American Psychological Association (APA) maintains a database of awards sponsored by APA and other related organizations (https://www.apa. org/about/awards). We strongly advise you to check out the individual websites of each of these organizations to view updated opportunities. Note that award programs can change over time on the basis of funding availability and other situational factors, so check the accuracy of any funding announcements with the award granting entity.

RESEARCH GRANTS

Research grants are monetary funding that applies to the direct and/or indirect costs associated with conducting your research. Direct costs relate immediately to your study. They are the expenses you incur as a result of engaging in research activities, like obtaining study equipment, paying study participants, renting laboratory space, or printing recruitment materials. Grant proposals typically ask you to describe exactly how you will use grant funds to cover your direct research costs. However, your budget should also account for indirect costs, which relate to general institutional overhead. Simply put, they are the expenses that the university incurs from providing the infrastructure for your research. For example, indirect costs can relate to things like general office supplies, maintenance of university grounds, and general support staff compensation. Funding agencies recognize that there are more than direct project costs associated with conducting research, so they negotiate with universities on rates of reimbursement for indirect costs; these are usually prespecified by each institution.

Benefits of Research Grants

For trainees who are passionate about research, obtaining a grant can be a huge milestone in their journey to becoming an independent scientist. In this section, we discuss the major benefits that research grants can offer to neuropsychology trainees and some other benefits of writing a grant proposal. First and foremost, the financial benefits that come from research grants can be substantial. Even the smallest, simplest human research studies incur costs for things like equipment, supplies, and recruitment tools. Neuropsychology and neuroscience research can have an especially high price tag, given that it tends to use expensive proprietary tests, neuroimaging and other neuro-diagnostic studies, analysis methods that can require special training and software, and a trained clinical staff. Unfortunately, academic institutions cannot always cover thesis or dissertation projects that have such high direct costs. With the support of grant funding, you may be able to conduct cutting-edge research that would previously have been impossible. Some programs provide additional funding that covers training and educational activities, conference travel, living expenses, health care, and tuition costs.

Applying for a research grant—whether or not it ends in funding—is a great accomplishment and learning experience. The process can be time consuming, but it forces you to think critically about your research. Designing a study from scratch is no easy task. You have to be very thoughtful about the feasibility of your project, from the perspective of time as well as resources. You will also have to think beyond the scope of your research: What are the clinical implications of your study? Does it change the way we think about a particular cognitive domain or neurological disease? Does it inform public health education or intervention? In the unfortunate (but not uncommon) event that your proposal is not funded, you still learn how to accept and incorporate critical feedback in future submissions.

Similar to awards, obtaining a research grant can be important for your overall professional development. Obtaining research funding can be an excellent way to demonstrate your commitment to a research career as well as your competitiveness for future funding opportunities. Having a history of funding success increases your visibility and credibility within the scientific community, and as you transition from graduate student to early-career neuropsychologist, a demonstrated history of funding success can facilitate professional advancement through hiring and salary negotiation, promotion, and tenure.

Types of Grants

In this section, we describe the major types of organizations that award research grants. We provide an overview of the U.S. National Institutes of Health (NIH) programs and mention some other organizations that have funding opportunities for neuropsychological and neuroscientific research (see Table 13.2).

Foundation Grants

A significant amount of research funding is available from foundations and other privately run organizations. These grants are typically made to support

TABLE 13.2. Sample Organizations Offering Research Grants

Category	Examples
Private foundations	Alzheimer's Research Foundation (https://www.alzheimersresearchfoundation.com)
	American Brain Tumor Association (https://www.abta.org)
	American Psychological Association (https://www.apa.org)
	Autism Speaks (https://www.autismspeaks.org)
	Brain and Behavior Research Foundation (https://www.bbrfoundation.org)
	BrightFocus Foundation (https://www.brightfocus.org)
	Dana Foundation (https://www.dana.org)
	Epilepsy Foundation (https://www.epilepsy.com)
	John A. Hartford Foundation (https://www.jhartfound.org)
	MacArthur Foundation (https://www.macfound.org)
	McKnight Foundation (https://www.mcknight.org)
	Michael J. Fox Foundation (https://www.michaeljfox.org)
	National Multiple Sclerosis Society (https://www.nationalmssociety.org)
	Robert Wood Johnson Foundation (https://www.rwjf.org)
NGO	American Association for the Advancement of Science (https://www.aaas.org)
	World Health Organization (https://www.who.int)
GO	Congressionally Directed Medical Research Programs (https://cdmrp.army.mil)
	National Science Foundation (https://www.nsf.gov)
	U.S. Air Force Research Laboratory (https://www.afrl.af.mil/)
	U.S. Army Research Laboratory (http://www.arl.army.mil)
	U.S. Department of Defense (https://dod.defense.gov/)
	U.S. National Aeronautics and Space Administration (https://www.nasa.gov)
	US. National Institutes of Health (https://www.nih.gov)
	U.S. Office of Naval Research (https://www.onr.navy.mil)
	U.S. VA Office of Research and Development (https://www.research.va.gov)

Note. NGO = nongovernmental organization; GO = governmental organization.

research that will further their organization's overall mission and objectives. This means that funding availability, application requirements, and the review process are unique to each granting organization—and can vary widely from year to year. The number of grant-giving foundations can be somewhat overwhelming, so two very helpful online resources for browsing and identifying relevant funding opportunities are the Foundation Directory Online (https://fconline.foundationcenter.org/) and the SPIN database (https://spin.infoedglobal.com). For perusing opportunities a little closer to home, another very helpful and searchable online database is the Community

Foundation Locator from the Council on Foundations (https://www.cof.org/community-foundation-locator).

Some grant funding can come from the MacArthur Foundation and related organizations whose mission is to support a variety of impactful projects. More common sources of funding dollars for neuropsychological and neuroscientific research are health care–related organizations. The broadest examples include foundations that focus on the field of psychology, including APA and the Association for Psychological Science, as well as those dedicated to neuroscience and brain–behavior relationships. A plethora of disease-based foundations also have grant programs that could be relevant if your research focuses on a specific patient population.

In addition to providing research awards, neuropsychological and neuroscientific organizations also have grant opportunities that are highly relevant to trainees and early career neuropsychologists. Examples include the National Academy of Neuropsychology's annual clinical research grant program and an annual outcome studies grant program from the American Academy of Clinical Neuropsychology's foundational arm. The Society for Clinical Neuropsychology also sponsors a number of annual master's thesis, dissertation, and early-career pilot research grants.

Nongovernmental Organization Grants

Nongovernmental organizations (NGOs) are typically nonprofit entities that operate independently of the government, such as the World Health Organization. They can provide some funding for research but are less likely to provide regular calls for submissions—meaning that funding could be offered on a case-by-case basis. That makes these a less common, but still possible, source of funding for neuropsychological and neuroscientific research.

Governmental Organization Grants

A substantial amount of funding is available through various governmental organizations. These organizations typically have long-standing, well-organized grant programs that offer regular calls for submissions at a variety of levels of funding support and professional experience—from graduate trainee to postdoctoral fellow to early-career scientist. Perhaps the most well-known federal grant programs come from the NIH (https://www.nih.gov); we cover these in more detail shortly. The National Science Foundation also offers grants opportunities, including a prestigious Graduate Research Fellowship Program that may be of interest to students early in their training.

National Institutes of Health Grants: Grant Types

Significant enough to warrant its own section in this chapter, the NIH comprises 21 different institutes and six affiliated centers. Each institute is dedicated to a specific field of study, has its own mission and research agenda, and offers funding for researchers at various stages of training. Examples that can be relevant to neuropsychology research include the National Institutes on Aging, Mental Health, Neurological Disorders and Stroke, Drug Abuse, and Minority Health and Health Disparities, which are only a few of the organizations that fund neuropsychology. If you are seriously considering applying for an NIH grant you should contact the program officer within the institute to which you will be applying. They can be an excellent resource to help you assess how well your project fits with the particular institute's mission and funding mechanisms.

Many NIH grant applications are solicited on the basis of a program announcement, which provides specific details on the scope of allowed projects and how the funds should be allocated. Other grants are unsolicited, meaning that you initiate and submit the application. When it comes to these grant mechanisms (NIH, 2020a, 2020b) there can be a bit of an alphabet soup, which can be overwhelming to students and trainees. Next, we provide a brief review of relevant opportunities (for a snapshot of opportunities over the course of one's career, see Figure 13.1).

National Research Service Award (F and T) Grant Mechanisms. The NIH Ruth L. Kirschstein National Research Service Award program has a number

FIGURE 13.1. Relevant National Institutes of Health Grant Mechanisms Over the Course of Your Career

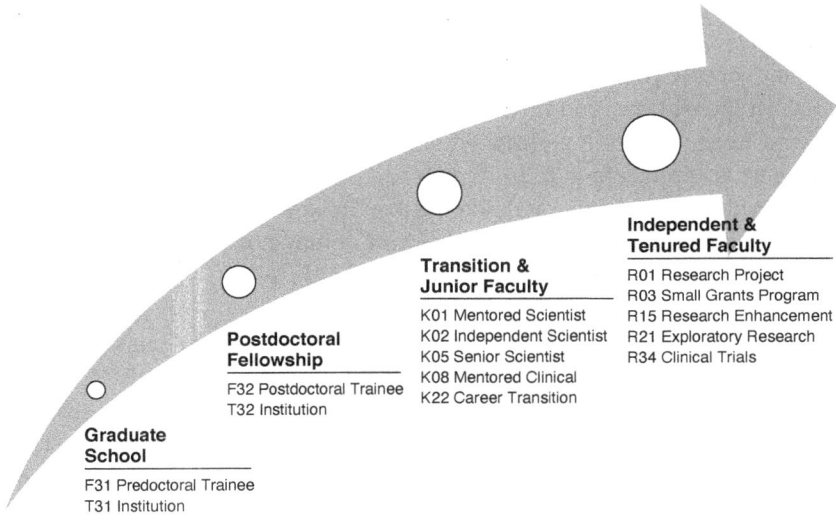

of grant mechanisms that provide support for trainees to develop the skills necessary to become independent research investigators. This specific program is dedicated to training junior scientists in the behavioral and health sciences, ranging from doctoral students up to postdoctoral fellows. Within the National Research Service Award program there are individual grants for predoctoral and postdoctoral trainees specifically—called the *F31* and *F32* awards, respectively. In addition to provision of funds for the proposed research project, awardees attend didactic and other training events where they have unique opportunities to network with trainees and faculty members within their institution. The goal of these programs is to provide mentored training that enables awardees to develop into productive, independent scientists. The F31/32 proposal is extensive and will include detailed descriptions of your research plan, background, training goals, institution, and mentorship. In fact, for early-career NIH awards the type and level of mentorship and training are just as important as the project itself. As such, we recommended that you work closely with your mentor(s) to begin crafting your proposal well in advance of the submission deadline. Also, check with your institution, because your department or college likely has a grant administrator that is available to provide assistance with developing a budget and submitting the application. As is the case for all NIH grants, the applicant submits materials through an online portal called eRA Commons (https://public.era.nih.gov/commons). Detailed information on the application process and tips for grant writing are also available on the NIH grants and funding website (https://www.grants.nih.gov).

Whereas the NIH F mechanism is granted to the individual, the T mechanism is granted to the institution. As a trainee, applying for a T31 or T32 grant is typically simpler and more straightforward than applying for an individual F grant because your institution will have already obtained funding from the NIH. For these grants, you submit a proposal directly to the faculty committee at your institution for a position within their larger training program. Being a student or trainee in a T32 program can provide the ideal stepping stone for individual grants later on down the line; however, the availability of such awards is limited—meaning your institution may not have an established T31/32 training program relevant to your field of study.

K Grant Mechanisms. Moving past your student and trainee years into your early career means that you should now be thinking about an NIH K-level grant. These are mentored career development grants, either for individual researchers seeking additional development of their research career (K01 and K02) or individuals from a primarily clinical background who wish to establish a research component in their careers (K08). For either, the NIH requires that at least 75% of your effort be devoted to your project and career development for 3 to 5 years. Similar to the F mechanism, K applications are just as much about the mentorship and educational plan as the project itself (NIH Research Training and Career Development, 2020). When ready to transition from a mentored, nonindependent investigator to an independent research grant, the Transition Career Development Award (K22) is the one for you. Once you're a senior scientist looking to support your own research and provide mentoring to new investigators, you should look into a senior Scientist Research Award (K05).

R Grant Mechanisms. As you transition out of the early career phase, your funding focus will move to the R-level grants. The NIH (2020b) reports that the R01 is their most commonly used grant mechanism, typically funding your project and anywhere from 20% to 40% of your investigator salary for 3 to 5 years; at the conclusion of the 5-year period a renewal application is required. If your project is on the smaller side and you can make do with limited resources, an R03 through the NIH's Small Grant Program may be ideal for you; this opportunity is limited to 2 years of funding and cannot be renewed. If your project is small and your institution is not typically a major recipient of NIH support, you may be eligible for an R15 grant. If your idea is so preliminary that you're looking to fund a pilot or feasibility study, your aim should be the NIH Exploratory/Developmental Research Grant (R21); funding for an R21 is generally provided up to 2 years. There is also the R34 grant, which is intended to support development of a clinical trial—normally over a period of 1 year, though some NIH institutes offer funding for a longer period of time.

National Institutes of Health Grants: Submission and Review Process

We won't lie to you: The NIH application and review process is neither quick nor easy. But it is a skill that can be learned and mastered. We give some resources and advice for preparing an application later on in the chapter. This section focuses on what happens to your application after it is submitted.

Center for Scientific Review. The initial step of the review process takes place through the NIH Center for Scientific Review (CSR; https://public.csr. nih.gov/), which checks your application to ensure that it meets administrative and formatting requirements. The CSR is also important in that it assigns your application to an NIH institute/center for review by experts who are knowledgeable about your field of study. For investigator-initiated R-level grant applications, the institute/center and review group assignments are based on your science; however, you can include an assignment request in your application that the CSR will consider. If your application is complete and formatted correctly, then the CSR assigns your application a lengthy identification number that denotes your application type, code (e.g., R01), organization to which it is assigned, and so on (see https://grants.nih.gov/grants/glossary.htm#ApplicationIdentificationNumbers).

Integrated Review Groups. Once your application clears the CSR, it is then assigned to an integrated review group (IRG). Led by a Scientific Review Officer, IRGs are essentially committees organized around one of a number of scientific areas that convene and review your application (NIH, 2020c). As an applicant, know that the NIH Office of Extramural Research (2020) publishes an online roster that lists the name and description of each review committee, committee Scientific Review Officer, and meeting schedules (https://public.era.nih.gov/pubroster).

The Priority Score. In general, you want to craft your proposal with the review process in mind. Applications are reviewed according to several core criteria (see Table 13.3). These include project significance, project innovation, project approach, the investigator(s), and the research environment. Once the application is received and reviewed by the committee, your proposal is rated on a scale that ranges from 1 (*exceptional*) to 9 (*poor*) for each of the core criteria. You also receive a total rating from each reviewer for the overall application. From all reviewer scores, a normalized average is calculated and then multiplied by 10 to yield a priority score.

Within a week of the review meeting, you will be informed about the review outcome via eRA Commons. There are three possible outcomes at this point. First, your application may receive a priority score that ranges from 10 (*exceptional overall proposal*) to 90 (*poor overall proposal*), with lower scores being more likely to move to the next phase of the review process. A priority score under 30 is considered ideal (National Library of Medicine, 2014). If your priority score falls at or around this level, your application will go through a second round of review during which the quality of the IRG review is assessed. Assuming your application passes this final round of review, you may receive a request for "just in time" information (e.g., institutional review board approval), which is usually a good sign that your application may be funded. Second, your application may receive a ruling of "not recommended for further consideration," in which case you can consider resubmitting. The third potential outcome is that your application is unscored because the review committee believed that its scientific merit placed it approximately

TABLE 13.3. National Institutes of Health Review Core Criteria

Criterion and definition	Key questions to address
Significance: The extent to which your proposed research is meaningful and impactful	What is the state of the field as it currently stands—its current working theories, knowledge gaps, barriers?
	How does your research plan to address any problem(s) within the field and for human health more broadly?
	What preliminary data do you have to demonstrate how your research is helpful in addressing these problem(s)?
Innovation: The extent to which your research project is original with regard to theory, hypotheses, methods, and/or tools	How unique is your proposed project, or is it a refinement of current concepts and practices?
	Will your research project challenge and seek to shift current paradigms through creation of novel hypotheses, methodologies, and/or measures?
Approach: The extent to which your study scope and methodology are sound and appropriate to the project aims(s)	Are your study design, methods, and statistical analyses well reasoned, well developed, and appropriate to the aims of the project?
	Did you consider potential problems and alternative strategies? This includes consideration of resolving any potential administrative or leadership conflicts.
Investigator(s): The extent to which you, collaborators, and any key personnel are relevant, well trained, and available	Are you (the principal investigator) trained to carry out the project? Do you have a history of accomplishments that have advanced the field already?
	Are key study personnel trained to carry out the project?
	Are each of your collaborators willing and available to provide support? Do they each offer valuable expertise or skills that are needed for your project?
Environment: The extent to which your institutional environment and resources support your project	Is your institutional support adequate and available?
	Are your institutional resources adequate and available?
	Is your project feasible? Do you have sufficient access to material resources and your population(s) of interest?

in the lower 50% of the applications under review (NIH, 2020b). Regardless of your outcome, within 8 weeks you should receive a summary statement reflecting the review committee's discussion and written comments by separate reviewers. The NIH (2020b) encourages applicants who did not receive a score to contact their program officer after reviewing the summary statement to discuss resubmission or next steps.

STRATEGIES FOR PREPARING A COMPETITIVE GRANT PROPOSAL

We now offer some advice for preparing a grant proposal. First and foremost, funding agencies want to know that you are a competent and committed researcher. In your proposal, make it clear that you have all the skills, experience, resources, and support necessary to carry your project from conception to presentation/publication. It can be helpful to incorporate data from a pilot study or preliminary analyses into the rationale section of your research plan. This can prove to reviewers that you have been thoughtful in planning your study (and that you know how to analyze data!). Grant reviewers like to see that applicants have a history of research success, including publications and presentations. For trainees early in their research careers, poster presentations and scientific talks, even at small conferences within your institution, can show that you are serious about your scientific pursuits.

As a trainee, it's important to think carefully about your own commitment to research before applying for any award. Many grants require awardees to dedicate a significant amount of time and effort to their research. Individuals funded by National Research Service Award grants, for example, are expected to be involved in research on a full-time basis (i.e., 40 hours per week). If you are more interested in spending time on clinical activities or teaching, then applying for this type of grant may not be the best option for you.

When preparing a grant application, specificity is a key ingredient for success. You should always tailor your application to the funding agency, making a case for how your specific project fits with their mission and goals. Funding agencies want to know how their money will be used, so make sure you prepare a detailed budget that accounts for all your costs. For grants that are aimed at providing you with the training necessary to become an independent researcher, it's important to identify three or four specific training goals. You should explain why each goal is important for your professional development and what you will do to accomplish each one. Your research plan should have clearly stated specific aims and hypotheses. Including a timeline in your proposal can be helpful in clarifying how you will accomplish your goals and make use of research funds during the award period.

Feasibility is another key ingredient to funding success. Funding agencies want to know that you will be able to accomplish your goals within the award period, make a strong case for your project's feasibility. Explain how your participant enrollment, study procedures, and design all reflect your dedication to completing your project within the given award period. Try to identify and troubleshoot potential barriers to completion as you design your project. In your proposal, explicitly discuss these barriers and how you will handle them if they arise.

Although specificity and feasibility are critical to any successful grant proposal, it's also important to convey how your project fits into the broader picture. For training grant applications, you should explain how each of your specific training objectives will further your ultimate career goal of becoming an independent researcher. Be sure to convey the significance and public health implications of your research project. No matter how narrow the scope of your study, explain how the findings will address gaps in the research literature and improve the field's scientific understanding.

Another factor that can make you competitive for funding is showing that you have a supportive training environment. In your proposal, discuss any qualities of your institution that may facilitate your training or the completion of your project. This can include having access to an established pool of research subjects, unique didactic opportunities, or access to statistical support. It is also important to show that you have a mentor who has similar research interests, is invested in your training, and meets with you regularly. The following are some important tips to keep in mind throughout the grant writing process.

Tip 1: Plan ahead. Be aware of deadlines, and get started early. Make a detailed list of all requirements, and make sure that you know the specific application procedures and components for the particular agency, organization, or NIH institute to which you are applying. Come up with a detailed and realistic schedule for completing each piece of the application. If you don't budget sufficient time for each, it will show in your application—and some funding entities, such as the NIH, allow you to resubmit a proposal only one additional time.

Tip 2: Keep it simple. Try to be as clear and concise as possible. Your reviewers probably have busy schedules and a stack of applications to review, so make it easy for them to read and understand your project.

Tip 3: Pay attention to detail. Ensure proper use of grammar, and use spell check (and even then, look everything over yourself). As we noted, make sure that you know the specific application procedures/components for the particular agency, organization, or NIH institute to which you are applying. Show your reviewers that you have crossed every "t" and dotted every "i."

Tip 4: Seek out and use your resources. Get feedback from as many people as possible. Ask your mentor, faculty members within your institution, colleagues, lab mates, and friends to review your application. Your own institution may offer a special seminar in grant writing, or there may be a workshop at an annual conference. There are plenty of print and online resources available to help you to craft a winning proposal. We recommend *The Grant Application Writer's Workbook* (Robertson et al., 2020) and *Writing the NIH Grant Proposal: A Step-by-Step Guide* (Gerin et al., 2017).

Tip 5: Be patient, and don't get discouraged. It may take 2 years from the start of an idea to actual funding, and the success rate of some award and grant programs can be on the low side. Remember: The process is a marathon—not a sprint. Keep focused on your goals, and remind yourself that rejection and constructive criticism are just a part of the process.

CONCLUSION AND FUTURE DIRECTIONS

We hope this chapter gives you a better sense of what research awards and grants may be available to you at this point in your training. Obtaining funding or recognition for your research is a wonderful feeling and can be incredibly beneficial for a trainee. We also hope that you now feel a bit more confident in where you can find grant and award opportunities and how you can prepare a strong application. We know the application process can seem daunting, but remember that the difference between the impossible and possible lies in your determination.

REFERENCES

Gerin, W., Kinkade, C. K., & Page, N. L. (2017). *Writing the NIH grant proposal: A step-by-step guide* (3rd ed.). Sage.

National Institutes of Health. (2020a). *Find funding: The NIH guide for grants and contracts.* https://grants.nih.gov/funding/searchguide/index.html#

National Institutes of Health. (2020b). *How to apply: Application guide.* https://grants.nih.gov/grants/how-to-apply-application-guide.html

National Institutes of Health. (2020c). *Study sections.* https://public.csr.nih.gov/StudySections

National Institutes of Health Office of Extramural Research. (2020). *NIH Scientific Review Group (SRG) roster index.* https://public.era.nih.gov/pubroster/rosterIndex.era

National Institutes of Health Research Training and Career Development. (2020). *Research Career Development Awards.* https://researchtraining.nih.gov/programs/career-development

National Library of Medicine. (2014). *Grants and funding: Extramural programs. Frequently asked questions.* https://www.nlm.nih.gov/ep/FAQScores.html

Robertson, J. D., Russell, S. W., & Morrison, D. C. (2020). *The grant application writer's workbook.* National Institutes of Health.

14 ETHICS, LEGAL STANDARDS, AND POLICY IN NEUROPSYCHOLOGY

DEDE UKUEBERUWA, CHRISTOPHER NGUYEN, AND DANIEL TRANEL

Ethics appears in neuropsychology in broad issues that demonstrate professional values and affect daily decisions regarding the provision of neuropsychological services. Knowledge of ethics is a core competency for neuropsychologists across settings focused on clinical practice, research, forensics, disability management, and other arenas. Moreover, neuropsychologists may be particularly well positioned within health and science systems to address issues of identity; vulnerability; and individual differences in cognition, mood, and personality that can inform ethical questions involving conflicting values among persons, organizations, and society. Imagine that you are an early-career neuropsychologist who is transitioning into a new role: Over the past few years, your clinical practice has focused on work with older adult patients; you have conducted dementia and capacity evaluations in a group memory clinic and informed patients and families of cognitive impairments and potential changes in functional independence and decision-making capabilities. Now you will lead evaluations in a community-based clinic that receives a range of referrals across the life span, from pediatric to adult, with a range of diagnostic histories. What ethical responsibility do you have to establish competency within each role, and what resources are available

https://doi.org/10.1037/0000250-015
The Neuropsychologist's Roadmap: A Training and Career Guide, C. Block (Editor)

for learning about conducting ethical practices? In this chapter, we review in detail the current guidelines and issues most relevant to neuropsychologists, including interactions with patients and research participants, assessment procedures, and mentoring relationships. We also review the intersection of professional ethics with legal concepts that are of significance to neuropsychologists, including historic legal standards, forensic practice, and independent neuropsychological evaluations. We conclude by offering recommendations and resources for further learning.

ETHICAL DEFINITIONS AND THE AMERICAN PSYCHOLOGICAL ASSOCIATION'S *ETHICAL PRINCIPLES FOR PSYCHOLOGISTS AND CODE OF CONDUCT*

To understand how ethics will be a part of your everyday practice as a neuropsychologist, you will first need to understand how the word "ethics" is defined, as well as the key principles that organizations endorse as important for psychologists and neuropsychologists.

Important Definitions

One definition of "ethics" is a set of rules or guidelines for right or wrong conduct among people or groups (Deigh, 2010). In other words, ethics helps clarify how people should act in a given situation. In addition, ethics may describe the analysis of moral principles and dilemmas. For example, which principles and values receive priority over others, and how do you act when values are in conflict? Ethics is important to neuropsychology because, even in the most technical emphasis areas, this field concerns people's well-being (see Figure 14.1). Guidelines are developed with an understanding of ethics in order to display professional competencies, foster protection of the public from harm, and optimize neuropsychologists' contributions to society. If you become a licensed psychologist or a member of many professional organizations and institutions, you will need to engage in specific ethical practices, which we outline in this chapter. In some instances, engaging in ethical practice and making ethical decisions will have "bottom-line answers" with a clear course of action (Bush & Drexler, 2002). For example, the American Psychological Association (APA) and most licensing boards prohibit psychologists from having sexual relations with patients with whom they are in a therapeutic relationship (Standard 10.04, Sexual Intimacies With Current Therapy Clients/Patients, in *Ethical Principles of Psychologists and Code of Conduct*;

FIGURE 14.1. Professional Ethics in Neuropsychology

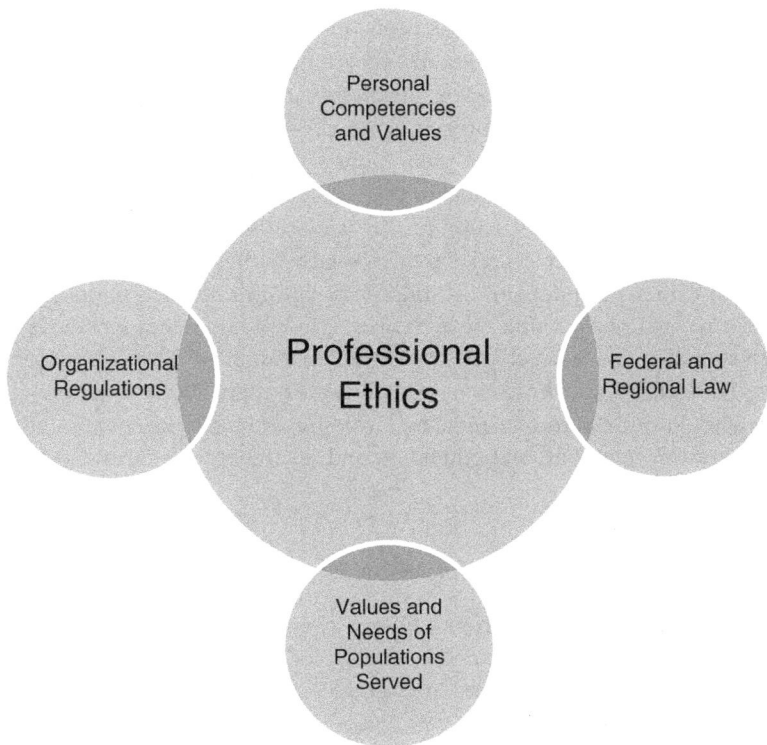

APA, 2017). Other ethical questions, though, have more ambiguous answers, and you will need to develop a process for determining how to act.

Ethical dilemmas occur when there is apparent conflict between ethical principles, personal and organizational ethics, ethics and laws, or other areas in which decision making has not been well defined. Psychologists often see various potential interactions with patients as falling in a gray area between clearly ethical and clearly not ethical, and thus they may benefit from an available model to help them work through such situations (Cottone, 2012). An ethical neuropsychologist may strive to optimize the needs of patients, requirements of law, and advancement of professional competencies. In this chapter, we discuss in detail the professional ethics and processes for resolving ethical dilemmas across clinical, research, and community contexts.

Ethical practice may involve a combination of rule following of required laws and professional guidelines along with a *positive* approach to best practices. In the opening example, you are a neuropsychologist transitioning to a broad community practice and may wish to promote a range of services that meet the highest standard of care available in the area. Here, "positive ethics" describes the process of conscious decision making about professional and personal behavior in order to actualize core values and improve the welfare of the patients in one's care as well as people in the larger society (Handelsman et al., 2002). This positive approach to ethical decision making is in contrast to *preventive* (negative) ethics (see Table 14.1), which comprises ethical behavior based on meeting professional expectations, avoiding harm to others, and preventing disciplinary action for rule violations. Neuropsychologists use both positive and negative/preventive approaches to ethical practice, and the choice of either may depend on individual values and situational factors. In order to facilitate making these choices, ethics scholars in psychology and neuropsychology have developed several models and flow charts for reasoning through ethical decision making (e.g., Johnson-Greene, 2005). Neuropsychologists should anticipate and plan for avoiding or resolving possible ethical challenges through continual education and awareness of ethics and how it applies to their specialty.

Know the Code: The APA *Ethical Principles of Psychologists and Code of Conduct*

Appropriate expertise in neuropsychology is a fundamental ethical issue in clinical practice, research, and the training of others, and it thus remains relevant to students and professionals at all levels as their roles and responsibilities continuously unfold. APA's *Ethical Principles for Psychologists and Code of Conduct* (2017) is a foundation of ethical practice of psychology in the United States. Commonly referred to as the "Ethics Code," this set of principles and standards applies to APA members and forms a guideline for all psychologists. The Ethics Code begins with the Preamble and General Principles (a set of aspirational goals) and then delineates a list of enforceable rules in the form of the Ethical Standards. The Ethics Code undergoes periodic revisions and updates according to an evolving understanding of the values and responsibilities of psychologists. In the current Ethics Code the Principles are as follows: (A) Beneficence and Maleficence, (B) Fidelity and Responsibility, (C) Integrity,

TABLE 14.1. Examples of Positive and Preventive Ethics for Neuropsychologists

Positive ethics	Preventive ethics
Culturally competent assessment practices	Mandated reporting of abuse
Evaluating and informing patients' goals	Keeping protected health information confidential according to federal law
Reflecting on core values and correcting biases	Meeting licensing board requirements

(D) Justice, and (E) Respect for People's Rights and Dignity. Readers located outside of the United States are encouraged to carefully review the details of their regional psychology organization's ethics code or guidelines for professional conduct.

Although the Ethics Code addresses many important aspects of professionalism, it frequently does not provide black-and-white guidelines on all matters that may arise for neuropsychologists. The Ethics Code also allows for professional discretion as well as the use of preventive or positive ethical principles. Although personal morals do not always lead to the best decisions, discarding them altogether is not entirely appropriate or even feasible (Handelsman et al., 2002). Ethical practice as a neuropsychologist will be an ongoing process of refinement throughout your career. You are encouraged to review the Ethics Code, as well as the recommendations for further education we discuss later in this chapter.

ETHICAL CONCEPTS IN NEUROPSYCHOLOGY

Ethics Regarding Clinical Patients and Research Participants

Ethical practice applies to work across different settings. The Ethics Code outlines standards and guidelines for practice that are expected to protect clinical patients, research participants, health care providers and systems, and society as a whole. In this section, we review these guidelines and highlight some tips for maintaining an ethics-informed neuropsychology practice.

Working With Patients, Participants, and the Public

Neuropsychologists are experts in the assessment of brain–behavior relationships; however, meeting the basic training requirements in neuropsychology or obtaining a professional psychology license does not imply that neuropsychologists are automatically competent in all areas of practice or research. Like all scientists, neuropsychologists must conduct an examination or consider appropriate evidence before drawing a conclusion. In the example in which you are a neuropsychologist transitioning to a community-based life span practice, you will need expertise in development, and the conducting of comprehensive evaluations, and an understanding of the cultural characteristics of the new community. In general, ethical practice involves considering possible ethical challenges and seeking necessary consultation when embarking on a new area of professional activity. Ethical issues also arise when neuropsychologists engage in activities outside clinical and research domains.

Tip 1: Refrain from making "armchair diagnoses." With the public and the media's rapidly increasing interest in neuropsychology topics, neuropsychologists should understand their role as experts. They should take particular care in regard to communications about diagnoses and ensure those communications are informed and based on solid evidence.

Tip 2: Clarify your role on public and social media. When commenting on public platforms or social media, neuropsychologists should clarify when there is no direct psychologist–patient relationship and ensure the public knows they are speaking with reference to general psychological information or publicly available data (APA, 2008).

Confidentiality

Maintaining confidentiality, or the limiting of information disclosed to third parties, provides important protections to patients' rights to privacy, test security, and avoiding misuse by nonexperts. Both the Principles and Standards of the APA Ethics Code review confidentiality as it cuts across multiple professional domains, including informed consent, managing risk, test data disclosure, and communication with third parties. Although confidentiality is a cornerstone of neuropsychological services, the public may not be aware that this privacy is not absolute. Public laws govern the specific details of when a psychologist must breach confidentiality, such as the mandated reporting of child abuse or threats of harm to self or others.

Tip 3: Be familiar with the mandated-reporting procedures for child abuse in your state. You can bookmark the procedures for your region on your computer so you will be ready if and when a situation arises (see, e.g., Child Welfare Information Gateway, 2019).

Informed Consent

Standard 3.10, Informed Consent, of the APA Ethics Code indicates that information pertinent to informed consent be provided as early as possible to a patient, and additional information may need to be reviewed or shared at multiple points throughout the provision of service. The Ethics Code contains explicit guidelines for *informed consent* in neuropsychology. Informed consent applies across many different professional activities of neuropsychologists who are providing a service to a patient, research participant, or legal representative of the person receiving the service. Informed consent involves a discussion between the neuropsychologist and another party (e.g., patient or participant) regarding the nature and process of the professional activity, uses of the data, billing practices, and confidentiality. In addition, neuropsychologists must obtain permission from the patient before audio- or video-recording any part of the service. It is important to recognize that informed consent is a process. Initial informed consent should be addressed at the outset of the service and must be obtained for most types of professional work across clinical and research settings that involve work with patients or participants. Exceptions include when the neuropsychological service is mandated by a judge. Neuropsychologists are also expected to encourage questions and provide responses in "reasonably understandable" language. This means that ethical neuropsychologists are thoughtful in their communication with patients and avoid complex professional jargon when explaining the evaluation; consent in the patient's primary language is preferred. You will need to take additional care when working with people who may have reduced decision-making capacity (i.e., probable dementia, delirium, intellectual disability) or when using language interpreters. Obtaining written consent will help you and the patient or participant thoroughly review expectations and maintain a record, and some employers may require neuropsychologist employees to obtain written consent from each patient. Nevertheless, oral consent may be appropriate in some settings when a person has difficulty providing a written response, such as in an inpatient hospital service.

Tip 4: Write an informed-consent document to clarify expectations for the neuropsychologist, the patient, and the procedures. You can then tailor use of the document to your particular setting and population. A publication by Johnson-Greene (2005) contains a flow chart for obtaining informed consent within neuropsychology practice.

In contrast to consent, *assent* occurs when a person agrees to receive an evaluation but cannot legally provide informed consent. For example, obtaining assent is appropriate for forensic evaluations or as part of routine educational or organizational practices (Johnson-Greene, 2005). Children are also presumed included under the category of people who are legally incapable of consent under most circumstances, and neuropsychologists must then obtain informed consent from a legal representative. Neuropsychologists working with minors should seek further information regarding best practices for obtaining assent and coordinating services with the parents. You may wish to use probing questions with the patient during the assent process in order to ascertain their level of comprehension of the planned service, such as asking them why they are taking part in a particular service and what they hope to take away from it.

Interpersonal Relations

Although the Ethics Code allows for professional discretion in the General Principles, the code also delineates 10 sections of Ethical Standards that are mandatory. Neuropsychologists are ethically bound to the same guidelines as all psychologists regarding avoidance of sexual contact and romantic relationships with current and former patients. *Any* physical, verbal, or nonverbal harassment that occurs in your role as a neuropsychologist is professionally unethical (Standards 3.01–3.04). Neuropsychologists are to avoid harm and the infliction of pain and suffering, and they are encouraged to follow institutional and legal guidelines specific to their practice or region. They may also encounter other relational situations that can lead to ethical dilemmas, such as when they form dual or multiple relationships with a patient—that is, interacting with a person both in a professional role and in another role outside of that (see Standards 10.04–10.08). For example, a neuropsychologist may serve on a parent–teacher association committee for a child's school and then find that a patient is also a parent on the same committee. Multiple relationships are not always unethical, but neuropsychologists should avoid entering into multiple relationships when they can because such relationships can contribute to bias, exploitation, or a conflict of interest (e.g., undue influence) that affects their ability to competently provide their services. This includes entering into a professional relationship with relatives or significant others.

Tip 5: Consult with other professionals when you feel unsure about a relationship conflict. The nuances of multiple relationships can be one of the most challenging and yet most common ethical concerns that arises for psychologists.

Safety and Risk Management

When providing neuropsychology services, you will need to take steps to ensure the safety of your patients, your practice, and the public. These steps will form your risk management strategy to minimize harm and optimize protection for you and others. Some aspects of risk management include maintaining confidentiality of patient information, developing an infection-control protocol for your office setting, or preparing for an emergency should your patient fall ill (e.g., has a seizure).

Maintaining confidentiality is a particularly central feature of ethical practice and risk management for neuropsychologists. At the same time, many neuropsychologists may have reasonable difficulty understanding when it may be necessary to breach confidentiality. When weighing such a breach, you may wish to start by considering which parties are at risk, such as the patient or a third party child or adult. You should be familiar with the case of *Tarasoff v. The Regents of the University of California* (1976), in which a student at the University of California, Berkeley, disclosed plans to kill another student to a psychologist he was seeing for psychotherapy. The psychologist reported the threat to the police but did not make attempts to contact the victim. The case led to a ruling indicating a *duty to warn* potential victims of a patient's credible and serious threat of harm. Additional rulings have further defined a duty to protect and have specified other details regarding expectations for psychologists in managing risk (Fulero, 1988). It is important to know that codification of these details into law varies regionally, and psychologists are expected to be familiar with the laws of their region. Although the duty-to-warn laws were born in the context of psychotherapy, they apply to neuropsychologists who are licensed psychologists in applicable states.

Tip 6: Remember, neuropsychologists protect patients and the public! Because neuropsychologists frequently obtain sensitive personal information from patients, they are mandated reporters. You may encounter a scenario in which you have learned of a patient's threats of violence, or of situations of child or elder abuse. You must then take reasonable steps to protect the patient or possible victim in accordance with the law.

Diversity and Culture Competency

As members of a person-oriented profession, neuropsychologists are tasked with developing competency with regard to diversity and culture. The Houston Conference Guidelines (Hannay et al., 1998) emphasize that clinical trainees should acquire knowledge regarding "cultural and individual differences and diversity" from their core of knowledge of general psychology and acquire clinical skills that recognize multicultural issues involved in assessment, treatment, and interventions. These guidelines suggest that clinical neuropsychologists providing services to culturally and linguistically diverse populations should have both the knowledge and skills to practice ethically and competently.

Tip 7: Across settings in which you train and work, you will need to develop cultural knowledge of and competence for interactions with a diversity of patients, participants, students, and professionals. Chapter 15 of this volume provides an overview of professional guidelines and ethical standards concerning neuropsychological services among culturally and linguistically diverse patients.

Assessment Procedures

Neuropsychologists provide assessments within their "boundaries of competence," with "competence" broadly defined as the skill and experience to undertake a task (Nagy, 2010). This undertaking requires a realistic assessment of your own strengths and weaknesses as well as a willingness to learn when faced with new tasks or expanding into a less well-developed area.

Tip 8: Obtain more interactive, didactic experiences (e.g., classroom, direct supervision, consultation) when learning a completely new area; independent study may be sufficient when fine tuning knowledge (Nagy, 2010). For example, reflection about your competence is recommended for the following assessment activities: working across cultural groups, ages, or developmental stages; making medical or psychological diagnoses; administering individual tests; and using various testing modalities (e.g., in person, telehealth). The Ethics Code states that psychologists must use reliable and appropriate assessment tools (Standard 9.02, Use of Assessments); more specifically, neuropsychologists should use tests that have established reliability, validity, and administration procedures, with a minimal risk of bias from unstandardized influences, such as environmental distractions during administration or a lack of culturally appropriate tools. These properties are also necessary for any tests the neuropsychologist develops or alters. Thus, this Standard indicates the need for careful development of neuropsychological tests that are appropriate for different populations, including those with varied cultural and linguistic characteristics.

Working With Technicians

Ethically competent neuropsychological practice extends to the conduct of staff under your management. Puente et al. (2006) supported inclusion of technicians in neuropsychology practice. By 2000, a majority of neuropsychologists employed technicians, that is, nonlicensed and/or non–doctoral level individuals who administer neuropsychological and psychological tests. The National Academy of Neuropsychology Policy and Planning Committee (2000) published a position statement affirming that neuropsychologists can supervise technicians and outlined recommendations for working with technicians in order to ensure standardized, unbiased, and efficient data collection. The VA also acknowledged and outlined the ethical use of technicians. These policies deemed ethical the use of well-trained technicians for the standardized administration of tests (Puente et al., 2006).

Tip 9: Review ethical standards with your staff and team members. Neuropsychologists supervising technicians are expected to ensure that their employees practice in an ethical manner.

Ethics Regarding Data and Reporting

Thus far, we have discussed ethical concepts as they pertain to the interactions of neuropsychologists and other people. In order to establish brain–behavior relationships, neuropsychologists collect, integrate, and describe data. You will need to attain competency in these areas to maintain an ethical neuropsychological practice and minimize ethical conflicts. We now review competency in data interpretation, appropriate disclosure of test and patient data, and maintaining security of test materials.

Qualifications to Interpret Data

When using outside test interpretation services, including automated scoring programs, the neuropsychologist remains responsible for the appropriate use of the information and the validity of the interpretation, and thus they rely on the competency they have gained in these areas. Neuropsychologists should consider all of the factors that can influence the assessment and results, including both patient and contextual information gained from medical records, clinical interview, and details about all the tests administered. Any significant limitations of test interpretation of which they are aware, such as deviations from standardized testing instructions and procedures, must be discussed with the patient, client, or referral source. After an evaluation, an explanation of the results should be given to the patient or the patient's representative, unless there are specific reasons prohibiting this, such as with a court-ordered evaluation.

Disclosure of Test Data

In addition to a patient's raw and scaled scores, professional test data include the neuropsychologist's notes, recordings and response records, reports, and test materials (e.g., stimuli, manuals). Neuropsychologists normally provide reports to patients, and patients typically have the prerogative to access reports in their own medical records. The extent to which actual test scores beyond the neuropsychologist's interpretation are included in reports is highly variable in the field, with some neuropsychologists including few scores and others providing a full summary of all scores (often included with the report as an appendix). Under Standard 9.04, Release of Test Data, psychologists may limit release of test scores to prevent harm to a patient, such as when the neuropsychologist has reason to believe that the patient may misinterpret or misunderstand test scores. For example, IQ scores may not be well understood by the general public and are especially vulnerable to such misinterpretation. Moreover, federal and state laws may further regulate the practice of releasing test scores and other raw data, such as when laws require adherence to the Ethics Code. As we have noted, the Ethics Code prohibits release of raw data to protect the patient's best interests (Tranel, 1994). In addition to patients, other people may request raw data—including attorneys, judges, and non-professional persons with a relation to the patient (e.g., family or guardian). This scenario frequently occurs in the context of legal cases brought by a plaintiff with an alleged brain injury, and legal concepts are further discussed in the Legal Concepts in Neuropsychology section.

Test Security

In addition to safeguarding test scores, neuropsychologists should maintain the integrity and security of all test materials, including manuals, protocols, and stimuli, in accordance with licensing contracts and relevant copyright laws. Problems may arise if test materials enter the public domain (Tranel,

1994) because of potential for interpretation of tests by unqualified persons and effects of prior exposure on the validity of some tests. In general, neuro-psychologists should not allow patients or third parties to audio- or video-record an evaluation and may wish to provide explicit guidelines with regard to recording feedback sessions. When administering tests electronically, neuro-psychologists should password-protect software, encrypt data, and limit access to other materials on the device. The growing availability of test materials online presents a particular challenge for neuropsychologists and stake-holders in test development and licensing given the widespread public access it entails. Copyright holders in the United States can take action by issuing a "take-down notice" to the internet service provider for the host site, and concerned neuropsychologists can send alerts to copyright holders when they become aware of potential breaches. Other tests are made publicly available by the owner or no longer have copyright restrictions, and many of these tests are now commonly shared via digital platforms. Neuropsychologists can take opportunities to communicate with the public regarding responsible use of these tests.

HIPAA and Billing Practices

As a neuropsychologist, you will have to comply with public laws that govern health services. The Health Insurance Portability and Accountability Act of 1996 (HIPAA) is a federal law that set national standards for securing health information and electronic health care transactions (U.S. Department of Health and Human Services, 2017). Updated rules about specific topics, including the privacy and security of protected health information, have since been published.

Neuropsychologists in clinical practice are expected to communicate with patients regarding competing interests between service to patients and the impact of billing reimbursement methods. For example, neuropsychologists can clarify a range of costs and any restrictions on services set by managed care organizations. Education regarding any new updates to the existing laws will be a necessary part of ensuring your neuropsychology practice remains in compliance and addresses areas of potential ethical conflict. Continuing education modules are available through the U.S. Department of Health and Human Services and other organizations.

Ethics Regarding Professional Development

Ethics competency in neuropsychology begins at the training level and will continue throughout your career. In this section, we discuss opportunities for the development of ethics competency within mentor and supervisor relationships and individual reflective practice, which is followed by a review of procedures for resolving ethical problems.

Mentorship and Supervision

As Stucky et al. (2010) noted, supervision is a central component of neuropsychology training and encompasses the teaching of a variety of skills, such as assessment, report writing, differential diagnosis, and treatment. However, these authors noted that "clinical competence does not equal supervisory competence and neuropsychology trainees and practicing clinicians who are considering or are new to supervisory roles must develop supervisory skills" (p.755). Although APA (2006) recommends clinical supervision as a core competency area for all psychologists, functional competency in teaching and supervision is a core domain in the training of clinical neuropsychologists (Smith, 2018). Thus, ethical neuropsychology supervision involves developing competency in appropriate supervision methods with respect to the supervisee and the service. A proposed model for neuropsychological supervision includes an individually tailored, process-based, developmental approach that engages with the supervisee at their level of professional development and provides graded responsibility (Stucky et al., 2010).

Reflective Practice and Self-Care

Use of ethical decision-making models may work best when professionals engage in reflective practice and commit to following ethical professional principles (Tjeltveit & Gottlieb, 2010). For example, paying attention to the social impact of your work may reorient the focus of your research. In addition, effective self-care practices may contribute to awareness of ethical behavior, clarification of values, and reduction of biases in professional judgment. Self-care could involve balancing your workload and personal life, developing strong social and professional networks, seeking and accepting help from other psychologists when needed, and offering help to others when appropriate. Handelsman et al. (2002) prudently stated, "In an era of regulation, managed care, litigation, and rapidly expanding opportunities and pitfalls, keeping our eyes on our own values may be especially difficult, but it is also more necessary" (p. 735).

Resolving Ethical Problems

Recognizing when ethical dilemmas are occurring and how to resolve them will be an important aspect of your professional work. Possible cues that an ethical problem has arisen include when a situation does not personally feel right, when receiving conflicting information from other professionals, or when someone has lodged a complaint. According to APA (2017),

> If psychologists' ethical responsibilities conflict with law, regulations, or other governing legal authority, psychologists clarify the nature of the conflict, make known their commitment to the Ethics Code, and take reasonable steps to resolve the conflict consistent with the General Principles and Ethical Standards of the Ethics Code. (Standard 1.02, Conflicts Between Ethics and Law, Regulations, or Other Governing Legal Authority)

Resolution of ethical issues may be a formal or informal process. Neuropsychologists can work independently or directly with colleagues to resolve minor ethical issues that occur, given that there is no risk of breaching confidentiality. For example, you may consult with colleagues regarding test selection for particular populations or for advisement on potential conflicts of interest in professional ventures. When necessary and appropriate, ethical violations (i.e., sexual misconduct, insurance fraud, plagiarism, and other violations of Ethics Code standards) can be referred to state and national ethics committees, and to state and provincial licensing boards, as well as to authorities for legal violations. When reporting an ethics violation, always prioritize patient confidentiality.

LEGAL CONCEPTS IN NEUROPSYCHOLOGY

A need to carefully consider ethical practice and resolve ethical conflicts is of particular importance for neuropsychologists working at the interface of health care and the legal system. Neuropsychologists have become increasingly involved in civil and criminal settings over the past decade (Kaufmann, 2016) and are increasingly being asked to provide expert opinions regarding cognitive and behavioral changes that could potentially indicate brain dysfunction after an injury sustained through the course of employment (i.e., a compensable injury) or in an accident (i.e., a motor vehicle crash or a slip and fall) where another party is at fault, as well as in civil actions or criminal proceedings. In this section we discuss several relevant legal concepts in neuropsychology (see Table 14.2).

Legal Standards

A number of historic legal standards pertinent to neuropsychology have been established. *Jenkins v. United States* (1962) established the precedent that psychologists who have proper training can be recognized in legal proceedings

TABLE 14.2. Key Legal Terms and Definitions

Term	Definition
Fact witness	Provides testimony regarding a direct assessment of a patient
Expert witness	Provides an opinion based on expertise of the subject
Capacity	A clinical status as determined by a clinician
Competency	A legal capacity to make certain decisions or perform certain acts, as determined by a judge
Independent neuropsychological evaluation	Evaluation of an individual completed by a neuropsychologist who has been retained by a third party; no doctor–patient relationship is established

as experts in diagnosing mental disorders (Packer, 2008). Psychologists, and neuropsychologists, are now almost universally accepted as potential expert witnesses in legal proceedings.

In regard to expert testimony, *Frye v. United States* (1923) established a "general acceptance" standard indicating that an expert's knowledge base and methods should be consistent with accepted clinical and scientific standards (DeMatteo et al., 2009). In addition, *Daubert v. Merrell Dow Pharmaceuticals* (1993) provided a set of factors for the court to make the determination regarding general acceptance of and admission into court testimony; in federal courts and certain states, the *Daubert* standard has replaced the *Frye* standard. General legal rules also govern the admissibility of testimony as evidence. For example, court testimony must limit hearsay and reports of statements made by a defendant that are not directly related to the introduced issue (e.g., brain dysfunction or mental health). Legal standards may also affect how neuropsychologists conduct their services. For example, you could provide advance disclosure to patients that an examination is being performed for a specific forensic purpose and is not meant to establish a doctor–patient relationship or lead to recommendations for treatment. Certain states require that psychology professionals obtain board certification before beginning to conduct forensic evaluations (DeMatteo et al., 2009).

Informed Consent in Legal Context

In clinical practice, informed consent is provided by the patient or their legal representative, but in some forensic contexts, such as when the evaluation is court ordered, this may not be required. However, neuropsychologists are expected to obtain assent from an individual by providing verbal or written documents that detail the purpose and scope of the evaluation (Fisher et al.,

2002). Nevertheless, people undergoing forensic evaluations may be precluded from receiving test results because the routine clinical (i.e., doctor–patient) relationship does not exist in this context (Johnson-Greene, 2005).

Types of Witnesses: Fact Witness Versus Expert Witness

Neuropsychologists are increasingly being asked to provide in civil actions or criminal proceedings expert opinions regarding cognitive and behavioral changes that potentially indicate brain dysfunction after compensable injuries. When a neuropsychologist evaluates a patient for the purpose of providing treatment or establishing a treatment plan, they often are referred to in the legal context as a *treating provider*. A neuropsychologist may become a *fact witness* if subpoenaed to testify about an evaluation they have conducted. As a fact witness, a neuropsychologist must limit their testimony to what they have personally observed from the assessment procedures, or to what is the accepted standard of care for relying on the observations of others (e.g., technicians).

When a neuropsychologist is retained to serve as a consultant and/or expert witness, they are generally referred to as an "expert." An *expert witness* is retained to render opinions regarding diagnosis, prognosis, or other issues to provide the court with information that may lie outside the common knowledge of the judge or jury. In contrast to a fact witness, a neuropsychologist expert witness would provide an opinion based on their expertise on the subject. These testimonies may occur in a deposition or at trial.

Capacity and Competency Evaluations

As health care experts in human cognition, neuropsychologists are uniquely qualified to participate in capacity and competency evaluations. The terms "capacity" and "competency" are often used interchangeably in clinical practice, but they actually have somewhat different meanings. Capacity has been conceptualized as *a clinical status as determined by the clinician* as to whether a person can perform a specific task (e.g., engagement in instrumental activities of daily living) or make a specific decision (e.g., opting to decline a medical procedure, changing a will; Moye & Marson, 2007).

Competency is a *legal construct established and governed by the courts* and refers to an individual's *legal capacity to make certain decisions or perform certain acts* (Moberg & Rick, 2008). Earlier in this chapter, we discussed neuropsychologists' competency as it pertains to engaging in professional activities. Here we refer to competency as a legal concept that applies to persons involved in legal proceedings. In a clinical context, a neuropsychologist may make a determination as to whether the person is capable of performing activities of daily living (e.g., medication and financial management, driving, independent living) or carrying out specific acts (e.g., consenting to medical procedures, entering into legal contracts). Competency rulings are also relevant in civil and criminal contexts; specifically, a decision about legal competency is made by a judge in regard to a person's ability to stand trial, waive Miranda rights, and bear the burden of criminal responsibility (e.g., being not guilty by reason of insanity; Moberg & Kniele, 2006). Such determinations can be highly influenced by results from a neuropsychological assessment.

Decisional agency, or *decision-making capacity*, is an element of competency (Moberg & Rick, 2008). When an illness or injury prevents a person from making decisions about financial, medical, or other personal matters, several legal authorizations can be designated to assist in these affairs. For example, *power of attorney* is a court-ordered authorization for an individual to act on another's behalf in a legal or business matter. *Guardianship* occurs when a court appoints one person to make health care and other nonmonetary decisions for another person, and *conservatorship* lends authorization for financial management. For illustrative case samples, review Kaufmann (2016), who provided a thorough discussion on the role of neuropsychologists in competency and capacity evaluations.

Independent Neuropsychological Evaluations

An *independent neuropsychological evaluation* (INE) refers to an evaluation in which a neuropsychologist is retained by a third party and in which no doctor–patient relationship is established.[1] Referrals for INEs typically come from an attorney, workers' compensation, public defender, or case manager, with the dual goals of (a) establishing whether the patient has anything wrong with them, from a neuropsychological perspective and (b) determining whether any such neuropsychological "injuries" were caused by the accident in question. An INE typically reaches a conclusion regarding "damages" (e.g., injuries) and causation (e.g., whether the accident caused the damages), and the neuropsychologist is typically asked to provide such opinions with a reasonable degree of neuropsychological certainty, in accordance with standard medical–legal practice.

---

[1] The term "INE" is adapted from medical practice, where the term "independent medical exam" [IME] is the coin of the realm. In fact, the term "IME" is used commonly to cover independent neuropsychological evaluations, too, even though the "INE" term is more precise.

ETHICS AND FORENSIC EDUCATION AND TRAINING

APA and the Canadian Psychological Association both require coursework in ethics for doctoral training programs in clinical psychology seeking to be accredited, and all students planning to practice within psychology are expected to develop competency in ethics. The Association of State and Provincial Psychology Boards is an alliance of the agencies in the United States and Canada that regulate professional licensure and certification of psychologists. The board administers the Examination for Professional Practice in Psychology (EPPP), an entry-level assessment required for licensure. In the current format (also known as "EPPP Part 1"), the exam includes knowledge of ethics within the breadth of psychology content, including topics covered in this chapter. In Part 2 of the EPPP, which is currently under development, examinees will undergo skill-based assessment, such as competency in ethical practices— the "how" of ethical practice rather than simply the "what" as tapped by the EPPP Part 1.

In addition to the EPPP, several state and provincial boards require a jurisprudence exam that covers federal and regional laws and ethics topics. Many psychology boards also require continuing education in ethics. Chapter 4 in this book provides further detail regarding licensing requirements to practice as a psychologist. For additional information regarding ethics training, or for resolution of ethics questions, consultation can be sought with a professional organizing body, such as the APA Ethics Office, the Society for Clinical Neuropsychology (APA Division 40) Ethics Subcommittee, state/provincial psychological associations, licensing boards, or institutional review boards and ethics services (see Table 14.3).

Neuropsychologists engaging in forensic and legal activities must attain additional skills beyond common clinical practice; specifically, additional education and training are necessary to become knowledgeable about the various court systems and legal proceedings, essential information regarding civil and criminal settings, jurisdictional guidelines, differences between burden

TABLE 14.3. Resources for Ethics Information and Consultation for Neuropsychologists

Organization	Website
APA Ethics Office	https://www.apa.org/ethics
APA Society for Clinical Neuropsychology, Public Interest Advisory Committee, Ethics Subcommittee	https://www.scn40.org/piac-es
Association of State and Provincial Psychology Boards	https://www.asppb.net/

Note. You may also consider contacting your particular state's psychology board. APA = American Psychological Association.

and standards of proof, potential outcomes, and trial procedures (Richards & Tussey, 2013). In addition, neuropsychologists providing services in these roles should have an understanding of the differences between court procedures in state and federal jurisdictions and a familiarity with seminal cases involving mental health law, as well as other unique issues, such as informed consent, contents of a forensic report, and reimbursement and profession fees (Leonard, 2015). Further primers on relevant court settings, ethical standards and guidelines, and other recommendations have been illustrated in specialized books (e.g., Richards & Tussey, 2013).

The important conclusion here is that forensic neuropsychological work is likely to call on skill sets and knowledge bases that go beyond what is normally acquired in the course of a clinical neuropsychologist's education and practice, and it is the neuropsychologist's responsibility to acquire the pertinent skill sets and knowledge before venturing into the forensic arena. Interactions with the legal system in the forensic arena and the occurrence of complex ethical questions make it all the more important for ethical neuropsychologists in that setting to be fully educated on relevant information. In addition to neuropsychology specialty organizations, guidelines and resources for training are available through the American Psychology–Law Society (APA Division 41; https://www.apa.org/about/division/div41) and American Academy of Forensic Psychology (https://aafpforensic.org/).

CONCLUSION AND FUTURE DIRECTIONS

Ethical neuropsychologists work to provide the highest standard of care and professionalism, identify· ethical conflicts, and resolve ethical issues. Ethical practice also allows space for professional judgment, values, and personality. Guidelines for ethical neuropsychology broadly apply to working with various people across the life span in health care, research, school, athletics, community, military/veteran, industry, and forensic settings. The nature of the practice and the setting may dictate the types of ethical issues neuropsychologists are most likely to face, and they should seek further education in areas of relevance to a particular professional role or case. Career transitions, when you are embarking on activities in a new area, are often appropriate times for reflection on ethical practice. As in other domains of neuropsychology, learning and developing competency in ethics continues when you leave the classroom and enter the professional world. Although challenges and stumbles will occur, seeking consultation may provide insight into limitations regarding a particular case or activity and prompt further education. Open discussion and exploration of ethics are encouraged.

REFERENCES

American Psychological Association. (2006, October). *Final report of the APA Task Force on the Assessment of Competence in Professional Psychology.* https://www.apa.org/ed/resources/competence-report

American Psychological Association. (2008). Reflections on media ethics for psychologists. *Monitor on Psychology, 39*(4), 46. https://www.apa.org/monitor/2008/04/ethics

American Psychological Association. (2017). *Ethical principles of psychologists and code of conduct* (2002, Amended June 1, 2010, and January 1, 2017). https://www.apa.org/ethics/code/ethics-code-2017.pdf

Bush, S. S., & Drexler, M. I. (Eds.). (2002). *Ethical issues in clinical neuropsychology.* Swets & Zeitlinger.

Child Welfare Information Gateway. (2019). *Mandatory reporters of child abuse and neglect.* https://www.childwelfare.gov/topics/systemwide/laws-policies/statutes/manda/

Cottone, R. R. (2012). Ethical decision making in mental health contexts: Representative models and an organizational framework. In S. J. Knapp, M. C. Gottlieb, M. M. Handelsman, & L. D. VandeCreek (Eds.), *APA handbook of ethics in psychology, Vol. 1. Moral foundations and common themes* (pp. 99–121). American Psychological Association.

Daubert v. Merrell Dow Pharmaceuticals, Inc., 509 U.S. 579 (1993). https://supreme.justia.com/cases/federal/us/509/579/

Deigh, J. (2010). *An introduction to ethics.* Cambridge University Press.

DeMatteo, D., Marczyk, G., Krauss, D. A., & Burl, J. (2009). Educational and training models in forensic psychology. *Training and Education in Professional Psychology, 3*(3), 184–191. https://doi.org/10.1037/a0014582

Fisher, J. M., Johnson-Greene, D., & Barth, J. T. (2002). Examination, diagnosis, and interventions in clinical neuropsychology in general and with special populations: An overview. In S. S. Bush & M. L. Drexler (Eds.), *Ethical issues in clinical neuropsychology* (pp. 3–22). Swets & Zeitlinger.

Frye v. United States, 293 F. 1013 (D.C. Cir. 1923). https://casetext.com/case/frye-v-united-states-7

Fulero, S. M. (1988). *Tarasoff*: 10 years later. *Professional Psychology: Research and Practice, 19*(2), 184–190. https://doi.org/10.1037/0735-7028.19.2.184

Handelsman, M. M., Knapp, S., & Gottlieb, M. C. (2002). Positive ethics. In S. J. Lopez & C. R. Snyder (Eds.), *Handbook of positive psychology* (pp. 731–744). Oxford University Press.

Hannay, H. J., Bieliauskas, L. A., Crosson, B. A., Hammeke, T. A., & Hamsher, K. (1998). The Houston Conference on Specialty Education and Training in Clinical Neuropsychology. *Archives of Clinical Neuropsychology, 13*(2), 160–166. https://doi.org/10.1093/arclin/13.2.160

Health Insurance Portability and Accountability Act of 1996, Pub. L. 104-191, 42 U.S.C. § 300gg, 29 U.S.C. §§ 1181–1183, and 42 U.S.C. §§ 1320d–1320d9

Jenkins v. United States, 307 F. 2d 637 (1962). https://casetext.com/case/jenkins-v-united-states-17

Johnson-Greene, D. (2005). Informed consent in clinical neuropsychology practice: Official statement of the National Academy of Neuropsychology. *Archives of Clinical Neuropsychology, 20*(3), 335–340. https://doi.org/10.1016/j.acn.2004.08.003

Kaufmann, P. M. (2016). Neuropsychologist experts and civil capacity evaluations: Representative cases. *Archives of Clinical Neuropsychology, 31*(6), 487–494. https://doi.org/10.1093/arclin/acw053

Leonard, E. L. (2015). Forensic neuropsychology and expert witness testimony: An overview of forensic practice. *International Journal of Law and Psychiatry, 42–43*, 177–182. https://doi.org/10.1016/j.ijlp.2015.08.023

Moberg, P. J., & Kniele, K. (2006). Evaluation of competency: Ethical considerations for neuropsychologists. *Applied Neuropsychology, 13*(2), 101–114. https://doi.org/10.1207/s15324826an1302_5

Moberg, P. J., & Rick, J. H. (2008). Decision-making capacity and competency in the elderly: A clinical and neuropsychological perspective. *NeuroRehabilitation, 23*(5), 403–413. https://doi.org/10.3233/NRE-2008-23504

Moye, J., & Marson, D. C. (2007). Assessment of decision-making capacity in older adults: An emerging area of practice and research. *The Journals of Gerontology: Series B, Psychological Sciences and Social Sciences, 62*(1), P3–P11. https://doi.org/10.1093/geronb/62.1.P3

Nagy, T. F. (2010). *Essential ethics for psychologists: A primer in understanding and mastering core issues.* American Psychological Association.

National Academy of Neuropsychology Policy and Planning Committee. (2000). The use of neuropsychology test technicians in clinical practice: Official Statement of the National Academy of Neuropsychology. *Archives of Clinical Neuropsychology, 15*(5), 381–382.

Packer, I. K. (2008). Specialized practice in forensic psychology: Opportunities and obstacles. *Professional Psychology: Research and Practice, 39*(2), 245–249. https://doi.org/10.1037/0735-7028.39.2.245

Puente, A. E., Adams, R., Barr, W. B., Bush, S. S., Ruff, R. M., Barth, J. T., Broshek, D., Koffler, S. P., Reynolds, C., Silver, C. H., Tröster, A. I., The NAN Policy and Planning Committee, & The National Academy of Neuropsychology. (2006). The use, education, training and supervision of neuropsychological test technicians (psychometrists) in clinical practice: Official statement of the National Academy of Neuropsychology. *Archives of Clinical Neuropsychology, 21*(8), 837–839. https://doi.org/10.1016/j.acn.2006.08.011

Richards, P. M., & Tussey, C. M. (2013). The neuropsychologist as expert witness: Testimony in civil and criminal settings. *Psychological Injury and Law, 6*(1), 63–74. https://doi.org/10.1007/s12207-013-9148-9

Smith, G. (2018). Education and training in clinical neuropsychology: Recent developments and documents from the Clinical Neuropsychology Synarchy. *Archives of Clinical Neuropsychology, 34*(3), 418–431. https://doi.org/10.1093/arclin/acy075

Stucky, K. J., Bush, S., & Donders, J. (2010). Providing effective supervision in clinical neuropsychology. *The Clinical Neuropsychologist, 24*(5), 737–758. https://doi.org/10.1080/13854046.2010.490788

Tarasoff v. Regents of the University of California, 17 Cal. 3d 425, 551 P.2d 334, 131 Cal. Rptr. 14 (Cal. 1976). https://law.justia.com/cases/california/supreme-court/3d/17/425.html

Tjeltveit, A. C., & Gottlieb, M. C. (2010). Avoiding the road to ethical disaster: Overcoming vulnerabilities and developing resilience. *Psychotherapy: Theory, Research, & Practice, 47*(1), 98–110. https://doi.org/10.1037/a0018843

Tranel, D. (1994). The release of psychological data to nonexperts: Ethical and legal considerations. *Professional Psychology: Research and Practice, 25*(1), 33–38. https://doi.org/10.1037/0735-7028.25.1.33

U.S. Department of Health and Human Services. (2017, June 16). *Health information privacy: HIPAA for professionals.* https://www.hhs.gov/hipaa/for-professionals/index.html

15 INDIVIDUAL AND CULTURAL DIVERSITY COMPETENCIES

CHRISTOPHER NGUYEN, OCTAVIO SANTOS, AND DARYL FUJII

The United States is becoming a diverse country, with the racial–ethnic minority population projected to increase to 56% by 2060 (Colby & Ortman, 2014). As a consequence, an understanding of how sociocultural factors influence people's behaviors is imperative to the competent delivery of health care services. When serving culturally and linguistically diverse (CLD) populations, neuropsychologists are ethically expected to consider patients' or research participants' biopsychosocial factors, psychometric characteristics and limitations of assessment measures, and boundaries of competence, among issues (American Psychological Association [APA], 2017; Casaletto & Heaton, 2017; Elbulok-Charcape et al., 2014; Fujii, 2017). The purpose of this chapter is to provide an overview of common challenges encountered in providing neuropsychological services to CLD populations. We discuss topics such as ethical and professional standards involving neuropsychological services for CLD populations, cultural competency in health care, the impact of language and culture on neuropsychological assessment, culturally responsive report writing, and culturally sensitive feedback, and we provide a summary of takeaway points. We must note that although an in-depth discussion of these topics is beyond the scope of this chapter, our goal is to present and introduce

https://doi.org/10.1037/0000250-016
The Neuropsychologist's Roadmap: A Training and Career Guide, C. Block (Editor)

relevant literature that is important to the topic of individual and cultural diversity in neuropsychology.

ETHICAL AND PROFESSIONAL STANDARDS INVOLVING NEUROPSYCHOLOGICAL SERVICES FOR CULTURALLY AND LINGUISTICALLY DIVERSE POPULATIONS

Although efforts in creating training guidelines in neuropsychology in the United States date back to the 1970s (Bieliauskas & Mark, 2017), it was only recently that a formal training model was proposed that includes training guidelines for cultural diversity. The Houston Conference Guidelines (Hannay et al., 1998) state that trainees should gain an understanding about "cultural and individual differences and diversity" from their core of knowledge of general psychology and acquire clinical skills that recognize "multicultural issues" involved in assessment, treatment, and interventions. The more recent Commission for the Recognition of Specialties and Subspecialties in Professional Psychology taxonomy conceptualized individual and cultural diversity as a core domain within the competency of professionalism (APA, 2020). According to the Houston Conference Guidelines and Commission for the Recognition of Specialties and Subspecialties in Professional Psychology taxonomy, clinical neuropsychologists who provide services to CLD populations should have both the knowledge and skills to practice ethically and competently (Hannay et al., 1998; Rey-Casserly et al., 2012). In addition, the APA (2017) *Ethical Principles of Psychologists and Code of Conduct* (hereinafter the "Ethics Code") provides guidance on the use of neuropsychological assessments with CLD populations.

The APA Ethics Code mandates that assessment methods and instruments be appropriate, validated, and reliable for patients or research participants, given their particular sociodemographic and cultural characteristics, including language preference and competence, thus requiring four overarching qualifications: (a) awareness of an instrument's psychometrics and normative samples (e.g., Standard 9.02, Use of Assessments); (b) documentation of limitations of the use of interpreters, test results, and interpretation (e.g., 9.03c, Informed Consent in Assessments); (c) avoidance of interpreters who have a dual relationship with the patient or who are inadequately trained and supervised to provide competent services (e.g., Standards 2.05, Delegation of Work to Others; and 3.05, Multiple Relationships); and (d) provision of clear explanations of any potential limitations to the individual being assessed or designated representative during informed consent and feedback (Standard 9.03, Informed Consent in Assessments). We also encourage you to review other APA professional practice guidelines, such as test user qualifications, multicultural practice, practice with transgender and gender nonconforming people, and assessment of and intervention with people with disabilities, among others (https://www.apa.org/practice/guidelines).

Concerns regarding culturally competent neuropsychological practices have often been raised (Ferraro, 2015) and motivated further efforts in advancing education, training, and organizational change, including

- recruiting and mentoring of racial–ethnic minorities into neuropsychology at the undergraduate level,

- implementing multicultural training standards,

- promoting institutional systematic changes,

- hiring bilingual psychometrists,

- increasing public awareness and dialogue between practitioners and test publishers,

- prioritizing evidence-based practice research with racial–ethnic minority populations by means of funded grants, and

- developing professional standards with the assistance of professional organizations (see Rivera Mindt et al., 2010, and Romero et al., 2009, for details).

A recent but initial step toward more standard practical guidelines to aid neuropsychology trainees and professionals who provide services to CLD populations emphasizes the importance of knowing oneself, one's clients, the assessment tools, and one's role as an advocate (see Díaz-Santos & Hough, 2016, for details).

Cultural Competency in Health Care

For health care professionals, the concept of cultural competence has become an important pillar of reducing disparities in health service delivery (Brach & Fraser, 2000). As defined by Cross et al. (1989), *cultural competence* is "a set of congruent behaviors, attitudes, and policies that come together in a system or agency or among professionals and enables the system, agency, or professionals to work effectively in cross-cultural situations" (p. iv). To be specific, *culturally competent care* involves understanding and integrating issues of diversity and sociocultural factors (e.g., communication styles, attitudes, and behaviors) among your patients or research participants.

Becoming a culturally competent clinician–scientist is an ongoing and dynamic process that may encompass several things (Sue & Sue, 2013). The first is awareness of your worldviews, which involves a critical self-examination of how your assumptions, values, and stereotypes about CLD populations could negatively influence how, when, where, and why you provide services. The second involves acquiring specific knowledge and an understanding of the culture(s) of your patients or research participants and how multiple factors (e.g., sociopolitical influences) can affect each person's worldview. The third requires ongoing learning of the culturally appropriate assessment, intervention, and skills necessary to effectively work with CLD populations. Finally, the acquisition of cultural knowledge leads to the development of core competencies based on theories, practices, and policies to ensure that the provision of services are responsive to CLD populations (Sue & Sue, 2013).

In the field of neuropsychology, cross-cultural studies have traditionally focused on comparing cognitive performance across people from "diverse backgrounds," typically on the basis of age, race, ethnicity, gender, language, national origin, and/or socioeconomic status (e.g., Fletcher-Janzen et al., 2000; Uzzell et al., 2007). Such studies have offered valuable insights that help contextualize assessment and inform practice issues. Recently, some researchers have proposed a cultural neuropsychology approach that is integrated, and involves direct examination of cultural practices, to better understand human brain function (Cagigas & Manly, 2014).

Although you as a neuropsychologist would typically attain formal training in diversity through your doctoral program, we highly recommended that you complete *continued* education about diversity in psychological practice to maintain your competence and to build knowledge that is based on the most current, emerging research. Becoming culturally competent in the provision of neuropsychological services to CLD populations means that you attain knowledge on both the concept of culture and the worldview of diverse people. Cultural competence has been postulated as one of the central components of health care to improve services and outcomes (APA, 2015). To ensure they are capable of providing culturally sensitive services or research, clinicians and researchers should also pursue ongoing training in diversity and cultural competence (APA, 2002; APA Office of Ethnic Minority Affairs, 1993).

Impact of Language and Culture on Neuropsychological Assessment

The impact of culture on neuropsychological assessments is multifaceted and varied, but it can be distilled into two dimensions: (a) collecting accurate data and (b) providing a context for interpreting data and making useful recommendations (Fujii, 2017). For example, cultural and language differences can influence one's ability to collect data from interviews or collateral sources; for example, a problem may arise because of miscommunication or an unwillingness on the part of the CLD person to disclose information. Such differences can also affect the accuracy of test results. Psychological tests are Western entities that reflect the values, knowledge, and experience of Western society (Greenfield, 1997), and thus the neuropsychological assessments you use may not be valid for people from cultures that do not necessarily share the same worldviews, values, and experiences as yours. To ensure that tests are fair for CLD populations, the American Educational Research Association, APA, and the National Council on Measurement in Education (2014) identified four general issues that must be addressed:

1. CLD populations must feel comfortable with both you as the neuropsychologist and the testing situation.

2. Tests must be free of measurement biases, including content and construct validity of test items, as well as what is considered a correct response.

3. Test items should be accessible to CLD populations (i.e., a CLD person should not be disadvantaged in processing and responding to test items).

4. Test results must yield valid interpretations for the intended use of a specific test, which means that all of the issues are addressed and that the person experienced a fair opportunity to learn the contexts and skills targeted by the tests.

Consideration 1: The testing situation. The testing situation, in which a patient sits alone for hours with a stranger who is asking them personal questions, questions about things that are not present, and questions that to which they, the examiner, knows the answer, is not a universally familiar one and can actually be quite discomfiting (e.g., many Latinas consider being alone in a room with a strange male as inappropriate; Ardila, 2007; Greenfield, 1997). Diminished neuropsychological test performance has been associated with a number of factors, including negative perceptions of the testing situation (e.g., stereotype threat; Thames et al., 2013); perceived discrimination by, and poor rapport with, the examiner (Thames et al., 2015); and anxiety (Dorenkamp & Vik, 2018). So, it is important that you as a neuropsychologist are aware of how CLD patients or research participants perceive the testing situation and maximize their comfort level (Fujii, 2017).

Consideration 2: Measurement bias. Measurement bias is also a significant problem when assessing a CLD patient because there is a general lack of appropriately translated and validated test instruments. In addition, many translated tests have questionable validity. For example, some measures have used a literal 1:1 translation approach from English into other languages. Unfortunately, this approach can fail to capture regional idiosyncrasies (e.g., varying dialects) or convey the same meaning in the target language, which can also affect scoring criteria. For best practices regarding test translation and adaptation, we refer you to the guidelines provided by the International Test Commission (https://www.intestcom.org). Ongoing efforts are being made to translate neuropsychological tests, but a major obstacle has been the cost of securing licensing fees from test publishers (Bender et al., 2010; Byrd & Manly, 2005; Manly, 2006; Vilar-López & Puente, 2010). Despite this, several textbooks and peer-reviewed articles include tests in several languages, with varying degrees of validation (e.g., Ferraro, 2015; Fletcher-Janzen et al., 2000; Fujii, 2017; Mitrushina, 2005; Strauss et al., 2006; Wong & Fujii, 2004).

In consideration of some of the limitations just discussed, you as the neuropsychologist may decide to select some tests with fewer language demands, such as measures of sensory function (e.g., the Tactual Performance Test, Tactile Form Recognition Test, visual form discrimination tasks), fine motor function (e.g., finger tapping, grooved pegboard), attention and concentration (e.g., cancellation tasks, trail-making tests, continuous performance tests), visual learning and memory (e.g., spatial span tests/Corsi blocks, Rey Complex Figure Test and Recognition Trial), and tests that assess some aspects of executive function (e.g., Tower of London, Wisconsin Card Sorting Test). However, be aware that even nonverbal tests are not completely free of cultural biases (Puente et al., 2013).

Consideration 3: Accessibility. Accessibility issues are most salient for CLD patients or research participants whose primary language is not English. Although a bilingual and bicultural neuropsychologist ideally should assess patients with a similar cultural and linguistic background, this is not always feasible (Echemendia & Harris, 2004; Elbulok-Charcape et al., 2014; Hill-Briggs et al., 2004; Mindt et al., 2010). Using an interpreter may be necessary because of language barriers; however, this may affect the standardized administration procedures when tests in different languages are used, which would significantly limit your ability to interpret test results (Searight & Searight, 2009). Whenever possible, we recommended using bilingual psychometricians or interpreters with experience in neuropsychological assessment and instruments that have been appropriately validated for the target language following standardized procedures.

Consideration 4: Validity. The selection of appropriate neuropsychological test norms is essential for valid test interpretations, but such norms may not be yet available for certain CLD populations (Boone et al., 2007; Brickman et al.,

2006; Manly & Echemendia, 2007; Vilar-López & Puente, 2010). Because most neuropsychological tests are normed on middle-class English-speaking White people, reliance on those data when assessing CLD populations may not only be inappropriate but could also result in unintended harm. Although age- and education-adjusted norms may assist you in the interpretation of the test results of CLD patients or research participants with whom you share similar characteristics, you should also consider a number of other variables, such as years residing in the United States, bilingualism, acculturation, and socioeconomic status. Test scores or behaviors cannot be interpreted without an understanding of the context in which they occur. For example, a low average score on the Boston Naming Test would have an entirely different meaning for a 62-year-old White attorney with early stage Alzheimer's disease versus a 62-year-old trilingual Hmong immigrant with a sixth-grade education. Similarly, an inability to write a check would be a red flag for cognitive decline for the White attorney, but not for the Hmong immigrant if he or she was not able to write in English (or never developed that skill in the first place).

Cultural Facets and ECLECTIC

Given the potential impact of culture on the neuropsychological assessment process, it is imperative that you be aware of cultural characteristics that can affect data collection and interpretation ahead of time. This information is crucial for guiding your examination process and maximizing fairness in testing. The knowledge base to help you gain familiarity with the background of a CLD patient can be acquired only through extensive research to prepare for the assessment. Specific facets of culture that are pertinent to neuropsychological assessment are identified by the acronym ECLECTIC are presented in Table 15.1: Education and literacy, Culture and acculturation, Language issues, Economics, Communication style, Comfort with the Testing situation, Conceptualization of Intelligence, and the Context of immigration (Fujii, 2018). An in-depth discussion of each facet and its impact on the assessment process is beyond the scope of this chapter; see Fujii (2017, 2018) for more details. Here we offer only a few examples for illustrative purposes, in particular with regard to the ECLECTIC facets of culture and acculturation, communication style, and comfort with testing situation.

Facet: Awareness of the effects of culture and acculturation. Culture is a multifaceted phenomenon that can be broken down into three components: (a) macrosocietal structures; (b) values, beliefs, and social structures; and (c) medical conditions and beliefs about illness (Fujii, 2017; Judd & Beggs, 2005). *Macrosocietal structures* include the physical, historical, and

TABLE 15.1. ECLECTIC Framework for Guiding the Neuropsychological Evaluation Process

ECLECTIC facet	Example
Education and literacy	CLD populations with low levels of education would lack opportunities to learn much of the content and skills measured by Western tests, thereby affecting valid interpretations of test scores.
Culture and acculturation	Macrosocietal structures of a CLD patient's country can provide clues to determine English proficiency or bilingualism, educational opportunities, or performance on Western intelligence tests.
	The values, beliefs, and worldview of a CLD patient can guide approaches to communication, rapport, and the generation of recommendations.
Language issues	Determining English proficiency will determine whether translated tests and an interpreter are needed.
Economics	The gross domestic product of a CLD patient's country likely is associated with learning resources and/or opportunities and correlated with performance on Western tests (see Fujii, 2018, for specific methodology).
Communication style	Understanding a CLD patient's idiom is important for diagnostic purposes and the facilitation of rapport.
	Incongruent communication styles between a neuro-psychologist and a CLD patient can affect testing and thus the validity of test results.
Comfort with the testing situation	Issues such as stereotype threat and stigmas associated with mental health services can influence a patient's comfort with and motivation for testing.
	Neuropsychologists should take caution when interpreting and using standard cutoff scores on performance validity measures.
Conceptualization of intelligence	Cultural differences in conceptualizations of intelligence contribute to measurement bias and the validity of test results.
Context of immigration	The timing of a CLD patient's immigration provides clues to their culture, has implications for the neuropsychologist's understanding of the patient's premorbid functioning, and provides information on potential psychiatric or medical conditions sustained during the immigration process.

Note. CLD = culturally and linguistically diverse. Data from Fujii (2017) and Fujii (2018).

economic contexts in which a people have lived over the course of centuries. These contexts can strongly influence a person's behaviors, worldview, and cognition. For example, historical events such as wars, colonization, and the philosophy and stability of government can affect a population's worldview, external cultural influences, and languages spoken. These events and structures, in addition to geography and a history of natural disasters, can significantly influence a country's economic development. A country's economy, in turn, has a profound influence on the quality of the educational system and access to learning tools, such as books, computers, and the internet (Fujii, 2018). Relatedly, low socioeconomic status is associated with increased exposure to stress and trauma (Ursache & Noble, 2016). In regard to fairness in testing, the ubiquitous influence of macrosocietal structures on the experience of a people can significantly affect one's familiarity with testing situations (comfort with testing), familiarity with the content of test items, such as what is considered a correct response (measurement bias), exposure to English (accessibility), and opportunities for learning (validity).

Facet: Awareness of cultural expressions of pathology and appropriate interventions. Knowledge of common medical and psychiatric illnesses and idioms of distress can provide important contextual information for differential diagnosis and case formulation. Both are key processes to guide assessment strategies and data collection. In addition, knowledge of traditional beliefs about illness and spiritual and medical interventions can help you as a neuropsychologist understand barriers to seeking Western treatments and increase your awareness of efficacious cultural treatments, as well as assist with communication styles between you and your CLD patients (Fujii, 2018; Judd & Beggs, 2005).

Facet: Awareness of religious and social norms. Religious institutions have important implications for a culture's values, attitudes, and worldview (Judd & Beggs, 2005). Social norms, such as expectations for interactions with family members or strangers of a different social status, and collectivist versus individualistic allegiance, have strong implications for what are considered appropriate behaviors and in which contexts. Awareness of these characteristics has clinical utility for developing rapport, guiding optimal approaches to communication, understanding a CLD patient's experience of the testing situation (e.g., their comfort with the situation), and making culturally consistent recommendations (Fujii, 2018).

Culturally Responsible Report Writing

Guidelines and methods for preparing evidence-based neuropsychological reports applicable to various settings and populations have already been reported elsewhere (see, e.g., Donders, 2016, and Fujii, 2017, for details). In brief, engaging in a culturally responsible report-writing process involves examining cultural influences on behavioral observations, assessment data, and documentation of any nonstandardized assessment procedures you may have used. For example, clinicians and researchers alike should consider cultural influences in nonverbal communication, such as facial expressions, eye contact, and body language, to avoid misinterpretations of their observations. Other assessment data, such as the patient's medical history, test results, and collateral reports (e.g., a friend or family member, work or school records) should be integrated and interpreted within the context of the assessment procedures and that person's cultural characteristics. You are also encouraged to rely on functional abilities described by collateral sources in the interpretation of assessment data. Most important, you should clearly document in the neuropsychological report all nonstandardized assessment procedures, and the rationale for the modifications, as well as limitations of test interpretations.

Culturally Sensitive Feedback

Strategies that are culturally specific within medical etiologies and patient populations have been proposed (see Fujii, 2017, 2018, and Postal & Armstrong, 2013, for details). In general, we suggest that a culturally sensitive feedback process includes the following six elements:

- openness to engaging in dialogue about the patient's culture by using culturally sensitive language familiar to them and their family members

- awareness of cultural norms, expectations, and types of communication as well as resources available to the patient that can be used to implement recommendations

- an understanding of the patient's sociocultural and linguistic background, approach to medical-related issues, psychological functioning, dependency, and family dynamics, to facilitate establishing rapport and maintain trust

- a discussion of the limitations of the assessment methods being used, the patient's receptiveness to proposed recommendations, and potential barriers to treatment

- an emphasis on individual cultural strengths for coping (e.g., family, community) and, when appropriate, introduction of religious concepts in the context of expressed beliefs and support

- identification of a spokesperson if a patient is accompanied by family or a member of their social support network; use of a professional interpreter when needed; and, with less acculturated patients, provision of visual aids

CONCLUSION AND FUTURE DIRECTIONS

In this chapter, we have provided an overview of issues that commonly arise in the neuropsychological assessment of CLD populations, including foundational concepts that are pertinent primarily to neuropsychologists in training, such as the notions of culture and cultural competency, ethical and professional standards involving the provision of neuropsychological services to CLD populations, and the impact of culture on neuropsychological procedures. Overall, a number of factors should be considered to provide a competent neuropsychological evaluation of CLD persons, such as considering patients' or research participants' biopsychosocial factors, the psychometric characteristics and limitations of assessment measures, and the boundaries of competence. Also important is the realization that becoming culturally competent is an ongoing and dynamic process that continues throughout the course of your training and professional career. As you move ahead from traineeship into your career, remember the following:

- Becoming culturally competent is a dynamic process that involves awareness of your assumptions and values, knowledge of the worldview of diverse individuals, acquisition of culturally appropriate interventions, and development of core cultural competencies.

- Patients' or research participants' level of acculturation and language proficiency can be assessed by examining the language(s) spoken in various settings, participation in social groups, health care utilization, activities and entertainment, and reading materials.

- Before the assessment, you as the neuropsychologist must research the CLD patient's culture to guide the process for collecting accurate data, interpreting the data within a cultural context, and making culturally consist recommendations. The ECLECTIC framework is a useful tool to identify facets of a particular culture and its potential impact on the neuropsychological assessment process.

- Consider the interface between cultural variables (e.g., acculturation, language proficiency) and the American Educational Research Association et al.'s (2014) standards for fairness in testing when selecting tests

EXHIBIT 15.1. Resources Related to Cultural Competence

American Academy of Clinical Neuropsychology Relevance 2050 Initiative: https://theaacn.org/relevance-2050-initiative

American Psychological Association Guidelines for Providers of Psychological Services to Ethnic, Linguistic, and Culturally Diverse Populations: https://www.apa.org/pi/oema/resources/policy/provider-guidelines

American Psychological Association Multicultural Guidelines: An Ecological Approach to Context, Identity, and Intersectionality: https://www.apa.org/about/policy/multicultural-guidelines

Asian Neuropsychological Association: https://www.the-ana.org

Hispanic Neuropsychological Society: https://www.hnps.org

National Academy of Neuropsychology Culture & Diversity Committee: https://bit.ly/2gjHAXi

Society for Clinical Neuropsychology Public Interest Advisory Committee, Ethnic-Minority Affairs Subcommittee: https://scn40.org/piac-ema/

and strategizing modifications in test administration for maximizing fairness and test validity; if necessary, select neuropsychological tests with less of a reliance on English language demands.

- When writing reports, describe nonstandardized test administration procedures and comment on the limitations of test interpretation, to amply qualify test results.

- Interpreters should receive adequate training in neuropsychological assessment so they can maintain standardized administration procedures.

For more education and support related to cultural competence, consult available resources, some of which are listed in Exhibit 15.1.

REFERENCES

American Educational Research Association, American Psychological Association, & National Council on Measurement in Education. (2014). *Standards for educational and psychological testing* (2nd ed.).

American Psychological Association. (2002). Ethical principles of psychologists and code of conduct. *American Psychologist, 57*(12), 1060–1073. https://doi.org/10.1037/0003-066X.57.12.1060

American Psychological Association. (2015). *APA dictionary of psychology.*

American Psychological Association. (2017). *Ethical principles of psychologists and code of conduct* (2002, Amended June 1, 2010, and January 1, 2017). https://www.apa.org/ethics/code/index.aspx

American Psychological Association. (2020). *Education and training guidelines: A taxonomy for education and training in professional psychology health service specialties and subspecialties.* http://www.apa.org/ed/graduate/specialize/taxonomy.pdf

American Psychological Association, Office of Ethnic Minority Affairs. (1993). Guidelines for providers of psychological services to ethnic, linguistic, and culturally diverse populations. *American Psychologist, 48*(1), 45–48. https://doi.org/10.1037/0003-066X.48.1.45

Ardila, A. (2007). The impact of culture on neuropsychological test performance. In B. Uzzell, M. Ponton, & A. Ardila (Eds.), *International handbook of cross-cultural neuropsychology* (pp. 24–44). Erlbaum.

Bender, H. A., García, A. M., & Barr, W. B. (2010). An interdisciplinary approach to neuropsychological test construction: Perspectives from translation studies. *Journal of the International Neuropsychological Society, 16*(2), 227–232. https://doi.org/10.1017/S1355617709991378

Bieliauskas, L. A., & Mark, E. (2017). Specialty training in clinical neuropsychology: History and update on current issues. In J. E. Morgan & J. H. Ricker (Eds.), *Textbook of clinical neuropsychology* (pp. 14–21). Taylor & Francis.

Boone, K. B., Victor, T. L., Wen, J., Razani, J., & Pontón, M. (2007). The association between neuropsychological scores and ethnicity, language, and acculturation variables in a large patient population. *Archives of Clinical Neuropsychology, 22*(3), 355–365. https://doi.org/10.1016/j.acn.2007.01.010

Brach, C., & Fraser, I. (2000). Can cultural competency reduce racial and ethnic health disparities? A review and conceptual model. *Medical Care Research and Review, 57*(Suppl.), 181–217. https://doi.org/10.1177/1077558700057001S09

Brickman, A. M., Cabo, R., & Manly, J. J. (2006). Ethical issues in cross-cultural neuropsychology. *Applied Neuropsychology, 13(2)*, 91–100. https://doi.org/10.1207/s15324826an1302_4

Byrd, D. A., & Manly, J. J. (2005). Cultural considerations in the neuro-logical assessment of older adults. In S. S. Bush & T. A. Martin (Eds.), *Geriatric neuropsychology: Practice essentials* (pp. 115–139). Taylor & Francis.

Cagigas, X. E., & Manly, J. J. (2014). Cultural neuropsychology: The new norm. In M. W. Parsons & T. A. Hammeke (Eds.), *Clinical neuropsychology: A pocket handbook for assessment* (3rd ed., pp. 132–156). American Psychological Association. https://doi.org/10.1037/14339-008

Casaletto, K. B., & Heaton, R. K. (2017). Neuropsychological assessment: Past and future. *Journal of the International Neuropsychological Society, 23*(9–10), 778–790. https://doi.org/10.1017/S1355617717001060

Colby, S. L., & Ortman, J. M. (2014). *Projections of the size and composition of the U.S. population: 2014 to 2060, Current Population Reports, P25-1143.* U.S. Census Bureau.

Cross, T., Bazron, B., Dennis, K., & Isaacs, M. (1989). *Towards a culturally competent system of care: A monograph on effective services for minority children who are severely emotionally disturbed.* Georgetown University Child Development Center. https://www.ncjrs.gov/App/Publications/abstract.aspx?ID=124939

Díaz-Santos, M., & Hough, S. (2016). Cultural competence guidelines for neuropsychology trainees and professionals: Working with ethnically diverse individuals. In R. Ferrero (Ed.), *Minority and cross-cultural aspects of neuropsychological assessment: Enduring and emerging trends* (2nd ed., pp. 11–33). Taylor & Francis.

Donders, J. (2016). *Neuropsychological report writing.* Guilford Press.

Dorenkamp, M. A., & Vik, P. (2018). Neuropsychological assessment anxiety: A systematic review. *Practice Innovations, 3*(3), 192–211. https://doi.org/10.1037/pri0000073

Echemendia, R. J., & Harris, J. G. (2004). Neuropsychological test use with Hispanic/Latino populations in the United States: Part II of a national survey. *Applied Neuropsychology, 11*(1), 4–12. https://doi.org/10.1207/s15324826an1101_2

Elbulok-Charcape, M. M., Rabin, L. A., Spadaccini, A. T., & Barr, W. B. (2014). Trends in the neuropsychological assessment of ethnic/racial minorities: A survey of clinical neuropsychologists in the United States and Canada. *Cultural Diversity & Ethnic Minority Psychology, 20*(3), 353–361. https://doi.org/10.1037/a0035023

Ferraro, F. R. (Ed.). (2015). *Minority and cross-cultural aspects of neuropsychological assessment: Enduring and emerging trends* (2nd ed.). Taylor & Francis. https://doi.org/10.4324/9781315708690

Fletcher-Janzen, E., Strickland, T. L., & Reynolds, C. R. (Eds.). (2000). *Handbook of cross-cultural neuropsychology*. Springer.

Fujii, D. (2017). *Conducting a culturally informed neuropsychological evaluation*. American Psychological Association. https://doi.org/10.1037/15958-000

Fujii, D. E. M. (2018). Developing a cultural context for conducting a neuropsychological evaluation with a culturally diverse client: The ECLECTIC framework. *The Clinical Neuropsychologist, 32*(8), 1356–1392. https://doi.org/10.1080/13854046. 2018.1435826

Greenfield, P. (1997). You can't take it with you: Why ability assessments don't cross cultures. *American Psychologist, 52*(10), 1115–1124. https://doi.org/10.1037/0003-066X.52.10.1115

Hannay, H. J., Bieliauskas, L. A., Crosson, B. A., Hammeke, T. A., & Hamsher, K. (1998). The Houston Conference on Specialty Education and Training in Clinical Neuropsychology. *Archives of Clinical Neuropsychology, 13*(2), 160–166. https://doi.org/10.1093/arclin/13.2.160

Hill-Briggs, F., Evans, J. D., & Norman, M. A. (2004). Racial and ethnic diversity among trainees and professionals in psychology and neuropsychology: Needs, trends, and challenges. *Applied Neuropsychology, 11*(1), 13–22. https://doi.org/10.1207/s15324826an1101_3

Judd, T., & Beggs, B. (2005). Cross cultural forensic neuropsychological assessment. In K. Barrett & W. George (Eds.), *Race, culture, psychology & law* (pp. 193–205). Sage. https://doi.org/10.4135/9781452233536.n10

Manly, J. J. (2006). Cultural issues. In D. K. Attix & K. A. Welsh-Bohmer (Eds.), *Geriatric neuropsychology: Assessment and intervention* (pp. 198–222). Guilford Press.

Manly, J. J., & Echemendia, R. J. (2007). Race-specific norms: Using the model of hypertension to understand issues of race, culture, and education in neuropsychology. *Archives of Clinical Neuropsychology, 22*(3), 319–325. https://doi.org/10.1016/j.acn.2007.01.006

Mindt, M. R., Byrd, D., Saez, P., & Manly, J. (2010). Increasing culturally competent neuropsychological services for ethnic minority populations: A call to action. *The Clinical Neuropsychologist, 24*(3), 429–453. https://doi.org/10.1080/13854040903058960

Mitrushina, M. N. (2005). *Handbook of normative data for neuropsychological assessment*. Oxford University Press.

Postal, K., & Armstrong, K. (2013). *Feedback that sticks: The art of effectively communicating neuropsychological assessment results*. Oxford University Press.

Puente, A. E., Perez-Garcia, M., Lopez, R. V., Hidalgo-Ruzzante, N. A., & Fasfous, A. F. (2013). Neuropsychological assessment of culturally and educationally dissimilar individuals. In F. A. Paniagua & A.-M. Yamada (Eds.), *Handbook of multicultural mental health: Assessment and treatment of diverse populations* (pp. 225–241). Elsevier. https://doi.org/10.1016/B978-0-12-394420-7.00012-6

Rey-Casserly, C., Roper, B. L., & Bauer, R. (2012). Application of a competency model to clinical neuropsychology. *Professional Psychology: Research and Practice, 43*(5), 422–431. https://doi.org/10.1037/a0028721

Rivera Mindt, M., Byrd, D., Saez, P., & Manly, J. (2010). Increasing culturally competent neuropsychological services for ethnic minority populations: A call to action. *The Clinical Neuropsychologist, 24*(3), 429–453. https://doi.org/10.1080/13854040903058960

Romero, H. R., Lageman, S. K., Kamath, V. V., Irani, F., Sim, A., Suarez, P., Manly, J. J., Attix, D. K., & The Summit participants. (2009). Challenges in the neuropsychological assessment of ethnic minorities: Summit proceedings. *The Clinical Neuropsychologist, 23*(5), 761–779. https://doi.org/10.1080/13854040902881958

Searight, H. R., & Searight, B. K. (2009). Working with foreign language interpreters: Recommendations for psychological practice. *Professional Psychology: Research and Practice, 40*(5), 444–451. https://doi.org/10.1037/a0016788

Strauss, E., Sherman, E. M., & Spreen, O. (2006). *A compendium of neuropsychological tests: Administration, norms and commentary.* Oxford University Press.

Sue, D. W., & Sue, D. (2013). *Counseling the culturally diverse: Theory and practice* (6th ed.). Wiley.

Thames, A. D., Hinkin, C. H., Byrd, D. A., Bilder, R. M., Duff, K. J., Mindt, M. R., Arentoft, A., & Streiff, V. (2013). Effects of stereotype threat, perceived discrimination, and examiner race on neuropsychological performance: Simple as black and white? *Journal of the International Neuropsychological Society, 19*(5), 583–593. https://doi.org/10.1017/S1355617713000076

Thames, A. D., Panos, S. E., Arentoft, A., Byrd, D. A., Hinkin, C. H., & Arbid, N. (2015). Mild test anxiety influences neurocognitive performance among African Americans and European Americans: Identifying interfering and facilitating sources. *Cultural Diversity & Ethnic Minority Psychology, 21*(1), 105–113. https://doi.org/10.1037/a0037530

Ursache, A., & Noble, K. G. (2016). Neurocognitive development in socioeconomic context: Multiple mechanisms and implications for measuring socioeconomic status. *Psychophysiology, 53*(1), 71–82. https://doi.org/10.1111/psyp.12547

Uzzell, B. P., Ponton, M., & Ardila, A. (Eds.). (2007). *International handbook of cross-cultural neuropsychology.* Psychology Press.

Vilar-López, R., & Puente, A. E. (2010). Forensic neuropsychological assessment of members of minority groups: The case for assessing Hispanics. In A. M. Horton & L. C. Hartlange (Eds.), *Handbook of forensic neuropsychology* (2nd ed., pp. 309–331). Springer.

Wong, T. M., & Fujii, D. E. (2004). Neuropsychological assessment of Asian Americans: Demographic factors, cultural diversity, and practical guidelines. *Applied Neuropsychology, 11*(1), 23–36. https://doi.org/10.1207/s15324826an1101_4

16 SELF-CARE AND WORK-LIFE INTEGRATION COMPETENCIES

LAURA FLASHMAN AND ROBIN HILSABECK

The use of competency models to evaluate training outcomes in specialties within neuropsychology has developed over time (Rey-Casserly et al., 2012; Smith, 2019), and one of the foundational domains in the most recent iteration of education and training competencies (Smith, 2019) is that of reflective practice/self-assessment/self-care. In our opinion, graduate and postdoctoral programs do not provide adequate training in this domain during the years while trainees focus on developing professional identities, knowledge-based competencies, and applied competencies. Juggling the demands of a career and developing a professional identity, as well as protecting time for a personal life, in terms of both relationships and physical and mental health needs, is an ongoing challenge (Feigon et al., 2018).

Students and early-career professionals in particular sacrifice time for their personal lives to promote their professional persona; however, even mid- and later career neuropsychologists struggle with balance challenges. Research has shown that occupational stress (aka "burnout") is increasingly a problem among academicians and teachers (e.g., Watts & Robertson, 2011). Among a number of stress-related measures, work–life balance and workload were the most consistent items predicting low job satisfaction,

https://doi.org/10.1037/0000250-017
The Neuropsychologist's Roadmap: A Training and Career Guide, C. Block (Editor)

stress, and negative health symptoms (Catano et al., 2010). Among the respondents in one study, the groups of academics most at risk of stress and strain were women, people between the ages of 30 and 59, and tenure-track faculty (Catano et al., 2010).

Throughout one's career, work–life balance is an important goal, and something that one should strive for to avoid burnout, maintain resilience, and promote a healthy lifestyle. There are several risk factors for burnout, including a high workload, a high need for perfection, and working in a helping profession such as clinical neuropsychology. Burnout differs from *stress*, which is a reaction to environmental factors, such as when engagement becomes too much and results in anxiety, fatigue, and/or emotional upset. *Burnout* refers to a state of mental or emotional tiredness that tends to occur as a result of continuous exposure to stress. Signs of burnout include feeling that you have to drag yourself to work, feeling less satisfied with your work even after an achievement, and lacking motivation to be productive at work. A 2020 article by Mayo Clinic staff lists the risk factors and signs of burnout.

Research has shown that optimal work–life integration is associated with improvements in resilience, life satisfaction, family functioning, physical health, and cognitive functioning (Watts & Robertson, 2011; Worley & Stonnington, 2017). But let's be honest here: If you are thinking that "work–life balance" means you are spending equal amounts of time each week working and not working, you should accept the fact that this work–life balance is a myth. It just doesn't exist. There are going to be moments in your life when you're more occupied with work because you're writing a grant proposal or paper or preparing for promotion, and there will be times when you are more focused on your personal life, including your family. You might have a vacation planned. You might have a new son or daughter (always a good way to make sure you spend more time at home!). Those life events have the tendency to change your priorities for a time. One of the advantages of academic life and/or private practice can be its freedom, autonomy, and flexibility—these allow us more opportunity for parenting (i.e., sneak out to catch a sporting event or school play, work at home with a sick child), for example, than other professions might.

In this chapter, we provide some guidance to help students, fellows, and even professionals achieve a good work–life integration. Perhaps the best way to do this is by changing your expectation from achieving "work–life balance" to "work–life integration"—this changes the vision of you on a teeter-totter, trying to keep both sides hovering in the air, to a vision in which you have flexibility and the opportunity to manage your availability at both work and at home. There are many ways to help bring integration to your workday and your life. Although no one can add more hours to the day, one can learn to make those hours count. One of the best ways to "make every minute count" is to plan your time and to develop efficient and effective routines while at the same time acknowledging the importance of "white space" in your calendar to help avoid overscheduling and overplanning. This may require an adjustment in your assumptions and expectations (and those of your colleagues/friends/family), an increase in organization and management of your time, and a concerted effort to set limits and schedule pleasurable and relaxing activities. The cost of ignoring balance may be physical or mental health issues, poorer work performance, and work dissatisfaction or job changes. Our assumption in this chapter is that your work–life integration is skewed in the direction of "too much work, not enough play."

STRATEGIES FOR SELF-CARE AND WORK-LIFE INTEGRATION

Here are our top suggestions to help integrate work and life outside of work. Although most of these things cross over or can be applied different ways, we have divided them broadly into work strategies, home strategies, and everywhere strategies (see Table 16.1).

Work Strategies

Strategy 1: Develop career goals and regularly assess progress toward them. An important step in the processing of developing work–life integration is identifying a clear career path and making a plan that will help you reach your career goals. In addition to your institutional resources, identify resources you might have through partner institutions, alumni societies, and professional and scientific organizations. Consider immediate goals, as well as longer term goals (think 2-year plan, 5-year plan, etc.). Putting your goals in writing can be helpful. SMART goals (Specific, Measurable, Achievable, Relevant, Time-bound; see Figure 16.1) can be used to address the domains of clinical work, teaching and supervision, scholarship, and/or service. Each of these areas is important in terms of preparing for promotion within your institution; however, these types of goals can also help you identify and create reasonable targets for participation in activities outside of work.

Strategy 2: Find good mentors. Ongoing mentorship in your personal goals is crucial. It is important to keep in mind that one person is not likely to be able to meet all your mentorship needs. You should feel free to seek out a variety of mentors to help address your professional development goals, your clinical goals, and your research goals. Mentorship is a useful way to learn, model, and implement one's work–life integration. Use your mentors

TABLE 16.1. Strategies for Self-Care and Work-Life Integration

Work strategies

✓ Develop goals and regularly assess progress toward them.

✓ Find good mentors.

✓ Build healthy relationships with peers.

✓ Learn about the work-related resources and supports available to you.

✓ Hit the ground running from Day 1.

✓ Prioritize. Strategize. Organize.

✓ Learn to say no.

✓ Know your work style, and problem-solve around that.

✗ You do not always need to find meaning in every aspect of your work.

Home strategies

✓ Have a baby—or a partner, or a friend, or a dog, or a cat, or a plant—who demands your time and attention.

✓ Build self-care activities into your schedule—and respect that schedule.

✓ Build resilience.

✓ Choose wisely, grasshopper.

✗ Do not waste time worrying about your workload.

Everywhere strategies

✓ Follow through on your commitments.

✓ Don't be afraid to ask for help.

✓ There is no such thing as a dumb question.

✓ Give yourself credit for the things you have accomplished.

✓ Remember that your to-do list will still be there tomorrow.

✗ Don't be afraid to ask for help.

and others in your department for any guidance on how and when to set limits and to help identify opportunities that will move you closer to your goals. (See Chapter 17, this volume, for a discussion of mentorship competencies.)

Strategy 3: Build healthy relationships with peers. In addition, get to know your peers. This will provide a built-in group of colleagues who are going through the same process and struggles as you are. In addition to providing support, they may be the people with whom you engage socially, particularly if you have recently moved to a new location and do not know many people outside of work. Be careful, however, to avoid the trap of upward and downward social comparisons. Set your own goals and benchmarks for evaluating progress. We all compare ourselves with others in our social worlds, whether it is comparing our looks with those of celebrities we see in the media or our talents and achievements with those of our coworkers.

FIGURE 16.1. Setting and Following SMART Goals

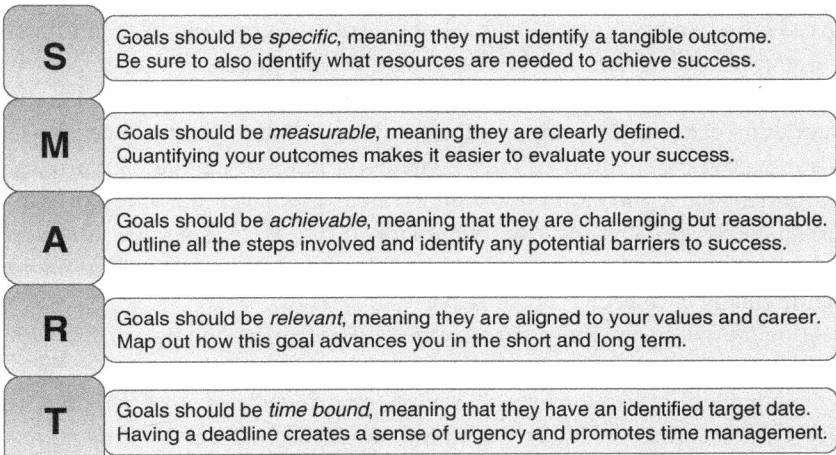

S	Goals should be *specific*, meaning they must identify a tangible outcome. Be sure to also identify what resources are needed to achieve success.
M	Goals should be *measurable*, meaning they are clearly defined. Quantifying your outcomes makes it easier to evaluate your success.
A	Goals should be *achievable*, meaning that they are challenging but reasonable. Outline all the steps involved and identify any potential barriers to success.
R	Goals should be *relevant*, meaning they are aligned to your values and career. Map out how this goal advances you in the short and long term.
T	Goals should be *time bound*, meaning that they have an identified target date. Having a deadline creates a sense of urgency and promotes time management.

Both upward social comparisons (when we compare ourselves with those who we believe are better than us with the desire to improve our current level of ability) and downward social comparisons (when we compare themselves with others who are worse off, often to make ourselves feel better about our abilities) can lead to unrealistic feelings of inadequacy or an inflated sense of self-worth. Social comparison, both upward and downward, has negative consequences. Avoid such comparisons if possible. And if you can't, learn to use social comparisons to provide motivation and enhance your self-esteem. If you find you are feeling chronically inferior, depressed, cocky, or pleased at the misfortune of others, look for better ways to put comparison in context, be realistic about who you are and what you have accomplished.

Strategy 4: Learn about the work-related resources and supports available to you. By knowing what resources and support are available to you at your institution, you can start making progress toward your goals in a way that efficiently allows you to be successful at work and allows time for the things you value outside of work. Are there work-study students who can help you pull together a database, are there "women in science" or other programs that might provide assistance on projects, are there departmental or institutional grants for young investigators that could provide seed money or data for future, larger projects? There will be a constant pull from your employer to do more, and they will often expect you to do this without additional resources or protected time. Check out any graduate or medical student organizations on campus, too. These may be good self-care resources.

Equally important is finding opportunities to collaborate. You can find mentors, advocates, research collaborators, and allies by taking the time to get to know your colleagues. This may help you find opportunities for growth without having to reinvent the wheel and provide guidance and support as you start your career. Remember that the whole can often be bigger than the sum of its parts, and putting together a strong collaborative team can make a stronger grant application, interdisciplinary clinic, or training opportunity. More hands also increase the likelihood that papers get submitted or published, skills are developed and incorporated into your repertoire, and you have the chance to contribute meaningfully to projects or patients that might not normally have been on your radar.

Don't forget to maximize your resources. Having a good relationship with administrators and support staff can allow you to confidently delegate tasks to free up additional time for either work or for outside-of-work activities. A good administrator will help you "think out of the box" and identify potential resources and opportunities for growth. There may be access to documentation, templates, administrative support, or even funding that you are unaware of but could be very helpful. In addition, never underestimate who might be your ally, and respect and gratitude demonstrated toward the support and administrative staff who help you ensures their future assistance when you need it!

Strategy 5: Prioritize, strategize, and organize tasks with time management techniques. Manage your time and pay attention to the tasks you need to do each day. Organize and prioritize what you must accomplish. Do what must be done, and let the rest go for another time. Time management is a skill that must be learned, and there are many strategies. One of the most well-known time management strategies is the Pomodoro technique, which involves pacing activities by using a timer to break down work into intervals, separated by short breaks. This helps you be super-attentive and productive for short, regimented periods of time, then take short breaks to regroup and reenergize, making large tasks more manageable. Other strategies that can be used as well (see, e.g., https://www.proofhub.com/articles/time-management-tips-for-work).

Sometimes you need to delegate. When possible, get others to help with tasks that do not need to be done by you. Many of us have a tendency to feel like it is easier, faster, or more efficient to just do the work ourselves, but the appropriate use of support staff, savvy technicians, or students can facilitate productivity and efficiency. Think about tasks that you can outsource—administrative duties, maintaining inventory, initial training of new personnel/

students, database management, and so on—and do it. Delegating is a skill that develops over time as one becomes familiar with and can leverage specific strengths of others in the group. It is a skill that will serve you well over the course of your career.

Strategy 6: Learn to say no to requests. Remember that it is all right to respectfully decline when you are asked to do something. The decision regarding what to accept and what to decline should be thoughtful and pro-active, with the target of advancing your career goals (i.e., increasing your sphere of influence, involvement at a national and international level, evidence of leadership, etc.). That being said, there are times when saying no to something that does not clearly advance your career may not be prudent (i.e., the chair of your department asks you to sit on a hospital committee). It is also the case that the benefits of an opportunity are not readily apparent. Before declining an opportunity, be sure to consult with your mentors.

Your stress level can benefit a great deal by setting expectations and boundaries early and clearly. Neuropsychologists have many skills, and thus you may be asked to become involved in projects that may be peripheral (or completely unrelated) to your career goals. Setting selective, reasonable, and appropriate expectations early in a position will improve the likelihood that boundaries are maintained. Having goals articulated in writing may help provide a reference guide and facilitate advocating for oneself when trying to set limits. Good communication, both at work and at home, can significantly enhance work–life integration. To achieve this, you must let people know what you want, what you will do, and what you won't do. Communicate with everyone who needs to know.

Strategy 7: Know your work style, and problem-solve around that. Try to find time at the beginning or end of the day (when fewer people are around) so you can work without interruption. We all have a time when we feel most effective (think early bird or night owl), and you will likely be able to get more done if you are able to protect some time during that window. Particularly if you have an open door policy at work, you will find yourself able to be more productive during a time when there are fewer people at work who might need you (and will be less likely to interrupt you).

Figure out when you need to keep going and when to call it quits. Some-times, you may opt to "grind it out." Although this phrase is often used to describe something that needs to be done that is tedious, laborious, or joyless, there are situations in which you need to just push yourself through the tasks you have set for yourself. Remember, this should last only a short time, and although the tasks themselves may feel arduous, the outcome of grinding it out is always satisfying. Your goal was met, and you (should) feel proud about your accomplishment. However, stop working when you are tired or stop being productive at work, at least for a little while. Take a break, take a walk, and call it good for the evening. Sitting at your desk spinning your wheels neither helps you move your work forward nor allows you to spend nonproductive work time meeting your personal needs.

Strategy 8: Know that you do not always need to find meaning in every aspect of your work. There are two ways to look at this. First, wellness gurus often tell us that to avoid burnout from hard or demanding work, we must find meaning in our work. This is not always true, however, and sometimes continuing to believe this can serve us badly. Always trying to find meaning in our work can be exhausting and often disappointing. Sometimes we just have to get through the administrative or mundane but necessary tasks, and then move on. On the other hand, if you are doing work you don't love, why are you doing it? If you feel your work is meaningless or frustrating more often than not, or you are now bogged down in the necessary but completely unenjoyable aspects of work, you might want to take another look at what you are doing, and see if you can recalibrate your job so the positive outweighs the negative.

Home Strategies

Strategy 1: Have a baby—or a partner, or a friend, or a dog, or a cat, or a plant—who also demands your time and attention. Okay, this one is kind of tongue-in-cheek, but there are things in your life outside of work that need your attention and caring. Figure out what that is for you. Even when you are not willing to make time for or prioritize yourself, you will likely be more willing to do it for your significant other (whomever or whatever that might be).

Strategy 2: Build self-care activities into your schedule—and respect that schedule. We make this recommendation frequently but are often guilty of not taking our own advice. It seems that when we feel we have too many demands placed on us, looking after ourselves becomes the first thing to get dropped. Eat a healthy diet, exercise regularly, and get enough sleep. Nurturing yourself results in a more efficient self and protects your brain (you ARE a neuropsychologist, for crying out loud!).

We all rely on our calendar to help us know where we need be every day at work, and we rarely miss meetings or cancel work activities we have scheduled. Treat your personal life in the same way. Formally schedule pleasurable or fun activities for yourself every day, as well as activities that you find relaxing. This could mean exercise, dinner with a friend, attending your child's ballet recital, and so on. Actually write it in your calendar; we find we rarely miss a "gym date" if it is "in the book." And respect your schedule. Respect it just like you do the time you allocate for work priorities.

Strategy 3: Build resilience. *Resilience* is the ability to adapt to life's changes. Studies show that increased resilience can enhance your quality of life and help decrease stress. You need to pay as much attention to your own needs and feelings as you do to those of your patients/clients. In addition to taking care of yourself, look at life through a positive lens, take time each day to reflect on things you are thankful for, and take time with family members and friends. This can be done in a number of different ways, including using mindfulness strategies, keeping a gratitude journal, or even just unplugging for an evening with your family with no outside distractions. There are many online resources about resilience factors and strategies, including one from the American Psychological Association (APA; 2012).

Strategy 4: Choose how you spend your time wisely, grasshopper. You have only a limited amount of time outside of work to do the many things that might be on your list. Constantly evaluate how you would like to use that limited resource. It is as important to do something pleasurable (exercise, spend time with your partner, play or read with your children) as it is to do all your household chores, so keep in mind that you don't have to finish all your "work" before you can "play." It is okay if your laundry remains undone or your house isn't cleaned for one more day, if that means you can go to a special family event or school activity. Conversely, if home chores are more important (your in-laws are coming!), try to make this a family activity or pass on the gym and take a long walk at lunch. Priorities will change, and you must make the choice that makes the most sense at that time.

Strategy 5: Do not waste time worrying about your workload when you are not at work. Work, or don't work. When you aren't working, don't think about work. Also, technology provides constant access to email and colleagues, which can make it easy to blur the line between work and home. This can be helpful in some situations but also can decrease your focus on where you are at the time. Try to separate the two as much as possible. Be as technology free as possible when you are not working.

A premise that you may have picked up from your parents, scout leader, or other well-intentioned authority figure is: You should not do anything fun until the work is done. This is just ridiculous. If you haven't realized it by now, there is ALWAYS work to be done. The best way to have good work–life integration is to be fully present wherever you are. Don't worry about work while you are not working, and don't regret being at work when you are there. Be as effective as possible in both roles, and embrace the moment for what it is.

Everywhere Strategies

Strategy 1: Follow through on your commitments. Whether this is focused on work or at home, you need to stick to what you say you are going to do. If you tell your wife and kids you're going to be home at 5:00, you better be home at 5:00. If your boss asks you to work this weekend and you've already communicated to him that you cannot work weekends, you need to stick to your guns and say no. When you commit to the things you said you would commit to, one of two things is going to happen: Either people will start respecting you more and you'll build trust and credibility, or you'll stop making so many commitments, which will free up the time to do what is actually important to you.

Strategy 2: Don't be afraid to ask for help. Mentally reframe asking for help as an efficiency strategy rather than a sign of weakness (or *fill in the blank* here). Asking for help is not a sign of lack of competence, lack of confidence, or laziness. Asking someone who can provide assistance, information, or guidance is a way to get things done more accurately and efficiently, allowing you to spend time on other projects or work and possibly even learn something new. Never hesitate to ask family and friends (at home) or colleagues or staff (at work) for their help and support if you need it.

Strategy 3: Remember that there is no such thing as a dumb question. People, in particular, those who are early in their career or have recently begun working in a new place, are often reluctant to ask directions to get guidance and learn the lay of the land. They are worried about being perceived as unqualified or in need of support. This results in a lot of time being wasted by figuring things out yourself or missing out on useful information. Try this positive reframe: The only dumb question is an unasked question. In addition to learning what you need to know, you will be modeling good behavior for your colleagues and trainees. This is equally true as you learn to negotiate through life challenges—such as marriage, parenting, and/or juggling a two-household career. Find out what others you trust have done in challenging situations, figure out whether store-bought cookies will suffice or if they must be homemade, learn time-saving techniques (think Instant Pot), and borrow some favorite recipes. This is considered efficiency, not inadequacy!

Strategy 4: Give yourself credit for the things you have accomplished. No one expects you to get the work–life integration act perfect every time. We have already admitted that it is hard to strike the perfect balance between the amount of time you spend working and the amount of time you spend engaging in other areas of your life. Imagine the effort of your balancing not as constantly having equal weight on both aspects of your life but as a series of course corrections whereby you shift between these two demands with an ultimate goal of having a strong foundation at work and at home.

It is important to remember that it is sometimes easier to measure progress and success at work. There are concrete milestones we can look at. It is much harder to measure being a good spouse/significant other/parent/child/friend. Assess yourself regularly, and make adjustments as needed. But don't forget to acknowledge the things you have completed, attended, and crossed off your to-do list, even when you have not accomplished everything, or as much as you would have like to have done. You would praise your child, your student, or your pet for jobs well done, so remember to give yourself a pat on the back for each thing you have accomplished. Baby steps move you forward just as well as hurdles, and we all do more and feel better when our accomplishments are acknowledged. Be your own cheering squad!

Strategy 5: Remember that your to-do list will still be there tomorrow. Despite your best efforts, you are not going to get everything you want to get done completed every day. This applies both at work and at home, and after you prioritize to get the "must be done" items completed, learn to get comfortable with the idea that unfinished tasks will remain. "Must be done" means a grant deadline, a tax deadline, a lecture or presentation, forms for a doctor's appointment, or a school permission slip. We all have things that we really would like to get done that don't fall into this must-be-done category. Strive to get all these items done, using all the strategies described above, but if finishing a paper or cleaning the house doesn't get done then there will be still another opportunity to do it the next day (or the day after that). Learning to live with things still on your to-do list is an important step in your personal growth and development.

COMMON CHALLENGES TO SELF-CARE AND WORK-LIFE INTEGRATION

No matter how hard you work, or how carefully you prepare, you inevitably will face challenges and encounter obstacles that seem insurmountable. Completing graduate and postdoctoral training in clinical neuropsychology is not for the faint of heart! Some of the most obvious challenges come in the form of degree requirements, such as passing your comprehensive examination and defending your dissertation. Other challenges come when you least expect them, such as interpersonal conflict with a colleague, illness of a close family member, or an existential crisis in yourself (e.g., "Am I really cut out for this profession?!"). Rest assured that with a few strategies in your back pocket, you can handle almost anything that comes your way, and for those times that you need help, refer to "everywhere" Strategy 2.

Common Challenge No. 1: Making Mistakes

First and foremost, when you make a mistake (and you surely will at some point!), remember that you are not alone and that the likelihood that someone else you know has been in a similar situation is high. As soon as a mistake becomes apparent, or even if you are not 100% sure but think you may have made a mistake, reach out to trusted colleagues and mentors for advice and a sympathetic ear. It will be important for you to be honest with yourself and fully understand and/or acknowledge your role in any given situation, whether it be at work or home. For example, if you have fallen behind on a deadline and it is clear that you cannot meet it, it is best for everyone involved if you 'fess up as soon as possible. Approach the person(s) affected with an apology and suggest a plan for getting back on track.

Of course, avoiding mistakes and uncomfortable situations in the first place is most desirable. As mentioned, beware of overextending and overpromising. Capitalize on your strengths and strategize about how to address areas needing improvement. Your mentors and colleagues, as well as close family and friends, can provide valuable insight and feedback toward these goals.

Common Challenge No. 2: Health Concerns

Although one never wants to be faced with health challenges that affect one's training, these situations are not uncommon, and it is important that you prioritize any such health issues. Reach out to your colleagues and mentors for support and advice. Your training director can assist you with developing alternative plans when time away from training is needed to attend to your health or someone else's and thus is a good resource to involve as soon as feasible. Although it may be difficult to disclose your particular situation, remember that everyone in the training program wants you to be successful, and sometimes the best option is to take some time off.

Common Challenge No. 3: Interpersonal Conflict

Encountering interpersonal conflict can be one of the toughest challenges you face during both your training and your career. Whether this conflict occurs with a fellow graduate student, colleague, mentor, or supervisor, you are likely to feel a range of emotions, from indignation to anger to sadness. Of course, seeking consultation from a trusted friend or colleague may be helpful, but when selecting your confidant be careful that you don't put someone else in an awkward position or unintentionally make the situation worse.

First, decide whether it is important to address the conflict or to let it go. Some questions to ask yourself are whether you will be interacting with this individual on a regular basis and whether they may have influence on any part of your training or career. If the answer to these questions is yes then, just as in professional practice, it is usually a good choice to begin by talking directly and confidentially with the person with whom you are experiencing conflict. Once again, you will need to be honest with yourself about your role in the conflictual relationship or situation. Remember that relationships are two-way streets, and both parties have a role in the dynamic. Do a careful self-assessment of potential biases that may be contributing to the conflict. Try to see the situation from the other person's viewpoint; enlist the help of your trusted confidant to look at the situation from different vantage points. Once you feel you can talk about the situation without too much emotion and can be truly open to finding resolution, even if the resolution is to acknowledge that you agree to disagree, set up a time to meet with the person. Suggest a meeting place that is quiet and private and, if possible, on neutral ground. Remind yourself that this individual is a human being and deserving of respect, just like you. Open the meeting by thanking this person for agreeing to get together and by sharing your desire to clear the air, get on the same page, and/or trying to find a mutually agreeable resolution. Allow the individual to share their thoughts without interrupting. Try to listen with an open mind. Whenever possible, acknowledge similarities and topics on which you agree. Work toward a compromise that is palatable to both parties. Of course, you may decide that you never want to speak to this person again, but at least you made an effort to resolve the issue in a professional manner. Finally, use of a neutral third party or mediator can be helpful in situations where you may need to continue to interact with this individual on a regular basis.

Common Challenge No. 4: Feeling Stuck

Another situation that sometimes happens is feeling stuck or worrying that you are not progressing at an appropriate pace or not performing up to par. Know that, no matter how calm and secure other people may appear, it is likely that anyone attempting work–life integration either is struggling or has struggled. Most of us feel this way at some point during our training and in our career development. The key is to determine whether your feelings are fleeting and likely to resolve with time and persistence or if they signal deeper discontent. It is important to explore your feelings fully and to enlist the help of a professional if they linger and begin to interfere with productivity. It is not uncommon at all for students and trainees to engage in psychotherapy. Graduate and postgraduate training can be stressful, and is it important to keep close tabs on your level of stress, happiness, sleep, and other aspects of mental and physical health. If you decide to seek professional help, trusted mentors, other faculty, professionals in the community, and/or the university counseling center may have helpful recommendations.

RESOURCES FOR SELF-CARE AND WORK-LIFE INTEGRATION

An important part of your professional journey is to identify and use any and all resources available to ensure your success (Table 16.2 lists some sample web and text resources). The roads to completing your training and developing your career are fraught with potholes, speed bumps, and detours, and you are wise to arm yourself with appropriate tools and strategies for maneuvering through these landscapes. Start with yourself. You are your best ally and resource. You know your strengths and limits. Listen to yourself and draw the line when needed so you can be the best "you" you can be, for your sake as well as the sake of those around you. It is imperative that you negotiate an optimal level of work–life integration. The level of integration optimal for you is not the same as the level optimal for your supervisor, your lab mate, or your friend. It is a very personal journey that is ever changing across stages of career and work settings. As we noted earlier, you should try very hard to

TABLE 16.2. Sample Web and Text Resources for Self-Care and Resilience

Domain	Resources
Online	APA Psychology Help Center: https://www.apa.org/helpcenter APA Committee on Colleague Assistance: https://bit.ly/2ZA6Kal Self-Compassion Guided Meditations and Exercises: https://bit.ly/2UjWGSk The Self-Care Project: https://bit.ly/2ZGqiKD
Text	Burchard, B. (2017). *High performance habits: How extraordinary people become that way.* Hay House. Hardy, J. (2017). *The self-care project: How to let go of frazzle and make time for you.* Orion Books. Skovholt, T. M., & Trotter-Mathison, M. (2016). *The resilient practitioner: Burnout and compassion fatigue prevention and self-care strategies for the helping professions.* Routledge. Teater, M., & Ludgate, J. (2014). *Overcoming compassion fatigue.* PESI. Willard, C., & Abblett, M. (2016). *The self-compassion deck: 50 mindfulness based practice cards.* PESI.

Note. APA = American Psychological Association.

avoid the trap of comparing your path with anyone else's. Set your own goals and benchmark, and adjust as needed. Feigon and colleagues (2018) offered several suggestions and recommendations when determining your personal work–life integration, including knowing thyself, setting expectations and boundaries early, avoiding comparisons, and seeking guidance; the authors also provide a very helpful resource list in their article.

Speaking of guidance, we cannot emphasize enough the importance of having both mentors and sponsors. *Mentors* provide valuable guidance and support, and *sponsors* make connections for you that advance your career. In the field of neuropsychology, and in particular, during training, there is much overlap between mentors and sponsors (Hilsabeck, 2018). Often your primary clinical neuropsychology supervisor is a main mentor and strong advocate who introduces you to key contacts and writes letters of recommendation. As much as possible, seek multiple mentors who can provide varying perspectives and introduce you to a variety of situations. Characteristics of mentors that are most valued by protégés include enthusiasm, compassion, a strong commitment to meet regularly, and being supportive of work–life integration (Cho et al., 2011). Although many mentors will become sponsors, do not hesitate to reach out to people you do not know, either at a conference or via email, to ask a question or share your interest in a similar topic. Many neuropsychologists are happy to help someone they do not know because it may benefit that person and the field as a whole (Hilsabeck, 2018). In addition, an interaction that starts as a simple conversation between two strangers with similar interests can sometimes turn into a long-term, meaningful relationship. Both mentors and sponsors note that one of the biggest benefits of mentoring/sponsoring is feeling proud and happy for protégés when they achieve their goals and feelings of reward and satisfaction for having played a part in that success.

Finally, take advantage of resources available from professional organizations such as APA, the National Academy of Neuropsychology, and the American Academy of Clinical Neuropsychology. APA, for example, devotes a web page to self-care, with recommendations for books and articles specifically for psychologists (https://www.apa.org/education/grad/self-care). APA also recognizes workplaces that foster employee well-being through their Psychologically Healthy Workplace Awards and provides resources for creating a healthy workplace environment. APA and its Division 40, Society for Clinical Neuropsychology, as well as the National Academy of Neuropsychology and the American Academy of Clinical Neuropsychology, have subcommittees or organizations for students that provide valuable support and information relevant to self-care and work–life integration. Last, but not least, is the never-ending resource that is the internet. Articles and books on self-care and work–life integration are plentiful, as are websites such as the University of California, Berkeley, human resource webpage (https://haas.berkeley.edu/human-resources/work-life-integration/). As part of your self-care plan, consider reading more about this topic and incorporating some strategies into your daily life.

CONCLUSION AND FUTURE DIRECTIONS

The importance of self-care and work–life integration has become recognized across health care specialties, including as a foundational competency in neuropsychology (Rey-Casserly et al., 2012; Smith, 2019). The purpose of this chapter was to provide practical guidance toward achieving work–life integration that may be helpful to students, postdoctoral residents/fellows, and even early- and midcareer professionals. Work–life integration inevitably will be challenging, and thus we encourage you to utilize the work, home, and everywhere strategies we have suggested and to refer to the many resources provided in this chapter. We hope the suggested strategies will resonate with you and spur additional conversation about and research into the possible benefits to health, productivity, and work–life satisfaction. Continued efforts to incorporate concepts supporting work–life integration into individuals' worldviews and organizational policies are needed and will take a concerted effort by all of us.

REFERENCES

American Psychological Association. (2012). *Building your resilience.* https://www.apa.org/topics/resilience

Catano, V., Francis, L., Haines, T., Kirpalani, H., Shannon, H., Stringer, B., & Lozanzki, L. (2010). Occupational stress in Canadian universities: A national survey. *International Journal of Stress Management, 17*(3), 232–258. https://doi.org/10.1037/a0018582

Cho, C. S., Ramanan, R. A., & Feldman, M. D. (2011). Defining the ideal qualities of mentorship: A qualitative analysis of the characteristics of outstanding mentors. *The American Journal of Medicine, 124*(5), 453–458. https://doi.org/10.1016/j.amjmed.2010.12.007

Feigon, M., Block, C., Guidotti Breting, L., Boxley, L., Dawson, E., & Cobia, D. (2018). Work–life integration in neuropsychology: A review of the existing literature and preliminary recommendations. *The Clinical Neuropsychologist, 32*(2), 300–317. https://doi.org/10.1080/13854046.2017.1411977

Hilsabeck, R. C. (2018). Comparing mentorship and sponsorship in clinical neuropsychology. *Clinical Neuropsychology, 32*(2), 284–299. https://doi.org/10.1080/13854046.2017.1406142

Mayo Clinic Staff. (2020, November 20). *Job burnout: How to spot it and take action.* https://www.mayoclinic.org/healthy-lifestyle/adult-health/in-depth/burnout/art-20046642

Rey-Casserly, C., Roper, B. L., & Bauer, R. (2012). Application of a competency model to clinical neuropsychology. *Professional Psychology: Research and Practice, 43*(5), 422–431. https://doi.org/10.1037/a0028721

Smith, G. (2019). Education and training in clinical neuropsychology: Recent developments and documents from the clinical neuropsychology synarchy. *The Clinical Neuropsychologist, 33*(3), 447–465. https://doi.org/10.1080/13854046.2018.1552437

Watts, J., & Robertson, N. (2011). Burnout in university teaching staff: A systematic literature review. *Educational Research, 53*(1), 33–50. https://doi.org/10.1080/00131881.2011.552235

Worley, L. L. M., & Stonnington, C. M. (2017). Self-care, resilience, and work–life balance. In K. J. Brower & M. B. Riba (Eds.), *Integrating psychiatry and primary care. Physician mental health and well-being: Research and practice* (pp. 237–263). Springer International. https://doi.org/10.1007/978-3-319-55583-6_11

17 MENTORSHIP IN CLINICAL NEUROPSYCHOLOGY

C. MUNRO CULLUM, SHAWN McCLINTOCK, AND LAURA LACRITZ

Our approach to writing this chapter involves providing examples of several facets of the mentor–mentee relationship. The senior author, Dr. Cullum (MC), has been a mentor for both coauthors at various stages of their careers. Indeed, Dr. Lacritz (LL) was a postdoctoral fellow of MC while Dr. McClintock was a graduate student and then a postdoctoral fellow with both MC and LL. In practice, we espouse a multidimensional mentoring model as one that offers the most and is ideal for the typical mentee (e.g., the person who is aiming to specialize in clinical neuropsychology and complete a 2-year postdoctoral fellowship). In this chapter, we provide an overview of some definitions of a mentor, review models of mentoring, and discuss the important roles that such individuals play in our professional and personal lives.

MENTORSHIP: DEFINITION, MODELS, AND CHARACTERISTICS

Mentors, advisors, consultants, oh my! Yes, these terms and others are often used interchangeably, which has created substantial ambiguity. Although there is some overlap of traits, qualities, and tasks among those roles,

We wish to thank all of our own mentors for their invaluable contributions to our careers and successes in this rewarding field.

https://doi.org/10.1037/0000250-018
The Neuropsychologist's Roadmap: A Training and Career Guide, C. Block (Editor)

there are also unique differences and aspects that distinguish them. As such, we will start by defining exactly what is a mentor and explain optimal mentoring models.

Definition of Mentorship

Really, what is a mentor? This is one of those million-dollar questions that has an endless array of answers. Interestingly, though, there has been a consistent theme to its definition across the centuries. The term "mentor" originated in the 8th century BC as it first appeared in Homer's *The Odyssey*. The character Mentor became a parental type figure to Telemachus, the son of Odysseus, and helped him manage and deal with life challenges. Fast-forward to the 21st century AD and that role still applies to a mentor.

Many terms are used interchangeably with the word "mentor" such as "advisor," "sponsor," "supervisor," "teacher," or "friend." Although those terms can be used to describe some of the functions of a mentor, they are not the same as a mentor (Sambunjak & Marušić, 2009). A mentor typically does not command or dictate; instead, a mentor is someone who cultivates, nurtures, and guides the mentee to be who they want to be and helps prepare them for the next stage of their career. A neuropsychology mentor helps provide the structure, vision, reality check, and encouragement for the mentee to successfully mature into an independent clinical neuropsychologist and launch into and sustain a fulfilling career. There are many influences a developing neuropsychologist will encounter along one's career path, but the mentor serves a unique goal.

As illustrated in Figure 17.1, the Mentorship Pyramid synthesizes the *goals* of the mentoring relationship along with the *role* and *involvement* of the mentor. For each goal, the mentor may play a slightly different role and have a different level of involvement. A mentor in some instances may serve each of those functions for their mentee: role model, teacher, advisor, and sponsor, depending on the setting, length, and context of the relationship and how the relationship evolves. For example, a graduate student may hold a particular faculty member as a role model and aspire to develop or assume similar attributes with very little involvement from the faculty member. However, the student may take a class from the neuropsychologist (mentor as teacher) and then seek them out for career advice (mentor as advisor), followed by joining their research lab and then ultimately asking for an introduction or recommendation as the student applies for a postdoctoral fellowship or a future job (mentor as sponsor). Alternatively, given that one mentor cannot do everything, a mentee may have a team of "mentors" who each serve only one or two of the goals in the Mentorship Pyramid, and it is important for

FIGURE 17.1. The Mentorship Pyramid

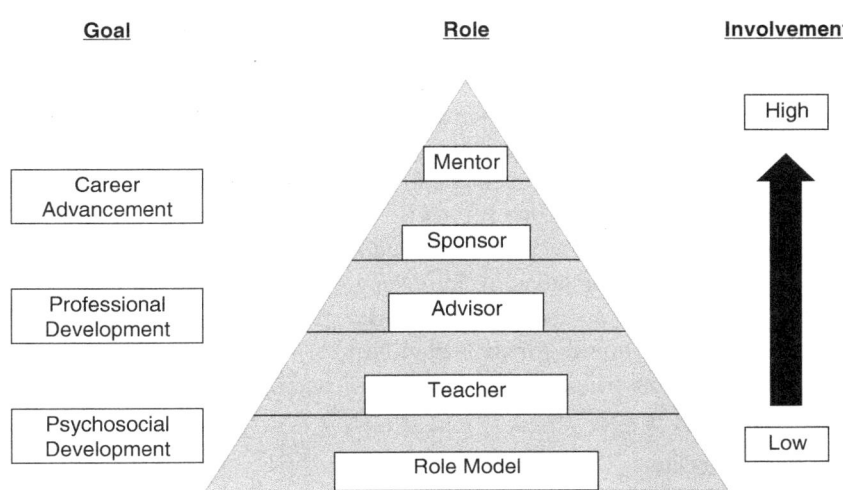

Note. From "What's a Mentor, Anyway?", by N. T. Mertz, 2004, *Educational Administration Quarterly, 40*(4), p. 551 (https://doi.org/10.1177/0013161X04267110). Copyright 2004 by Sage Publications. Adapted with permission.

the mentee to gauge who in their settings can best help them achieve specific goals. For example, a mentee who would like to learn a particular skill set to propel their research or clinical acumen may seek out people with whom they can learn those skills (e.g., advanced statistical approach, test development, neuroimaging analysis, and/or type of rehabilitation intervention).

It is important to remember that a mentor does not serve only as a sponsor. Although there is some overlap, sponsorship and mentorship are not the same. *Mentoring* involves providing guidance and expertise to help the mentee reach their goals; *sponsoring* consists of making connections that will advance the mentee's career. This may involve introducing them to people who are in positions of influence, recommending them for positions or promotions, and connecting them with opportunities to help meet their career goals. In essence, the sponsor is putting themselves and their reputation on the line for the mentee, and thus have a vested interest in their success. Although having a good mentorship has been shown to enhance job satisfaction, improve self-efficacy in professional activities, and increase faculty productivity (e.g., number of publications or amount of funding), sponsorship is also essential for career advancement. Sponsors have key knowledge about how organizations or institutions operate and can use their political savvy, knowledge, and personal influence to break down barriers and/or facilitate connections with those in power or who have influence within a particular system. This may be as simple as sending a curriculum vitae and providing a personal recommendation to the hiring manager for a position that has many applicants or being proactive in advocating for the mentee in a situation or for a position that would help their career. In fact, some sponsors seek out opportunities for their mentees, garner support for them, and provide mentorship to help ensure their success. Indeed, sponsors frequently have also served as mentors for the person they are helping to promote, though not always, and not all mentors will be sponsors. Just as mentees must be proactive in seeking out mentors, so too must they be willing to ask for sponsorship. Similarly, sponsors need to be vigilant for relevant opportunities for their mentees. For additional information on mentoring and sponsoring, see Hilsabeck (2018) and Ayyala et al. (2019).

Mentorship Models

From a simplistic standpoint, there are two primary mentorship structures: informal and formal (Cornelius et al., 2016). The *informal mentoring model* involves a relaxed, less committed, use-as-needed, arrangement between the mentor and mentee. Whereas this arrangement works for some people, or in instances when an ancillary mentor is desired (e.g., for consultation more than helping the mentee move toward specific career goals), the more limited structure, communication, collaboration, and established goals of the relationship may be less effective for others. Conversely, the *formal mentoring model* implies an arrangement and commitment between the mentor and mentee, or among the mentoring team, whereby there is shared agreement regarding the timeline and goals of the mentoring relationship. As the mentoring relationship is forming, all parties should discuss what type of mentoring relationship they envision. Formal rather than informal mentoring may be more effectual in some respects, with long-lasting career development benefits, though informal mentoring has its place as well, depending upon the mentor as well as the mentee's needs and aspirations.

Within the formal mentoring structuring, there are multiple mentoring models, and one size does not fit all. The models tend to be formed on the basis of the number of people and the goal. Regarding numbers, there is one-on-one mentoring, team mentoring, peer mentoring, and transgenerational mentoring. One mentor cannot typically provide all that is needed, and team mentoring may be useful so that multiple areas of expertise are represented on which the mentee can draw for growth. Peer mentoring involves mentoring among peers. Although this is useful, because the people are at similar career development stages and may be going through the same trials and tribulations, peer mentoring is usually more limited because there may be a lack of wisdom that can better be provided by a more senior mentor who can provide a different vantage point to inform decision making.

Transgenerational Mentoring

To augment peer and team mentoring, *transgenerational mentoring* uses a team-based mentoring approach with a mixture of mentors and mentees at various career stages, including senior, midcareer, and early career. This affords bidirectional exchanges, thereby allowing all parties to be mentors; that is, the senior-career mentor can mentor the mid- and early-career mentee, and at the same time the early-career mentee can mentor the mid- and senior-career mentees. For instance, an early-career mentee may be aware of new information, insights, technology, and models in the field that can be shared with the mid- and senior-career members. Think about this: When a new neuropsychological test comes out, who usually is the first person to master it? We'll give you a hint—it's usually not the senior mentor. With this transgenerational model, the person is forming a triumvirate of mentors who can address different needs and help the person develop as a mentor in their own right.

Tripod Model of Mentorship

A modification of the transgenerational model is the *tripod model of mentorship*, whereby, irrespective of career stage, the person has senior and junior mentors with whom they receive or provide mentorship, while having a peer with whom to discuss career experiences and challenges that can occur (see Figure 17.2).

FIGURE 17.2. The Tripod Model of Mentorship

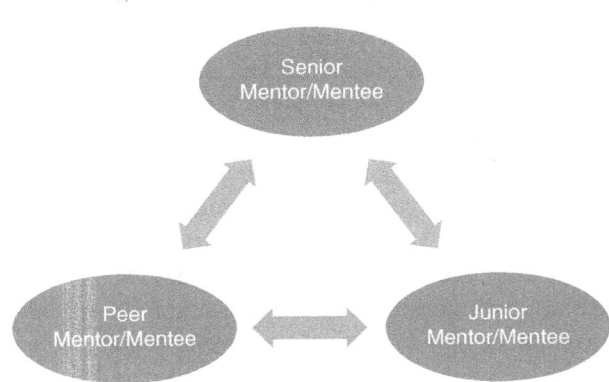

The tripod model of mentorship emphasizes that mentors at each level can learn from and contribute to the development of mentees at different professional levels. The role of a senior mentor is more obvious in relationship to junior colleagues; they can provide career-specific guidance across a number of areas, including job search/promotion support, research and publishing, networking, skill refinement, and so on, and peer mentors can provide support (e.g., empathy, active and reflective listening) and share their experiences (e.g., career journey, applying for fellowship or job, negotiating authorship on a paper), allowing each party to benefit from the other's approaches to similar problems and dilemmas. Peer mentors can also help with networking and become valuable collaborators. Last, the junior mentor (i.e., someone at an earlier career stage) can provide valuable knowledge and perception in areas such as office climate, procedures, personnel dynamics, and new technologies that might not be as readily apparent to more senior mentors. The American Psychological Association (2006) generated *Introduction to Mentoring: A Guide for Mentors and Mentees*, which includes examples of how mentors at different developmental stages can provide support along a variety of career and psychosocial domains; it may serve as a useful resource.

The goal of the mentoring relationship also affects the mentoring model. The mentee needs to define their goals as they relate to clinical work, research, education, service, and self-care and consider whether the goals are short-term, mid-term, or long-term in nature; the number and type of goals will dictate the time frame and structure of the mentoring model to conform to meet the end goal. If a mentee has set only one goal, and it is a short-term goal to be accomplished within 3 to 6 months, the mentoring model will be built to focus only on that goal for that brief duration of time. However, if the mentee has set multiple short- and long-term goals, then the mentoring model will be built to best accomplish those goals and include a lengthy time with multiple mentors. The optimal structured mentoring model is one that has input from all involved in the mentoring relationship, with a mutually agreed-upon structure, format, and timeline. Thus, less informality and greater formality may benefit many individuals in order to maintain momentum and meet goals sooner than might occur with a more informal model. It is also worth noting that mentoring teams do not need to be geographically together; neither does the team need to necessarily meet as a group, although communication can certainly be beneficial. Mentees who are particularly well organized and have mutually defined goals with their mentors may be the "drivers" of the process, in fact, seeking different mentors at different times for different issues, which we discuss shortly. For a review of other mentorship models and benefits of mentorship for both the mentor and mentee, see Henry-Noel et al. (2019).

Characteristics of Mentorship Relationships

Pop quiz: What is a mentor, and what is a mentee? Note that your answer will be rated a 0, 1, or a 2 depending on the details. Just kidding. But seriously, by now in this chapter you should know what a mentor and mentee are. Knowing the definition and model is a critical first step, and now it is time to get down to the nitty-gritty of the characteristics of the mentoring relationship.

Mentor and Mentee Expectations

Deciding to engage in a mentoring relationship represents a commitment on the part of both the mentor and mentee. Prospective mentors need to decide if they have the time needed to help the mentee meet their goals and whether they have the required expertise. One of the mentor's first tasks is educating the mentee about the mentoring process and discussing the degree to which the relationship will be formal or informal. As part of this, the mentor sets the tone for the relationship and helps promote success by setting clear expectations for both parties, which should include outlining goals, setting up the frequency and length of meetings, identifying a timeline, and establishing the modes of communication. Likewise, the mentee should express their desires and goals for the mentoring relationship. These are all points that should be discussed and decided upon at the start of the relationship to avoid unrealistic or unmet expectations.

Lineage

Having good mentors is essential to success in many professions and certainly in academic neuropsychology. Much like the closely aligned field of behavioral neurology, one's training lineage is important and a source of pride for many. The question "Where did you train?" often comes up in introductions, and "With whom did you train?" is equally, or more, important. Although neither is a guarantee of clinical nor research proficiency or excellence, training with acclaimed experts in our field carries with it prestige that is acknowledged within and outside our profession. Attorneys seeking neuropsychology experts, for example, often research potential candidates' curriculum vitae in detail, including their training lineage, in order to bolster the status of their experts in the eyes of attorneys, judges, and juries. In situations where good mentorship is not available, potential mentees may turn to mentorship programs and involvement in professional organizations, which may provide access to mentors that might otherwise be difficult to arrange.

It can be interesting and fun to trace one's academic lineage, much like many people seek to know their familial ancestry these days. Although there is no at-home kit to determine neuropsychology family lineage, simply asking mentors and using online resources (e.g., https://academictree.org) can be helpful. For example, MC was a graduate student of Erin Bigler, who can trace his academic roots back to the experimental laboratory of Wilhelm Wundt!

Throughout our years of training, many of us have the opportunity to work with excellent mentors, although, as discussed elsewhere in this chapter, different mentors can be useful in different ways, and we may want to emulate certain characteristics of one mentor for certain applications and the characteristics of another, who might be a better "fit" or have greater appeal, in other situations. As with clinical and research supervisors, we should take the best from each mentor and incorporate those qualities that best suit our individual personalities.

Not every mentor's personal approach is going to be one that we can or should try to emulate, because we are all unique, but working with a variety of mentors at various stages of our training and careers has many benefits. MC had the privilege of being supervised and mentored by some of the most distinguished clinical neuropsychologists in the world, including Erin Bigler, Nelson Butters, Dean Delis, Ron Ruff, Bob Heaton, and Igor Grant, and each has been a tremendous influence on MC's career. Like parenting (though not to suggest mentors are even necessarily older than mentees, as they do not have to be!), mentoring never ceases, as even senior neuropsychologists such as MC to this day have thoughts along the lines of "WWED?" or "WWND?" (What would Erin do? What would Nelson do?) as situations arise. Reflecting on the likely response of a mentor and/or reaching out to contact them for their advice can be most useful and reassuring while keeping strong relationships alive.

Number of Mentors

Another million-dollar question that often arises is whether one mentor is enough. A parallel to this question can be found in graduate training clinical supervision. How many people had only one clinical supervisor? The answer, most likely, is none. Similarly, a person can have more than one mentor; in fact, a wise mentor might make such a recommendation. To this end, having multiple mentors, or even a mentoring team, can be extremely useful. As we have acknowledged, one mentor is never enough. Trust us, it takes a team of mentors. As in many other types of relationships, a single mentor is probably unable to provide everything needed at a particular point in time, but a mentoring team can provide guidance across many areas, such as career development, prioritizing and juggling a busy schedule, diplomate preparation, clinical expertise, leadership and governance, negotiation skills, research, and publishing. Thus, it is prudent to build a mentoring team composed of mentors who will help the mentee have a successful career development experience and career.

Inclusion and Diversity

Inclusion and diversity are important topics that can have an impact on career development and the mentoring relationship. *Inclusion* refers to the aspect of actively creating a safe and welcoming space/relationship; *diversity* refers to characteristics that make us unique and spans a multitude of areas, such as age, sex, gender, nationality, race, ethnicity, culture, sexual orientation, and religion. Specific to clinical neuropsychology, diversity can also include career stage, type of doctoral degree, specialization, professional organization membership, approach to assessment, and diplomate status. The mentoring relationship can serve as a safe space to discuss and process the many aspects of inclusion and diversity, and these dimensions should be discussed early and openly in the relationship.

Given the different qualities that may be desired in a mentor, how important is it for your mentor to be similar to you in terms of demographic or diversity characteristics? Although there are clear advantages for mentees from a psychosocial perspective to having mentors who share some common features and past experiences, those factors are not as important as simply having access to a mentor. Mentoring can improve the success of many people and may be even more important for those who are underrepresented in academic health careers (Henry-Noel et al., 2019) irrespective of individual differences between the mentor and mentee (Hill-Briggs et al., 2004; Sachs et al., 2018). However, depending on personal circumstances or specific needs it may be important for a mentee to have a mentor who is similar to them in particular ways (e.g., race–ethnicity, gender, similar clinical or research interest). As we've noted, this is a case where having a mentoring team can be beneficial; a team can help ensure inclusion and diversity among the mentors, given that different mentors bring different personal qualities and experiences to the table, in addition to their "official" role in mentoring.

MENTORSHIP RELATIONSHIP: INITIATING, CULTIVATING, AND CONCLUDING

As in a real mentoring session, we will review what we have accomplished thus far and then move forward. Defined the mentor and the mentee: Check. Learned about formal mentoring and mentor and mentee characteristics that help make mentoring successful: Check. Now it is time to talk about initiating and cultivating the mentoring relationship.

Step 1: Initiating a Mentorship Relationship

How does one find a mentor? Sometimes this is a naturally evolving relationship, as when someone is assigned as a supervisor and the relationship builds into one of mentor–mentee, which, as noted, goes beyond supervision. In other cases, one needs to actively search for a mentor to provide assistance with a specialized area of training such as neuropsychology.

Tip 1: Look within your training program. In applying to graduate programs, internships, and postdoctoral residencies, applicants should identify programs that best match their interests and training needs, which means having at least one affiliated neuropsychologist and a potential opportunity for one or more mentors. Surveying others about their experience working with a potential mentor is useful, as is examining that mentor's track record with respect to not only what their training lineage was but also what their mentees and supervisees have gone on to do in their careers.

Tip 2: Look outside your training program. In situations where a good mentor may not be readily available, trainees must search beyond their immediate environment. Although no app has yet been designed specifically for finding a neuropsychology mentor, our field fortunately is still relatively small and blessed with many individuals willing to help others in their careers, and mentoring at a distance is viable, in particular with modern teleconnectivity options. Finding the right mentor for the right need is key to establishing a productive mentor–mentee relationship. Mentoring to promote career development via organizational involvement is somewhat of a specialty area, because not everyone in our field pursues these endeavors. As such, a mentee who wants to get involved in organizational leadership (e.g., elected positions such as member-at-large, secretary, treasurer, president) may need to identify mentors with governance and leadership experience whom they admire and who have a track record of helping others along these lines. Some organizations (e.g., the American Psychological Association's Society for Clinical Neuropsychology, the National Academy of Neuropsychology) now provide active and rather formal mentoring opportunities, and many mentors are willing to have mentees shadow them during professional meetings and discuss their own paths to leadership.

Tip 3: Join an organization, and attend an organizational meeting. Becoming involved as a member of one or more of our professional organizations and attending meetings or conferences is an excellent way not only to develop one's network but also to avail oneself to potential mentors, and it provides valuable learning opportunities. For instance, when at a professional conference, participate in mentoring sessions when they are offered and actively seek out the person or persons with whom you would like to meet regarding mentorship. Sometimes attending a poster session can be a win–win because it provides a great space to talk about your current work and identify and engage with potential mentors. Other opportunities for contacting mentors include attending talks by potential mentors, sitting in on organizational business meetings, interacting with other mentees or students of potential mentors, and attending social hours and informal gatherings. Regularly engaging in these activities allows for one's informal network to develop and grow, which in turn can make it easier to approach potential mentors or ask for an introduction by a mutual acquaintance/colleague.

Step 2: Cultivating the Mentorship Relationship

When thinking of strategies to enhance the mentoring relationship (see Table 17.1), keep in mind some of the lessons learned in your Cognitive–Behavioral Therapy 101 class, such as creating a schedule and agenda, setting goals, and checking in. Like every effective relationship, a mentoring relationship also requires commitment, dedication, respect, and time. We now offer some tips for both the mentee and mentor to enhance the mentoring relationships.

Tip 1: Make a clear commitment. Commitment ensures that the mentor and mentee are aware of the responsibilities that come with each role. When entering into the relationship, each person dedicates themself to the role and agrees to carry out the responsibilities.

TABLE 17.1. Strategies for a Successful Mentor–Mentee Relationship

Mentor	Mentee
Have adequate time to devote to the mentee	Take the initiative
Set clear expectations	Clarify your goals and expectations
Help set realistic priorities	Communicate your needs clearly
Establish timelines	Respect your mentor's time
Communicate clearly	Set the agenda for meetings, and send in advance
Be honest, but respectful	Be on time for meetings
Challenge when necessary, but be supportive	Be organized
Motivate and encourage	Show commitment to the process
Foster independence	Demonstrate reliable follow-through
Maintain confidentiality	Be efficient
Acknowledge success	Look for opportunities to give back
Recognize when other mentors are needed	Express your appreciation
Recognize if/when relationship has met the mentee's goals	

Tip 2: Determine needs and goals for the mentoring relationship. Mentees must determine what needs they intend the mentoring relationship to fill. Figuring out their needs will guide them in approaching the right mentor for a particular goal.

Tip 3: Establish the mode and frequency of communication. Will communication occur in person, via email, and/or by phone or video? How often should meetings be scheduled? It's typically the mentee's responsibility to initiate meetings, set the pace, and ask for input. To do this, the mentee can initially check with the mentor regarding optimal communication methods and frequency of meetings. Once confirmed, the mentee can preschedule the meetings and provide reminders as needed.

Tip 4: Schedule well in advance. In general, it is advisable to preschedule mentoring sessions 3 to 6 months ahead of time and, at least in the early stages, it may be helpful to try and keep a consistent day and time so that the meetings become routine. It is important to ensure the schedule is on each person's calendar, with reminders in place as needed.

Tip 5: Be respectful of all members in the mentoring relationship. It is essential that the members of the mentoring relationship have respect for each other in order to support an exchange of ideas, openness to refinement of those ideas, and mutual areas of agreement and disagreement. Feedback should be provided in a constructive and respectful fashion, providing a safe environment that promotes honesty and directness.

Tip 6: Be patient—a mentoring relationship takes time to grow. Time is also an essential ingredient for the relationship. Everyone must provide time for the relationship to begin and thrive.

Tip 7: Develop (and follow) an agenda. For each session, create ahead of time a mutually agreed-on agenda in order to maximize the allotted time (see Exhibit 17.1). Both the mentee and the mentor should collaboratively create and set short- and long-term goals to be worked toward in the mentoring sessions. Such goals may be centered around the career development stage, need to be operationalized/defined, and have an established time frame for completion. For example, tangible goals for the mentoring agenda for a first-year postdoctoral fellow might include preparation for licensure, starting the diplomate process, and publishing at minimum one peer-reviewed manuscript. Listing the goals on the agenda helps to ensure that the mentee and mentor have a focus and roadmap for the mentoring sessions.

Tip 8: Create a career development matrix. To optimize structure of the mentoring sessions and assist with goal setting, the mentee in collaboration with the mentor can create a *career development matrix* (CDM). The CDM is a tool to orchestrate a portfolio, like a business or retirement portfolio, and integrate it with the objectives of the early career clinical neuropsychologist.

EXHIBIT 17.1. Examples of Discussion Topics During Mentorship Meetings

- Getting licensed to practice
- Getting board certified
- Navigating appointments and promotions at an academic institution
- How to start your own clinical practice
- How to handle medicolegal cases
- Maintaining a strong curriculum vitae
- How to publish articles, books, and book chapters
- How to write and/or review a grant
- How to be a good collaborator
- Learning the politics of the field
- Learning the "who's who" in neuropsychology and related disciplines
- How to create a better presentation and present at a conference
- Becoming a better speaker/presenter
- Becoming a leader in a professional and/or scientific organization
- Learning how to balance personal and professional life goals
- Negotiating a salary
- How to successfully navigate a career
- How to become an effective mentor
- Inclusion and diversity
- Ethics

The portfolio includes two categories: *inputs* and *outputs*. The inputs may include resources (e.g., referral sources, practice and/or research infrastructure, funding sources, time, personnel support, trainees) that will support the operations of the early-career trainee in their environment, whereas the outputs include the tasks that are necessary to carry out the career objectives (e.g., licensure and diplomate preparation, manuscript and grant writing, teaching, patient services). The CDM provides a concise visual tracking system to monitor the input source and resources that are currently or will be available, as well as the allocation of those resources. With this type of information, the mentee and mentor can use the CDM to help guide mentoring sessions and inform the next steps for successful career development, as well as identify what additional inputs are needed to reach their output goals.

Step 3: Concluding the Mentorship Relationship

To use an example from the 1970s TV show *Kung Fu* (okay, younger readers and mentees may need to Google that!), the master Shaolin priest holds a pebble in his open hand, and his mentee's task is to try to take it before he is able to close his hand. The classic line said to the young priest in training, who is referred to as "Grasshopper" by Master Kan, is "When you can take the pebble from my hand, it will be time for you to leave." The goal of mentoring is to help the mentee get to the next level of achievement they seek, and it is usually apparent to the mentor when this level is reached and when at least the basics of "training" (or some aspect thereof) is "complete" and it may be time for young Grasshopper to move on, or to allow the young trainee to realize they may now be well on their path to becoming (to use another, more contemporary, reference) a neuropsychology Jedi. The humble mentee usually does not feel as though they are done being mentored, and they really are not in the broader sense, because we all need and continue to benefit from mentors throughout our careers. Even after the clear goals of mentorship have been met, some mentoring relationships last, sometimes throughout one's career, such as a graduate mentor who continues to serve as a resource for decades after graduation, while others will transition to friendships and working relationships, and still others may fade after the goals have been met. These are all acceptable outcomes depending on the goals and type of relationship that develops between the neuropsychology mentor and mentee.

MENTORSHIP RESOURCES

Access to appropriate mentors can vary depending on goals and setting. As we mentioned, mentors do not need to be local, and in fact some mentoring may come from printed materials. The American Psychological Association (2006) mentoring guide we mentioned provides a nice additional overview for mentors and mentees and the National Institutes of Health offers a variety of valuable resources for research mentors and mentees (see, e.g., https://oir.nih.gov/sourcebook/mentoring-training and https://training.nih.gov/mentoring_guidelines). Checking with an academic institution may also yield resources. As an example, the University of Wisconsin offers mentoring training resources for clinical and translational researchers as part of the National Research Mentoring Network (https://ictr.wisc.edu/mentoring). Many of the national neuropsychological organizations have mentoring programs at different levels and for different purposes (see Table 17.2). Unfortunately, some of these resources go underutilized. One should not let an application process deter them from seeking out these opportunities as well as asking for someone (e.g., program director, supervisor) to endorse them, if appropriate, to support their application.

CONCLUSION AND FUTURE DIRECTIONS

The mentoring relationship is one of the most important and rewarding in academic neuropsychology, regardless of which approach to mentoring one chooses or how the process evolves. Seeing the accomplishments of mentees

TABLE 17.2. Sampling of Mentorship Resources

Domain	Resources
National Institutes of Health (NIH)	The NIH and its Office of Intramural Research offers multiple resources for research mentors and mentees.
American Psychological Association	Leadership Institute for Women in Psychology
	Office on Early Career Psychologists
	Committee on Early Career Psychologists
American Psychological Association of Graduate Students	LGBT Graduate Student Mentoring Program
American Academy of Clinical Neuropsychology (AACN)	AACN Student Mentorship Program
American Board of Clinical Neuropsychology	Mentorship program for candidates seeking board certification
National Academy of Neuropsychology	Women in Leadership/Student and Postdoctoral Committee Sponsorship Program
	Leadership and Ambassador Development Program
Hispanic Neuropsychological Society	Mentorship program for members

Note. LGBT = lesbian, gay, bisexual, and transgender.

and the fruits of their labors rewarded provides a sense of great pride for mentors as well as a feeling of accomplishment for mentees. Having pride in one's academic "family tree" and carrying on the tradition of mentoring future generations means that, as a mentor, one's impact on the field is magnified, greatly expanding the number of lives touched, whether it be in terms of scientific advancement and knowledge, betterment of current and future patients, and/or evolution and progression of the field. For the mentee, having different mentors for different facets of one's career provides a strong background and system of support and guidance that can be useful throughout one's career.

REFERENCES

American Psychological Association. (2006). *Introduction to mentoring: A guide for mentors and mentees.* https://www.apa.org/education/grad/mentoring

Ayyala, M. S., Skarupski, K., Bodurtha, J. N., González-Fernández, M., Ishii, L. E., Fivush, B., & Levine, R. B. (2019). Mentorship is not enough: Exploring sponsorship and its role in career advancement in academic medicine. *Academic Medicine, 94*(1), 94–100. https://doi.org/10.1097/ACM.0000000000002398

Cornelius, V., Wood, L., & Lai, J. (2016). Implementation and evaluation of a formal academic–peer-mentoring programme in higher education. *Active Learning in Higher Education, 17*(3), 193–205. https://doi.org/10.1177/1469787416654796

Henry-Noel, N., Bishop, M., Gwede, C. K., Petkova, E., & Szumacher, E. (2019). Mentorship in medicine and other health professions. *Journal of Cancer Education, 34*(4), 629–637. https://doi.org/10.1007/s13187-018-1360-6

Hill-Briggs, F., Evans, J. D., & Norman, M. A. (2004). Racial and ethnic diversity among trainees and professionals in psychology and neuropsychology: Needs, trends, and challenges. *Applied Neuropsychology, 11*(1), 13–22. https://doi.org/10.1207/s15324826an1101_3

Hilsabeck, R. C. (2018). Comparing mentorship and sponsorship in clinical neuropsychology. *The Clinical Neuropsychologist, 32*(2), 284–299. https://doi.org/10.1080/13854046.2017.1406142

Mertz, N. T. (2004). What's a mentor, anyway? *Educational Administration Quarterly, 40*(4), 541–560. https://doi.org/10.1177/0013161X04267110

Sachs, B. C., Benitez, A., Buelow, M. T., Gooding, A., Schaefer, L. A., Sim, A. H., Tussey, C. M., & Shear, P. K. (2018). Women's leadership in neuropsychology: Historical perspectives, present trends, and future directions. *The Clinical Neuropsychologist, 32*(2), 217–234. https://doi.org/10.1080/13854046.2017.1420234

Sambunjak, D., & Marušić, A. (2009). Mentoring: What's in a name? *Journal of the American Medical Association, 302*(23), 2591–2592. https://doi.org/10.1001/jama.2009.1858

18 INTERDISCIPLINARY SCIENCE, PRACTICE, AND EDUCATION COMPETENCIES

JOANNE R. FESTA AND CHRISTINA A. PALMESE

Patients present with a complex of physical, emotional, and cognitive symptoms. For many years, they have been served in specialty silos, left to coordinate the complexities of findings from multiple providers and the implications for their own care. In this new age of health care, optimal patient care integrates the expertise of multiple disciplines to enhance patient diagnosis and treatment. A growing number of providers from all specialties, including psychologists and neuropsychologists, are now working more collaboratively in patient care. Evidence demonstrates that integrating behavioral health into primary care improves quality, efficiency, and outcomes (Balasubramanian et al., 2017). The newest generation of neuropsychologists will have a greater likelihood of participating in interdisciplinary teams and ultimately may serve on multiple teams in their professional practice.

Many terms have been used to describe how a variety of different providers treat a single patient, such as "multidisciplinary," "interdisciplinary," "transdisciplinary," and "integrated care," to name a few. Although all of these indicate that multiple specialties are involved in patient care, *interdisciplinary* or *interprofessional* care is defined by a focus on collaboration

https://doi.org/10.1037/0000250-019
The Neuropsychologist's Roadmap: A Training and Career Guide, C. Block (Editor)

and communication among all health professionals. The American Psychological Association's Center for Psychology and Health further describes integrated health care as characterized by "the sharing of information among team members related to patient care and the establishment of a comprehensive treatment plan to address the biological, psychological and social needs of the patient," with the team composition determined by the needs of the patient (https://www.apa.org/health/integrated-health-care).

A recent survey of neuropsychologists in integrated-care practices revealed three primary themes for integrating with multidisciplinary teams: (a) advocacy, (b) collaboration, and (c) communication (Kubu et al., 2016). It referred to the following definition of integrated care teams, which

> bring together health care professionals who work collaboratively to treat the whole person. Physicians, psychologists and neuropsychologists, nurses, and other allied providers work in tandem to diagnose physical and psychological health problems, plan and provide treatment, and evaluate whether treatment is effective. (Novotney, 2010, p. 40)

NEUROPSYCHOLOGY AND INTERDISCIPLINARY CARE

The U.S. Department of Veterans Affairs has set standards for integrating psychologists into the care teams of all veterans (Pomerantz et al., 2014), and neuropsychologists were, perhaps, one of the first groups of specialists who were truly integrated into treatment teams in the rehabilitation setting. Their functions can be quite diverse, ranging from assessment and treatment planning to interventions and discharge determinations (Johnson-Greene, 2018). Interdisciplinary neuropsychological practice is, fundamentally, rooted in evidence-based medicine and shared decision making about brain–behavior relationships. In the following sections, we address how neuropsychologists, on the basis of their education and clinical training, offer the following knowledge and skills to integrated-care teams.

STRUCTURAL AND FUNCTIONAL NEUROANATOMY

Integral to neuropsychology is a working knowledge of structural and functional neuroanatomy as well as neuropathology. For many patient populations, clinical diagnosis and treatment depend on the neuropsychologist's ability to adeptly localize and lateralize dysfunction in the brain. To do this, the neuropsychologist must be aware of the anatomic substrates that support specific cognitive functions, and this knowledge must be used to select appropriate tools to measure brain functions of interest. Furthermore, neuropsychologists must appreciate the vast array of potential causes of brain dysfunction (i.e., VITAMINS: Vascular, Infectious/Inflammatory, Traumatic/Toxic, Autoimmune, Metabolic, Iatrogenic/Idiopathic, Neoplastic, and Social factors) in medical decision making. Chapter 11 of this volume offers more information on neuroanatomy.

Sociocultural Considerations

Cultural factors for patients who do not speak English or who speak it as a second language should be taken into account, and culturally appropriate measures and normative data should be used whenever possible. For example, because of cultural differences, it is not uncommon for Spanish speakers to call a "pretzel" a "snake" on a commonly used picture naming test. In other cultures, multiple sounds or words may be needed to convey the name of each individual item on list learning tests, which can affect encoding and retention. Still, in other cultures there can be a melodic quality whereby a slight variation in intonation affects what is being communicated. All of this affects how we interpret test scores, as well as how well we are able to truly measure the cognitive skills of interest, localize dysfunction in the brain, and offer a diagnosis. In situations where cultural norms are unavailable, careful consideration must be given to the referral question and best interest of the patient. For patients undergoing brain surgery, neuropsychological assessment is a required part of the preoperative workup. In these situations, conclusions about cognitive status sometimes can be made by using raw scores or by looking at changes in standard scores, rather than overall impairment level. Alternately, it may be appropriate to move forward with the assessment simply to document a baseline of functioning based on what is available, with a caveat that the measures were developed for native English speakers and that test results should be interpreted with caution. It is critical to perform a risk–benefit analysis of conducting versus not conducting a neuropsychological assessment in these populations.

Neuropsychological Measures and Normative Data Sets

A scientifically based and problem-focused neuropsychological battery with appropriate psychometric properties optimizes patient care and outcome. The number of available neuropsychological measures is extensive, and care must be taken to use only those relevant to the patient and referral question. This includes using assessment tools with appropriate normative samples and good validity, reliability, sensitivity, and specificity for identifying brain dysfunction.

Early neuropsychological batteries, such as the Halstead–Reitan Battery, were broad-based assessments sensitive to brain damage. Often performed over multiple days, lasting 8 or more hours, the batteries could localize lesions, determine degree of impairment, and provide extensive detailed analysis of brain functioning. With the evolution of the field and development of psychometrically sound measures that can be administered as stand-alone assessment tools to localize and lateralize brain dysfunction, assessment batteries can now be more problem focused to assess brain function as it pertains to a specific problem or referral question, such as assistance with the determination of a surgical target or the postoperative prognosis, qualification of diagnosis and impairment level, or extent of care coordination necessary for cognitive optimization or to ensure patient safety. Although some predefined batteries may last 2 hours, many are as brief as 30 to 60 minutes. Of the brief assessment tools, these generally have been developed to assess specific disease processes, such as those published by CERAD (Consortium to Establish a Registry for Alzheimer's Disease) for dementia and the MACFIMS (Minimal Assessment of Cognitive Function in Multiple Sclerosis) for multiple sclerosis, but often neuropsychologists will use a flexible battery whereby assessment measures are added or removed from the examination to optimize investigation of the referral questions. Determinations about the depth and breadth of the assessment also should be based on the patient's ability to withstand assessment, time constraints, and insurance limitations. Useful data can be gleaned from even very brief batteries.

Diagnostic Formulation

As part of an integrated-care team, the neuropsychologist adds tremendous value to the conceptualization of a disease process and patient prognosis. It is important to understand whether clinical strengths and weaknesses are long standing or represent new areas of deficiency. Neuropsychologists determine what the primary versus secondary areas of impairment are and what the diagnostic and prognostic implications of this might be. Given that certain neurological and other medical disorders are associated with specific neurocognitive profiles, this, too, should be considered during test selection and integration into diagnostic formulations.

Neuropsychologists' extensive knowledge of statistics and psychometrics can be of great benefit in practice and research. If a patient has completed serial neurocognitive exams, a reliable change analysis can help determine whether a clinically meaningful change (i.e., a change in function that is rare in the general population) is present versus simply a statistically significant difference. As neuropsychological data are increasingly integrated into medical workups, algorithms are being developed for cognitive risk identification across various patient and disease populations. These predictive models can lead to early intervention and have a positive impact on medical decision making with the ultimate goal of enriching patient care. Continued development and use of empirical instruments to reliably measure outcomes will remain important to document the value of our field and to further our understanding of disease processes and intervention efficacy.

Targeting Recommendations

The results of a neuropsychological assessment can lead to the generation of interdisciplinary interventions to optimize cognitive, emotional, and/or behavioral functioning. When customizing the treatment program for individual patients, neuropsychologists must consider the overall value and feasibility of each recommendation. For example, factors such as financial constraints (e.g., insurance coverage and out-of-pocket expenses) and the patient's access to the services might require additional care coordination. Alternately, it is important to consider whether a patient is motivated to engage in a particular recommendation, especially when it might involve engagement of other health care providers, such as may be necessary when proposing various medication options, exercise and diet modifications, or various interpersonal therapies (e.g., speech therapy, cognitive remediation, supportive psychotherapy). The patient's ability to make appropriate decisions and to follow through with recommendations are integral to their success. In some cases, practical safety issues, such as following a medical protocol (e.g., dietary restrictions, medication management), driving skills, and oversight of activities of daily living, must be the focus of interventions. For others, vocational issues or future-planning directives may be predominant. It is critical that neuropsychologists actively engage with specialists across multiple health care fields to provide patients with the most up-to-date information about location, cost, and accessibility of available resources, from support groups; to psychotherapists; cognitive, speech, and occupational rehabilitation; driving evaluations; social workers; sleep specialists; and more. The neuropsychologist prescribes the right treatment and the right dose to fit the patient: These are not one-size-fits-all recommendations.

SPECIALIZED TRAINING IN NEUROPSYCHOLOGY

Guidelines for specialized education and training in neuropsychology have been established by the Houston Conference and recognized by the American Academy of Clinical Neuropsychology as core requirements for professionals in our field (Hannay et al., 1998). These guidelines advocate a model of training that begins in graduate school and continues at each subsequent level of training, with incremental increases in exposure to clinical assessment, interdisciplinary care, and professional ethics. It encourages that trainees be offered opportunities to supervise other trainees beginning early in their training as well, o prepare them for becoming supervisors when they are engaged in their own clinical practices.

Once a fundamental knowledge base has been established and the clinical experiences achieved at the graduate school level, students are ready to begin their fellowship, preferably at an institution accredited by the American Psychological Association or the Canadian Psychological Association. Subsequent completion of a 2-year neuropsychology fellowship also should be pursued. Should opportunities be unavailable to a postdoctoral candidate at a particular location, then creating an appropriate training experience is at the discretion of the trainee. For example, the advent of technologies, including telehealth, have increased opportunities for distance learning that can co-occur within a nonaccredited training position. Students similarly can make sure their nonaccredited training meets the requirements for state licensure and then independently pursue supplemental learning experiences outside their fellowship that fulfill the Houston criteria. The ultimate achievement of board certification will confirm one's expertise and competence in neuropsychology regardless of the conventionality of the path taken to get there.

COMMUNICATION FOR INTERDISCIPLINARY TEAMS

Neuropsychologists traditionally have conveyed their findings, diagnoses, and treatment recommendations in long, well-crafted reports that focused on metrics and contained great detail. Recent survey information has confirmed what many have come to realize: Few, if any, health care professionals read those lengthy reports but instead refer to last summary sentences of the report for the pertinent neuropsychological information (Postal et al., 2018). Furthermore, lengthy reports necessitate extended time for preparation, thereby delaying communication of results, often for many weeks.

Neuropsychology has also suffered the vestiges of a well-earned reputation for using complex, professional jargon and, perhaps at times, impractical recommendations. Whether engaging in a screening, brief examination, or comprehensive assessment, in this new age of interdisciplinary practice communications are greatly streamlined, reports are shorter, language is simplified, and recommendations are practical. Often neuropsychologists are serving a very specific function on the team: Does the patient have neuro-cognitive sequelae from a specific disorder, or is the patient an appropriate neurosurgical candidate? Neuropsychologists must clearly answer the question at hand as concisely as possible. In some cases, results are communicated to the team on the same day of the exam.

Electronic medical records (EMRs) often facilitate communications between providers, and thus having access to the EMR is essential for capturing important history and conveying the neuropsychologist's contri-bution to the team. Interdisciplinary team members may communicate in many ways: through reports posted on the EMR or otherwise sent to team members, at clinical meetings, in brief email communications, or in passing hallway communications, all while remaining highly attentive to protecting patient confidentiality in compliance with regulations set for by the Health Insurance Portability and Accountability Act of 1996 (HIPAA). Communica-tions of findings may be conducted directly with patients in your office or clinic, with family members, or with new professionals to whom patients are being referred. In addition to providing patient diagnosis, prognosis, and recommendations, neuropsychologists may communicate strategies to other team members to optimize interactions with the patient, the family, or other team members. The variety of neuropsychologists' contacts requires different methods of communication, from the shorthand nomenclature of professionals, to straight talk with patients and families (especially those with cognitive impairments), to therapeutic counseling. Interdisciplinary communications can vary greatly and are most effective when the practi-tioner is flexible in their approach.

NEUROPSYCHOLOGY IN THE 21ST CENTURY

In an era of increased technological advancement, the field of neuro-psychology must demonstrate adaptability in a rapidly changing health care environment. Telehealth is one of the fastest evolving areas of medical care that helps clinicians bring their clinical expertise to places where it does not exist. This includes the use of telehealth to provide hospital in-services, remote clinical training, and community education. At the patient level, telehealth also can be used for clinical intakes and even remote neuropsychological evaluations using a combination of standard neurocognitive measures and computerized assessment tools (Brearly et al., 2017; Cullum et al., 2014). Note, though, that the provider must be licensed in the state in which the patient is sitting.

Advancements in computerized assessment can increase accessibility to care in both primary and specialty care settings. There is a push for innovative test development for enhanced data capture to help with diagnosis and treatment. For example, it has been suggested (Miller & Barr, 2017) that psychometrically sound and ecologically valid computerized measures include technologies such as accelerometry for patients with movement disorders, voice recognition software, and virtual reality platforms. Assessment of passive data, such as those gained through measurement of affect, also could yield useful clinical and research information. Elements of item response theory could be increasingly incorporated into computerized tools as well. An increase in this electronic data collection could be useful for data pooling because the information could easily be stored and shared with encryption among providers and medical centers. This said, with increased consideration of telehealth and computerized assessment come questions about data security, privacy, and data collection, and special steps must be taken to ensure that protected health information is kept secure.

Among the goals of data pooling are enhancement of normative samples, cost reduction, and outcome data collection. The National Institutes of Health (NIH) Toolbox (https://www.healthmeasures.net/explore-measurement-systems/nih-toolbox), a nationally sponsored collection of psychometrically sound cognitive and emotional measures available to neuropsychologists at minimal or no cost, currently offers access to objective life span measures across several cognitive and health domains that can be applied to various patient populations to track current medical status and long-term outcome (Carlozzi et al., 2017). Measures from the Toolbox already have been integrated into EMR so that patients can access and complete various mood and health inventories through patient portals. Patient responses can trigger interactive and real-time feedback with clinical care support when necessary to enhance quality of, and access to, care. Patient endorsements also can be imported to research databases and analyzed in conjunction with various other aspects of their medical health. This can be particularly useful for the construction of brain maps such as those sponsored by the National Institutes of Health BRAIN (Brain Research through Advancing Innovative Neurotechnologies) Initiative (Koroshetz et al., 2018) and the Allen Brain Atlas (http://portal.brain-map.org/). These brain mapping projects integrate neurocognitive data with gene maps and neural networks to improve our understanding of disease etiology, prognosis, and prevention.

With the rise and evolution of EMR, it is important to keep in mind that many medical centers offer patients full and immediate access to medical notes, including neuropsychological reports. Care must be taken to protect private health information in reports and to make sure that patients receive appropriate counseling before viewing the results online. This might mandate the need for briefer evaluations and the use of technology for rapid scoring, provision of face-to-face feedback immediately after exam completion, and generation of shorter reports that are highly symptom and treatment focused.

PRACTICAL ISSUES FOR INTERDISCIPLINARY CARE

Neuropsychologists have been blazing trails to become integral members of interdisciplinary teams for many years: Although some roles are well established, such as working on epilepsy and neurosurgical teams, others are still in progress, as those currently developing in the primary care setting. Opportunities for interdisciplinary practice may exist in nearby medical practices or may require development, and it is generally the neuropsychologist who is proactive in establishing the need and service stream. Colleagues have demonstrated that pilot programs can be created within an existing interdisciplinary service to embed a neuropsychologist on a part-time basis, perhaps as little as half a day a week. As the benefits of our services are realized and the demand increases, the service will likely grow. When embedded on site, be prepared for curbside consultations with other professionals and for referrals to come as part of the "warm handoff," a referral practice in which a medical provider introduces the patient to the neuropsychologist in real time. Same-day services, which ensure that the patient obtains all services needed to optimize care, are the hallmark of interdisciplinary care in some settings. This is often how interdisciplinary care is provided, but before pursuing these practices, a neuropsychologist should determine if this model is the right fit for them. In the next sections, we address a number of variables that should be considered in pursuing interdisciplinary practices.

Practice Location

Integrating one's professional work into a hospital, clinic, or practice may be the ideal, but the degree to which neuropsychologists are colocated in institutions across the United States is not well documented. Although some may be housed with other team members, neuropsychologists may continue to evaluate patients in a consultative service or in telemedicine but with a shift to increased participation in team meetings and group treatment decision making, perhaps via a HIPAA-protected Skype or other internet format. These operational elements are still evolving.

Case Identification

Creating opportunities may require enhanced identification of potential cases. Some neuropsychologists have used a screening technique of *stepped care*, an approach of screening in a stepwise fashion from the least to the most intensive, with the most complex assessment reserved for more extreme cases (Lanca, 2018). Others have developed innovative tablet technology to reliably increase the detection of cognitive dysfunction in a clinic setting, thereby facilitating rapid, early identification of patients at risk for cognitive dysfunction and in need of neuropsychological services (Rao, 2018). The patient population and setting will guide the methodologies to be used. Paramount to the development of these services is being abreast of the literature, recent findings, and latest treatments in the field.

Payment Models

As patient care evolves to increasingly include interdisciplinary care, there will also be a shift in payment models from volume to value. The change will likely be from fee-for-service to bundled payments for overall care by professionals from multiple specialties treating a specific condition for which integrated multidisciplinary care is optimal (Pliskin, 2018). Be prepared for changes in procedure codes and reimbursements, and be willing to adjust as current terminology and policies change.

Impact and Efficacy

Neuropsychology team members must continually measure their impact and return on investment to maintain their team standing. Often, the benefits may be less obvious than those of other professionals' contributions. Benefits of your team membership may include improved medication adherence, appointment compliance, health outcomes, and overall patient satisfaction. A measure of these parameters must preexist your participation as a team member in order to assess your initial impact. Periodic review of these quality outcome measures, overall impact, and efficacy may ultimately lead to modification of practices.

Service Satisfaction

For all health care professionals, patient satisfaction is a key parameter used to determine professional competency and success. For a variety of reasons, patient satisfaction may not be an accurate marker of our service effectiveness given the possible negative consequences patients may encounter given the findings of a neuropsychological evaluation (e.g., restrictions on driving). Thus, Press Ganey surveys (https://en.wikipedia.org/wiki/Press_Ganey_Associates), a hospital's standard measure of patient satisfaction with their health care experiences, may not reflect the true impact of neuropsychological services on patient care. Other measures of outcome and quality have been developed and may be more appropriate to assess the unique contributions of neuropsychologists to patient satisfaction and outcomes (Westervelt et al., 2007). Be prepared to offer more appropriate measures to administrators for a fair assessment of your contribution.

CONCLUSION AND FUTURE DIRECTIONS

As a trailblazer of interdisciplinary care, be prepared for bumps in the road and the need to modify practices, fight for inclusion, and highlight your contributions. An important measure of satisfaction will ultimately be your professional fulfillment given your participation in interdisciplinary teams. In this chapter we have provided information on the important areas in which neuropsychology has contributed to interdisciplinary teams as well as some relevant practical issues to consider throughout your training and career.

REFERENCES

Balasubramanian, B. A., Cohen, D. J., Jetelina, K. K., Dickinson, L. M., Davis, M., Gunn, R., Gowen, D., deGruy, F. V., Miller, B. F., & Green, L. A. (2017). Outcomes of integrated behavioral health with primary care. *Journal of the American Board of Family Medicine, 30*(2), 130–139. https://doi.org/10.3122/jabfm.2017.02.160234

Brearly, T. W., Shura, R. D., Martindale, S. L., Lazowski, R. A., Luxton, D. D., Shenal, B. V., & Rowland, J. A. (2017). Neuropsychological test administration by videoconference: A systematic review and meta-analysis. *Neuropsychology Review, 27*(2), 174–186. https://doi.org/10.1007/s11065-017-9349-1

Carlozzi, N. E., Goodnight, S., Casaletto, K. B., Goldsmith, A., Heaton, R. K., Wong, A. W. K., Baum, C. M., Gershon, R., Heinemann, A. W., & Tulsky, D. S. (2017). Validation of the NIH Toolbox in individuals with neurologic disorders. *Archives of Clinical Neuropsychology, 32*(5), 555–573. https://doi.org/10.1093/arclin/acx020

Cullum, C. M., Hynan, L. S., Grosch, M., Parikh, M., & Weiner, M. F. (2014). Teleneuropsychology: Evidence for video teleconference-based neuropsychological assessment. *Journal of the International Neuropsychological Society, 20*(10), 1028–1033. https://doi.org/10.1017/S1355617714000873

Hannay, J., Bieliauskas, L., Crosson, B. A., Hammeke, T. A., Hamsher, K., & Koffler, S. (1998). Proceedings of The Houston Conference on Specialty Education and Training in Clinical Neuropsychology. *Archives of Clinical Neuropsychology, 13,* 157–250. https://doi.org/10.1186/1472-6920-6-5

Health Insurance Portability and Accountability Act of 1996, Pub. L. 104-191, 42 U.S.C. § 300gg, 29 U.S.C. §§ 1181–1183, and 42 U.S.C. §§ 1320d–1320d9

Johnson-Greene, D. (2018). Clinical neuropsychology in integrated rehabilitation care teams. *Archives of Clinical Neuropsychology, 33*(3), 310–318. https://doi.org/10.1093/arclin/acx126

Koroshetz, W., Gordon, J., Adams, A., Beckel-Mitchener, A., Churchill, J., Farber, G., Freund, M., Gnadt, J., Hsu, N. S., Langhals, N., Lisanby, S., Liu, G., Peng, G. C. Y., Ramos, K., Steinmetz, M., Talley, E., & White, S. (2018). The state of the NIH BRAIN Initiative. *Journal of Neuroscience, 38*(29), 6427–6438. https://doi.org/10.1523/JNEUROSCI.3174-17.2018

Kubu, C. S., Ready, R. E., Festa, J. R., Roper, B. L., & Pliskin, N. H. (2016). The times they are a changin': Neuropsychology and integrated care teams. *The Clinical Neuropsychologist, 30*(1), 51–65. https://doi.org/10.1080/13854046.2015.1134670

Lanca, M. (2018). Integration of neuropsychology in primary care. *Archives of Clinical Neuropsychology, 33*(3), 269–279. https://doi.org/10.1093/arclin/acx135

Miller, J. B., & Barr, W. B. (2017). The technology crisis in neuropsychology. *Archives of Clinical Neuropsychology, 32*(5), 541–554. https://doi.org/10.1093/arclin/acx050

Novotney, A. (2010, January). Integrated care is nothing new for these psychologists. *Monitor, 41*(1), p. 40. http://www.apa.org/monitor/2010/01/integrated-care.aspx

Pliskin, N. H. (2018). The economics of healthcare shape the practice of neuropsychology in the era of integrated healthcare. *Archives of Clinical Neuropsychology, 33*(3), 260–262. https://doi.org/10.1093/arclin/acy008

Pomerantz, A. S., Kearney, L. K., Wray, L. O., Post, E. P., & McCarthy, J. F. (2014). Mental health services in the medical home in the Department of Veterans Affairs: Factors for successful integration. *Psychological Services, 11*(3), 243–253. https://doi.org/10.1037/a0036638

Postal, K., Chow, C., Jung, S., Erickson-Moreo, K., Geier, F., & Lanca, M. (2018). The stakeholders' project in neuropsychological report writing: A survey of neuropsychologists' and referral sources' views of neuropsychological reports. *The Clinical Neuropsychologist, 32*(3), 326–344. https://doi.org/10.1080/13854046.2017.1373859

Rao, S. M. (2018). Role of computerized screening in healthcare teams: Why computerized testing is not the death of neuropsychology. *Archives of Clinical Neuropsychology, 33*(3), 375–378. https://doi.org/10.1093/arclin/acx137

Westervelt, H. J., Brown, L. B., Tremont, G., Javorsky, D. J., & Stern, R. A. (2007). Patient and family perceptions of the neuropsychological evaluation: How are we doing? *The Clinical Neuropsychologist, 21*(2), 263–273. https://doi.org/10.1080/13854040500519745

19 LEADERSHIP DEVELOPMENT COMPETENCIES

CYNTHIA S. KUBU

Leadership is not necessarily a title or a defined role; instead, it relates to *influence*. Although many neuropsychologists, in particular, trainees or early-career neuropsychologists, may not view themselves as leaders, there are several reasons why patients, peers, or colleagues would consider you a leader (e.g., attainment of a degree, advanced training in brain–behavior relationships). Thus, it is important to recognize and develop your leadership abilities to better serve patients, trainees, science, and the profession as well as ensure that you are thriving in your career.

In today's rapidly changing environment there are myriad opportunities to develop, expand, and strengthen your leadership abilities and the inner belief that you are a leader. Successful leaders are aware of this. The literature identifies some of the successful actions that characterize leaders who continue to develop and thrive while inspiring their teams and colleagues to do the same. The goal of this chapter is, in broad strokes, to review some of the literature on leadership and provide real-world, pragmatic suggestions for moving along the professional development leadership path. In addition, I briefly touch on the important topic of women and leadership.

https://doi.org/10.1037/0000250-020
The Neuropsychologist's Roadmap: A Training and Career Guide, C. Block (Editor)

DEFINING LEADERSHIP

The academic literature was dominated for over 40 years by Burns's (1978) model of leadership, which distinguished between transactional and transformational leadership styles. *Transactional leadership* is characterized by the exchange of something of value (i.e., a transaction); workers are rewarded with wages for providing services to the leader. According to Burns's model, transactional leadership focuses on time, efficiency, and minimizing risk. In contrast, *transformational leaders* model a set of values that inspire people to go beyond their own needs (i.e., salary) for the sake of the organization or group. Transformational leaders articulate a clear vision for the future, are attentive to individual differences, and intellectually stimulate workers (Bass, 1985). Transformational leaders are not risk averse and see opportunities in risks or challenges. They prefer to identify the most effective answer, even if it is not the most efficient, and may challenge the status quo. In his original conceptualization, Burns characterized transformational leaders as those who engage with others to raise everyone to a higher level of motivation or morality.

Multiple studies have documented that transformational leadership styles are related to positive organizational metrics (e.g., Lowe et al., 1996). It is important to note, though, that both transactional *and* transformational leadership styles can be effective, depending on the context. In fact, in Bass's (1985) conceptualization these two leadership styles were viewed as complementary (and not orthogonal). Effective leaders are curious and open to experimenting with the leadership styles that are most effective to achieve to goal at hand.

BASIC COMPETENCIES IN LEADERSHIP DEVELOPMENT

It is virtually impossible to read a book or paper on leadership that does not reference the concept of *emotional intelligence*. Emotional intelligence is most often attributed to Daniel Goleman (1995) and is characterized by a 2×2 grid that encompasses four skills (Bradberry & Greaves, 2009): (a) self-awareness, (b) self-management, (c) social awareness, and (d) social management. These are skills that many clinical neuropsychologists use in their clinical work and are equally important in applying to professional relationships to facilitate communication and create growth opportunities that are mutually beneficial. In addition, these are also skills that can be developed and improved over time.

Emotional Intelligence Skill 1: Self-Awareness

Self-awareness is the ability to perceive your own emotions in the moment and understand your patterns of response or tendencies across situations. Self-awareness does not require deep analysis of your faults but simply a clear understanding of what a developing leader finds inherently rewarding and results in positive emotions as well as the kind of situations that result in negative emotions. People high in self-awareness have good knowledge of what is intrinsically motivating to them and what kinds of situations are most likely to push their buttons. Negative emotions are not bad in and of themselves given that they provide valuable feedback. Sometimes those negative emotions (e.g., anxiety, fear) can suggest that you are stepping outside of your comfort zone into an opportunity that provides an opportunity for growth. Other times, negative emotions can indicate that your current situation is interfering with other aspects of your life and that it is time to reconsider your situation so that those emotions do not sabotage other important life goals and values. Similarly, being attentive to positive emotions provides powerful feedback that you (the developing leader) are on the right path and can increase your ability to see and embrace new opportunities that lead to further growth and positive emotions. Self-awareness is *foundational* to all other skills.

Emotional Intelligence Skill 2: Self-Management

Closely related to self-awareness is the concept of *self-management*. Self-management is the action part of self-awareness. It entails the ability to use clear knowledge and awareness of your emotions to stay flexible and take positive action. Self-management ensures that your (the developing leader's) actions are intentional and on course. Self-management avoids having your negative emotions drive behavior in unhelpful ways and helps ensure that forward momentum is maintained. Self-management does not necessarily mean that emotions are kept under wraps and unaddressed; instead, your awareness of your own emotions is very powerful feedback that can be used to identify when a new strategy or approach should be considered. Self-awareness and self-management comprise the *personal competencies* of emotional intelligence.

Emotional Intelligence Skills 3 and 4: Social Awareness and Social Management

The next two skills are focused on others and include social awareness (e.g., empathy) and social or relationship management (e.g., conflict resolution and communication). Together, these comprise the *social competencies* of emotional intelligence. Many psychologists have the clinical training to apply these skills with patients; and these same skills are critical outside of the clinic to identify common values and motivate others to achieve specific goals.

Social Awareness

Social awareness requires curiosity about others and very basic observational skills, such as listening and watching others. To be successful at social awareness, you as a developing leader need to be present in the moment and not caught up in your internal monologue or thoughts.

Social Management

Also thought of as *relationship management*, *social management* is the action piece of social competence and requires good knowledge of one's own and others' emotions to promote successful interactions. Clear communication is essential, as is the ability to effectively address conflict. Leaders who are skilled in social management connect and work effectively with diverse people, including those whom they may not particularly enjoy. Strong relationships are critical to success and, in the best case, are based on the norms of reciprocity, trust, and genuine regard. I expand on this point later when I discuss social capital.

OTHER IMPORTANT CONCEPTS IN LEADERSHIP DEVELOPMENT

As Ibarra et al. (2013) noted, "People become leaders by internalizing a leadership identity and developing a sense of purpose" (p. 62). Perhaps the most important task you as a developing leader will need to address is to identify and clearly articulate your sense of purpose and write a concrete statement that impels you (the leader) to action (cf. Craig & Snook, 2014; Ibarra et al., 2013). On the face of it, this seems to be a relatively easy task, but it is not trivial and requires a significant amount of honest, reflective work followed by action.

Concept 1: Knowing What You Value

Before articulating a purpose statement, it is essential for you, as a developing leader, to know what you value, because time is finite and "One life is too short for doing everything" (cf. Massimo Vignelli); consequently, you need to have a clear, honest understanding of what is important to you. The concentric-circles exercise is a helpful tool to clarify what you value. In brief, the developing leader draws a series of concentric circle (see Figure 19.1). The smallest and central circle represents all the things, people, activities, that are most important to you. The middle circle represents the things and activities that are also valued, but not as much as those in the center circle. The outer circle also includes other valued activities or goals that are important, but not as important as those in the central or middle circled. This exercise forces the developing leader to identify what is truly most important and to make very difficult decisions because, literally, everything that is important cannot fit in the central circle. There is no right or wrong arrangement of various values in the circle, and some values may shift slightly over time with life changes (in fact, I recommend that people routinely revisit this exercise over the course of their careers).

Concept 2: Understanding Your Personal Strengths and Weaknesses

Just as important as having a solid knowledge of your values, developing leaders have an accurate understanding of their strengths and relative

FIGURE 19.1. Concentric-Circles Values Exercise

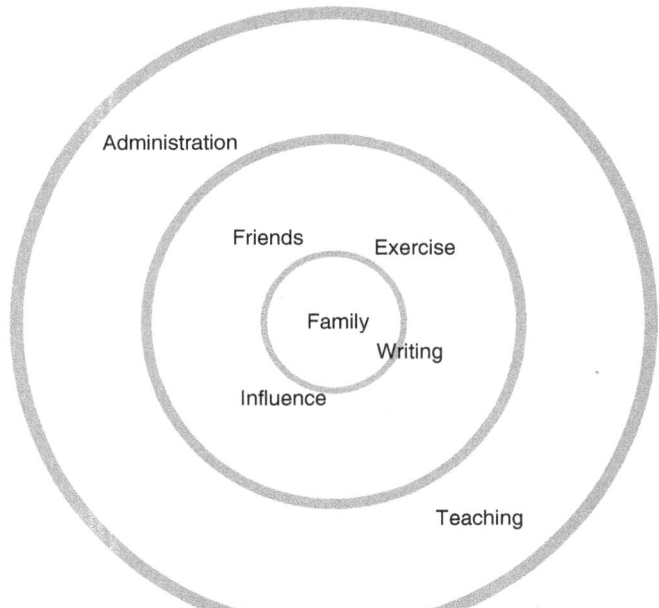

weaknesses. There are various tools to help you identify those strengths and weaknesses. The Strengths Finder (Rath, 2007) is one such tool that is based on decades of data collected by The Gallup Organization (Asplund et al., 2014). The Strengths Finder process is based on the assumption that energy should be put into leveraging and capitalizing on your innate strengths so that you as a developing leader attain expertise in those areas rather than expending energy to remediate relative weaknesses. Another useful tool for developing leaders is participation in a 360-degree evaluation in which direct reports, colleagues, and supervisors provide feedback using quantitative scales and fields for verbatim comments to help the developing leader identify relative leadership strengths and areas to target for improvement (e.g., Antonioni, 1996).

Concept 3: Having a Sense of Purpose

Effective leaders also have a clear sense of their purpose and can succinctly articulate that. Craig and Snook (2014) defined this as a *purpose-to-impact statement* and outlined a process in which developing leaders reflect on times when they were at their best. They recommended that a developing leader reflect on their own personal life story to identify common themes or experiences that help clarify those values, goals, passions, and lifelong pursuits that resulted in the experience of "flow" (cf. Csikszentmihalyi, 2014).

After completing this important reflective work to identify the "why" of why you are here in this world, at this point in time, the next crucial step is to distill that into a clear action statement that impels you to act, for example, "My leadership purpose is to. . . ." The language in the statement should be highly personal and motivate you to act. Friends and family should immediately understand your leadership purpose-to-impact statement and unequivocally agree that is who you are and how you act in this world. For example, my purpose to impact statement is: "I make connections to help people flourish." Now, I don't have the time to make infinite connections to help all people flourish. In order to be maximally effective and leverage my unique resources, I focus my efforts in two domains: (a) faculty development and (b) transdisciplinary research in clinical neuroethics. Clarity of your valued activities or goals, strengths, and purpose in life helps you as a developing leader identify people and opportunities to help accomplish your goals. It is easier to identify opportunities that enable us to grow and accomplish our purpose if we know where we want to go.

For example, my purpose-to-impact statement is that I make connections to help people flourish. To do this, I intentionally focus on professional development and my research, both of which entail making connections among people, ideas, and disciplines. A few years ago, I was invited to serve on, and then cochair, the promotion and tenure committee for the medical school with which I am affiliated. This is a very labor-intensive committee requiring a 3-year commitment and would take time away from my ability to do the amount of research writing I usually do. One of my close friends asked why I was considering this role in light of all of my other responsibilities. After careful consideration, I decided that the benefits associated with serving on the promotion committee (i.e., developing new leadership skills, increased visibility and influence in the institution, greater knowledge of the promotion/tenure process to help faculty with the process) would outweigh the short-term costs associated with less time to write. In contrast, imagine if I were offered the opportunity to teach a new course on neuro-ethics with the expectation that the course would ultimately develop into an ongoing national course. In this example, the necessary expenditure of time to develop, run, manage, and continually update a new program would take time from my other, more valued activities and people for an indefinite period of time; as a consequence, I would choose to respectfully decline the opportunity. My last point illustrates the importance of saying "No, thank you." Jim Collins (2001) advised that great leaders have a "stop doing" list: "Most of us lead busy but undisciplined lives . . . with ever-expanding 'To Do' lists" (p. 139). Those who are most successful show "a remarkable discipline to unplug all sorts of extraneous junk" (p. 139). In order to unplug the extraneous junk, you need clarity on your purpose-to-impact statement which is based on what is important to you (i.e., your values).

Collins (2001) recounted the philosopher Isaiah Berlin's essay (2013) of the fox and the hedgehog, which is based on a Greek parable: The fox knows many things, but the hedgehog knows one big thing. The fox develops all sorts of schemes to try to trap the hedgehog and is undeniably cunning and fast. As he lies in wait to attack the hedgehog, the hedgehog quickly realizes the plan and relies on the same defense over and over, by simply curling into a ball with his sharp spikes splayed, deterring anyone from attack. The fox is foiled and plots a different attack only to face the hedgehog's same defense. Berlin divided people into two groups: foxes and hedgehogs. Foxes see the world in its complexity and pursue many ends simultaneously without synthesizing knowledge into a unifying whole. Hedgehogs focus on one big idea and simplify the complexity of the world into one unifying, elegant idea. If something is not relevant to the unifying idea, it does not hold their interest. Collins argued that the most successful leaders, and those who have developed some of the most profoundly important ideas, were hedgehogs.

Collins's (2001) team went on to elaborate on the *Hedgehog concept* as it applies to the business world and stated that the hedgehog concept stems from the intersection of three circles: (a) what you can be the best at in the world (and, equally important, what you cannot be the best at in the world), (b) what you are deeply passionate about, and (c) what drives your economic engine. Collins went on to clearly indicate that the first circle—what you can be best at in the world—is not what you want or desire to be best at but a clear understanding of what you can be best at. Once again, his work in the business sector illustrates the importance of an accurate appraisal of strengths and weaknesses coupled with passion and clarity regarding the big idea on which you choose to focus (i.e., your purpose-to-impact statement).

In summary, across diverse literatures, including psychology, philosophy, and business, the same themes emerge: good leaders have clarity regarding their values, strengths and weaknesses, and purpose in the world. Although self-reflection is important, all the self-reflection in the world doesn't help you achieve your goals unless you act.

Concept 4: Exhibiting Purposeful Action

As I noted, a purpose-to-impact statement should impel you as a developing leader to act. The importance of action is emphasized in Ibarra's (2015) book *Act Like a Leader, Think Like a Leader*. She relied on psychological research (as well as decades of detailed case studies) to illustrate the importance of action in developing a sense of oneself as a leader. Developing leadership skills is like developing any other skill—it benefits from reflective practice and action. Ibarra and colleagues (2013) stated that leadership development is an iterative process that involves purposeful, intentional action. The developing leader's actions may be affirmed or resisted by others (e.g., colleagues, subordinates, bosses) that will lead to either increases or decreases in the likelihood of engaging in similar actions. The developing leader's sense of self as a leader is shaped by those responses. If the leadership actions and steps are affirmed, the opportunities to develop new leadership skills expand with more challenging roles, which contributes to an upward spiral of increased recognition from senior leadership, even greater opportunities to expand and grow leadership abilities, and so on. This upward trajectory provides more opportunities to expand and stretch to learn different leadership skills and capabilities. Conversely, if the developing leader's actions are resisted, the developing leader is less likely to seek out leadership growth opportunities, which leads to fewer opportunities to be viewed as a leader and, ultimately, to a diminished sense of oneself as a leader. It is inevitable that some leadership actions will not be successful, but those unsuccessful actions also provide learning opportunities. Leadership requires action and putting yourself out there. The challenge is to identify when and which leadership opportunities to pursue at what point in your career to maximize the likelihood of success. The concepts of social capital and strong negotiation skills are integral to understanding when and which professional opportunities to pursue.

Social Capital
Social capital comprises social networks with shared norms and values that facilitate cooperation within or among groups. Social capital is not synonymous with your *social network*, although a strong, diverse social network is critical to social capital. Your social network should include people within and outside your immediate work setting with different skill sets, backgrounds, ages, and life experiences. A diverse social network can help you as a developing leader identify potential leadership opportunities outside of your immediate work environment and/or provide advice on when and how to move forward with specific leadership actions. A developing leader should include mentors and sponsors in their social network and not ignore the possibility that people who are more junior may serve those advisory roles with respect to specific skills. This group of advisors can be invaluable in professional development (e.g., Ragins & Kram, 2007).

The concept of social capital differs from a social network in that social capital is based on the shared norms of reciprocity and trust such that it is known throughout your social network what you stand for and that you are reliable, trustworthy, and cooperative (Paldam, 2000). Effective leaders establish social capital by having good emotional intelligence, developing strong genuine relationships with others; showing up; and accomplishing the job in way that fosters trust, reciprocity, and cooperation toward a shared goal. Social capital takes time to develop, and typically, more senior people in a group (not necessarily older, but senior with respect to involvement in the organization) can assume greater leadership risks by, for example, applying for higher profile positions or publicly taking an unpopular stand. In very practical terms, developing leaders increase their social capital by expanding their social networks and developing relationships on the basis of shared goals and values as well as acting in trustworthy ways with integrity.

Negotiation
For many people, negotiation is often associated with negative emotions that can effectively derail any likelihood of success. Common negotiation

situations include asking for more resources (e.g., salary, office space, time). Developing leaders are aware of their emotional responses to negotiating situations (i.e., self-awareness) and have identified and practiced the skills to manage their emotions (i.e., self-regulation). They are aware of gender- or race-based assumptions that can accompany negotiations and how their own behaviors may conform to those role expectations.

Successful negotiators are also aware of their audience and the organizational culture and demands (i.e., social awareness, social management). This awareness does not mean that the negotiator has already identified a scripted scenario to the upcoming negotiation; it is critical to avoid falling into the trap of the ladder of inference when preparing for a negotiation. In brief, the *ladder of inference* states that a person tends to selectively pay attention to the data that support their own inferences or hypothesis about the other person's motivations in the negotiation. Those inferences are used to predict behavior that may be completely inaccurate (i.e., assume that our boss will automatically say no to our request). When people climb up the ladder of inference they misinterpret behaviors to support their inferences and respond accordingly, which can interfere with genuine, open communication and sabotage successful negotiations. The best way to climb down the ladder of inference is to be curious and open to the other's point of view while advocating for your own personal stance.

Successful negotiation also relies on knowing precisely what you want. The request should be succinct and have a clear rationale that aligns with the organization's goals and values. Successful negotiators orient the audience to the topic and don't make assumptions. When making the request, fewer words are generally more effective so that the message is clear. Successful negotiators identify before a meeting what their best alternative outcome is and have a good understanding of what the other's best alternative outcome is as well. Successful negotiators identify common values and goals to help create win–win negotiations and advocate from a principle base (i.e., goal) rather than a position base (i.e., my way or nothing else). Successful negotiators realize that it is acceptable to postpone the negotiation discussion when the negotiation is not going the way they planned and request more time to consider additional information before finalizing the negotiation. They provide a specific time when they will resume the discussion. Finally, successful negotiators seek out opportunities to develop their negotiating skills (e.g., appeal for a temporary reduction in clinical or teaching responsibilities in order to apply for a grant, request for financial support to attend a conference, propose a plan to share training responsibilities to benefit all supervisors) and diligently prepare.

Concept 5: Exerting Influence

I started this chapter by asserting that leadership is influence. It is not necessarily a title or the exercise of power. *Power* is the ability or official capacity to exercise control or authority. It is a top-down process based on a hierarchical structure. In contrast, *influence* relies on interpersonal skills and relationships to help change behaviors and/or attitudes. The skills that underlie influence include effective communication skills, persuasion, the ability to positively impact others, and, ultimately help motivate people to achieve desirable outcomes. Influence is a critical skill for transformational leaders and can be applied regardless of your official role in an organization.

Baldwin and Grayson (2004) identified three kinds of influencing activities. The first relies on logic that seeks to align people on the basis of rational and intellectual arguments. These *logical appeals* focus on two types of benefits: (a) organizational and (b) personal. Logical appeals objectively outline the rationale for the requested action and include specific behaviors (see Table 19.1). Successful influencers who adopt logical appeals are very well prepared and know the data, have researched other options, anticipated the potential problems and identified solutions, consider benefits to others, and engage others in a dialogue. The second process Baldwin and Grayson identified was *emotional appeals*. Emotional appeals involve framing requests around an important emotional motivator (e.g., one that promotes feelings of well-being, a sense of belonging). Finally, the authors described the third process: *cooperative appeals*. Cooperative appeals build connections between the influencing leader and the team as well as the stakeholders that, ultimately, results in support for the proposal. Cooperative appeals are a way of leveraging the teams' expertise while creating a stronger team. Successful leaders flexibly and nimbly use all these strategies to exert influence. They also routinely engage in reflection to identify what was effective in their influencing behaviors and what was not as effective so they can continue to grow and develop as leaders.

Neuropsychologists are fortunate in that there are multiple opportunities to develop leadership skills by volunteering to serve on institutional, community, national, and international working groups or committees (see Table 19.2, as well as Chapter 20, this volume). In particular, the American Psychological Association recognizes the value of trainees and early-career psychologists and has specifically dedicated slots for members of these groups on many committees. As a developing leader puts their names forward for various leadership opportunities, they can further develop their social capital, which provides a growing base from which to exert even greater influence.

TABLE 19.1. Baldwin and Grayson's (2004) Influencing Strategies

Strategy	Description
Logical appeals	Objectively and logically explain the rationale for the action.
	Provide evidence that the proposal is feasible.
	Explain clearly and logically why the proposal is the best option.
	Detail the logical process by which potential organizational problems or concerns will be addressed.
	Explain how the proposal will have long-term benefits for the organization.
	Provide opportunities for people to learn new skills through the proposal.
Emotional appeals	Show how the proposal meets the team members' individual goals and values.
	Describe the task with enthusiasm and express confidence in the team's ability to accomplish it.
	Link the proposal to a clear and appealing vision that the team can support.
Cooperative appeals	Provide the necessary resources to accomplish the task.
	Remove barriers to success.
	Volunteer to help the team accomplish the task.
	Offer to help people with their regular work.
	Solicit suggestions on improving the proposal to create a win–win outcome for everyone.
	Solicit input from the team on how to accomplish the task, and incorporate those suggestions into the process.
	Thoughtfully reflect on and respond to people's concerns and suggestions (i.e., listen).
	Before making a specific request, ask for opinions on the general topic.
	Create coalitions with people who support the requested action.
	Inform people about credible stakeholders who support the proposal.
	Involve credible stakeholders in the influencing effort.
	Develop strategic alliances by networking with key stakeholders who can help.

Note. Data from Baldwin and Grayson (2004).

A NOTE ON GENDER AND LEADERSHIP DEVELOPMENT

Before I end this chapter, it is worth briefly mentioning some of the literature on gender and leadership, in particular because women trainees outnumber men in neuropsychology.

The meta-analyses data on gender and leadership clearly show that there are no significant gender difference in leadership effectiveness (e.g.,

TABLE 19.2. Leadership Resources for Psychology and Neuropsychology Trainees

American Psychological Association (APA)

General leadership resources: https://www.apa.org/members/your-growth/leadership

APA Develop Your Leadership Skills webinar: https://www.apa.org/careers/early-career/get-connected/get-involved

APA Supercharge Your Presence webinar series: https://www.apa.org/members/content/online-professional-presence-series

APA Emerging Leadership Academy: https://pages.apa.org/emerging-leaders

APA Council of National Psychological Associations for the Advancement of Ethnic Minority Interests Leadership Development Institute: http://www.cnpaaemildi.org

APA Leadership Institute for Women in Psychology: http://www.apa.org/pi/women/programs/leadership

APA Practice Leadership Conference: https://www.apaservices.org/practice/advocacy/state/leadership

Other leadership resources

National Academy of Neuropsychology Leadership Ambassador Development Program: https://bit.ly/2nXfk6j

Society for Neuroscience Leadership Development Program: https://bit.ly/2IKF59d

Association of American Medical College leadership development courses: https://bit.ly/2nkssCg

Clifton Strengths Assessment: https://www.gallup.com/cliftonstrengths/en/home.aspx

DiSC Assessment Program: https://www.discprofile.com

Eagly et al., 2003; Eagly & Johnson, 1990; Paustian-Underdahl et al., 2014). However, women are still underrepresented in leadership positions (see Kubu, 2018).

Eagly and Johannesen-Schmidt (2001) critically examined the literature on gender and leadership in the context of *social role theory*. They argued that leaders elicit a set of expectations based on their gender roles or "the shared beliefs that apply to individuals on the basis of their socially identified sex" (p. 783). Agentic and communal attributes are clearly related to gender roles. *Agentic attributes* are behaviors that are typically ascribed to men, such as being assertive, controlling, and confident. These attributes are most often associated with leadership roles. In contrast, *communal attributes*, including kindness, empathy, nurturing, and interpersonal sensitivity, are more often associated with women. Although leaders may exhibit communal attributes, those attributes are not as strongly associated with leadership roles. Gender role expectations provide an "implicit, background identity" and are shared by subordinates, peers, and leaders, and they are often internalized. The challenge occurs when gender role expectations conflict with leadership role expectations. Eagly and Karau (2002) argued that the incongruity between female gender role expectations and leadership expectations results in prejudice against women leaders. As a consequence, women leaders are put in a double bind in which maintenance of their gender role may result in a failure to meet the leadership role expectations, whereas maintenance of leadership role expectations may result in a failure to conform to their gender role, both of which, according to Eagly and Karau, may have negative consequences for women. Ibarra and Petriglieri (2016) referred to this phenomenon as "our impossible selves." The conflict between gender and leadership role expectations is influenced by organizational factors as well such as the extent to which an organization is male dominated.

Gender role expectations are closely related to *organizational citizenship behavior* (OCB), a type of social exchange behavior (Organ, 1988). OCB includes behaviors that help support the social and psychological work environment and include actions such as helping others, doing volunteer work, and socializing with new employees. OCBs are discretionary and not part of the official job description and consequently are not formally recognized by the formal reward system. The data illustrate that OCBs, in particular, communal OCB, are expected more of women. Women are penalized if they do not engage in communal OCB versus men (see Heilman & Chen, 2005, for more details). Yet OCB comes at a cost: More time spent engaging in behaviors that are not part of the formal job description (and, hence, not rewarded) comes at the expense of those job behaviors that are part of the job responsibilities and formally rewarded (Bergeron et al., 2012, 2013). Thus, women are placed in a double bind in which they are viewed less favorably if they do not engage in OCB, yet engaging in OCB takes time from essential job duties. Navigating these different role expectations is challenging and can be even more difficult for persons of color (which requires a separate chapter). However, I believe that by having clarity about why (i.e., what is important to you) and what they want to achieve as a leader (i.e., your purpose-to-impact statement), as well developing a deep reservoir of social capital and a sound advisory board, women can more easily navigate conflicting role expectations as they develop into leaders. (For a more detailed discussion of leadership and gender, please see Eagly & Carli, 2007, and Kubu, 2018.)

CONCLUSION AND FUTURE DIRECTIONS

Effective leaders have a clear understanding of their values, strengths, and purpose. They are aware of their own emotions and able to manage those emotions. They also empathize with others' emotions and demonstrate a clear understanding of the organizational context. Effective leaders are skilled at negotiation and know how to use influence to make change. Effective leaders rely on a diverse network and have deep social capital that is based on the norms of trust and reciprocity (i.e., effective leaders have integrity and do what they say they will). Effective leaders seek out opportunities to flex their leadership muscles by volunteering in professional organizations, submitting papers and grant proposals, mentoring students or junior colleagues, and sharing their desire to develop leadership skills by making specific requests to other leaders (i.e., requesting to serve on a search committee). Effective leaders learn from their successes and failures and persist and continue to strive to be the best they can be. Last but not least, they take advantage of all the resources available to them for continued learning and professional growth.

REFERENCES

Antonioni, D. (1996). Designing an effective 360-degree appraisal feedback process. *Organizational Dynamics, 25*(2), 24–38. https://doi.org/10.1016/S0090-2616(96)90023-6

Asplund, J., Agrawal, S., Hodges, T., Harter, J., & Lopez, S. J. (2014). *The Clifton StrengthsFinder® 2.0—2014 update.* https://www.strengthsquest.com/193766/clifton-strengthsfinder-technical-report-2014-update.aspx

Baldwin, D., & Grayson, C. (2004). Positive influence: How leaders get others to see it their way. *Leadership in Action, 24*(1), 8–11. https://doi.org/10.1002/lia.1052

Bass, B. M. (1985). *Leadership and performance beyond expectations.* Free Press.

Bergeron, D. M., Schroeder, T. D., Martinez, H. M., Amdurer, E. E., & Van Esch, C. (2012, August 3–5). *The stability of organizational citizenship behavior over time: Women as good citizens* [Paper]. Academy of Management Conference, Boston, MA. https://doi.org/10.5465/AMBPP.2012.14833abstract

Bergeron, D. M., Shipp, A. J., Rosen, B., & Furst, S. A. (2013). Organizational citizenship behavior and career outcomes: The cost of being a good citizen. *Journal of Management, 39*(4), 958–984. https://doi.org/10.1177/0149206311407508

Berlin, I. (2013). *The hedgehog and the fox: An essay on Tolstoy's view of history.* Princeton University Press.

Bradberry, T., & Greaves, J. (2009). *Emotional intelligence 2.0.* TalentSmart.

Burns, J. M. (1978). *Leadership.* Harper & Row.

Collins, J. (2001). *Good to great.* Harper Collins.

Craig, N., & Snook, S. (2014, May). From purpose to impact: Figure out your passion and put it to work. *Harvard Business Review, 92*(5), 104–111, 134. https://www.hbs.edu/faculty/Pages/item.aspx?num=47372

Csikszentmihalyi, M. (2014). *Flow and the foundations of positive psychology: The collected works of Mihaly Csikszentmihalyi.* Springer. https://doi.org/10.1007/978-94-017-9088-8

Eagly, A. H., & Carli, L. L. (2007). *Through the labyrinth: The truth about how women become leaders.* Harvard Business School.

Eagly, A. H., & Johannesen-Schmidt, M. C. (2001). The leadership styles of women and men. *Journal of Social Issues, 57*(4), 781–797. https://doi.org/10.1111/0022-4537.00241

Eagly, A. H., Johannesen-Schmidt, M. C., & van Engen, M. L. (2003). Transformational, transactional, and laissez-faire leadership styles: A meta-analysis comparing women and men. *Psychological Bulletin, 129*(4), 569–591. https://doi.org/10.1037/0033-2909.129.4.569

Eagly, A. H., & Johnson, B. T. (1990). Gender and leadership style: A meta-analysis. *Psychological Bulletin, 108*(2), 233–256. https://doi.org/10.1037/0033-2909.108.2.233

Eagly, A. H., & Karau, S. J. (2002). Role congruity theory of prejudice toward female leaders. *Psychological Review, 109*(3), 573–598. https://doi.org/10.1037/0033-295X.109.3.573

Goleman, D. (1995). *Emotional intelligence.* Bantam Books.

Heilman, M. E., & Chen, J. J. (2005). Same behavior, different consequences: Reactions to men's and women's altruistic citizenship behavior. *Journal of Applied Psychology, 90*(3), 431–441. https://doi.org/10.1037/0021-9010.90.3.431

Ibarra, H. (2015). *Act like a leader, think like a leader.* Harvard Business Review Press.

Ibarra, H., Ely, R., & Kolb, K. (2013, September). Women rising: The unseen barriers. *Harvard Business Review,* pp. 61–66. https://hbr.org/2013/09/women-rising-the-unseen-barriers

Ibarra, H., & Petriglieri, J. L. (2016, March 4). *Impossible selves: Image strategies and identity threat in professional women's career transitions.* INSEAD Working Paper No. 2016/12/OBH. https://doi.org/10.2139/ssrn.2742061

Kubu, C. S. (2018). Who does she think she is? Women, leadership and the "B"(ias) word. *The Clinical Neuropsychologist, 32*(2), 235–251. https://doi.org/10.1080/13854046.2017.1418022

Lowe, K. B., Kroeck, K. G., & Sivasubramaniam, N. (1996). Effectiveness correlates of transformation and transactional leadership: A meta-analytic review of the MLQ literature. *The Leadership Quarterly, 7*(3), 385–425. https://doi.org/10.1016/S1048-9843(96)90027-2

Organ, D. W. (1988). *Organizational citizenship behavior: The good soldier syndrome.* Lexington Books.

Paldam, M. (2000). Social capital: One or many? Definitions and measurement. *Journal of Economic Surveys, 14*(5), 629–653. https://doi.org/10.1111/1467-6419.00127

Paustian-Underdahl, S. C., Walker, L. S., & Woehr, D. J. (2014). Gender and perceptions of leadership effectiveness: A meta-analysis of contextual moderators. *Journal of Applied Psychology, 99*(6), 1129–1145. https://doi.org/10.1037/a0036751

Ragins, B. R., & Kram, K. E. (2007). *The handbook of mentoring at work: Theory, research and practice.* Sage.

Rath, T. (2007). *Strengths Finder 2.0.* Gallup Press.

20

ADVOCACY COMPETENCIES

SCOTT SPERLING, BETH C. ARREDONDO, STEPHANIE D. BAJO, AND LUCAS D. DRISKELL

It is impossible to describe the full history of advocacy efforts within the field of neuropsychology in a single chapter. It is also beyond the scope of this chapter to outline all of the professional psychological and neuropsychological organizations, and their various committees and subcommittees, whose mission and/or objectives in some way focus on advocacy. Instead, in this chapter we aim to introduce and define *advocacy*, provide a brief historical and current context to illustrate professional advocacy work and demonstrate its importance, and share reasons why we believe that you, your fellow students, and all neuropsychologists should be actively engaged in advocacy. To this end, we also provide practical guidance as to how you can effectively engage in various types of advocacy. You are also encouraged to review a special issue of *The Clinical Neuropsychologist* (Howe & Pliskin, 2010) to further your knowledge about advocacy in neuropsychology, and Chapter 19 of this volume, for guidance on becoming involved in leadership, which by its nature involves advocacy for the profession.

https://doi.org/10.1037/0000250-021
The Neuropsychologist's Roadmap: A Training and Career Guide, C. Block (Editor)

WHAT IS ADVOCACY?

Advocacy, defined as "the act of pleading for or actively supporting a cause or proposal" (Garner & Black, 2009, p. 64), comes in many different forms. Though often conceptualized as taking place within government structures, it frequently occurs on an person-to-person basis. Advocacy can be manifested in a person's effort to spark change in legislative policy or in the minds and practices of colleagues and patients. It can occur in reaction to a specific event; via response to a threat to the field; in proactive work aimed at increasing the profession's standing across institutions; or as reflected in improvements in local, state, and federal policies, referral and reimbursement rates, and public perception.

It is critical to the livelihood of the profession, and arguably a responsibility of each individual neuropsychologist, to regularly engage in professional advocacy. As eloquently stated by Howe et al. (2010), we as neuropsychologists are "the current stewards of our profession, and it is our responsibility to protect and enhance the profession so that its benefit to individual patients and to society can continue to be realized and expanded" (p. 375). Although you as a student may feel less knowledgeable or empowered to engage in professional advocacy during this time in your professional career, or even intimidated by the prospect, it is important to remember that you possess expertise as well as unique and valuable perspectives. Your knowledge and insights can be quite powerful, in particular when accompanied by a sheer willingness to advocate for your patients, the public, and the profession. As such, we argue here that students be included in the conceptualization of "current stewards" and supported in their development as professional advocates.

Unfortunately, the majority of psychology training programs do not directly encourage, let alone prepare, students to become successful advocates. This not only does a disservice to your development as a future advocacy leader but also constrains the grassroots or organization driven person-power capital that can be generated behind any rising advocacy effort requiring expedient action. It also diminishes a potentially powerful pipeline of students who—if provided with the appropriate education, mentoring, and leadership opportunities—might otherwise serve as strong advocates in diverse sectors across their professional careers. Until programs integrate advocacy training into their curricula, the onus will continue to fall on you to proactively seek training and mentorship in advocacy skill development.

ADVOCATING FOR PSYCHOLOGY

You should be aware that advocating for the practice of clinical psychology, and psychology as a science, is a prerequisite to the vitality of neuropsychology as a *specialty*. Significant legislative and regulatory changes that affect the scope of practice for nondoctoral–trained psychologists, insurance coverage and reimbursement, and funding for psychological research are often experienced by a wide range of practicing psychologists, not just neuropsychologists. For historical context, we now describe a few key and critical advocacy issues relevant to the current and future generations of clinical psychologists.

Centers for Medicare & Medicaid Services Physician Designation and Reimbursement Rates

The Centers for Medicare & Medicaid Services (CMS; https://cms.gov) is a government agency that manages federally funded health insurance programs and provides benefits to more than 100 million people nationwide. Medicare covers people age 65 years or older and those with certain disabilities under age 65, and Medicaid is available to those who meet eligibility because of low income. The extensive network of CMS beneficiaries inherently includes people with high health care needs that are due to conditions associated with aging, certain disabilities, and/or barriers to accessing quality care secondary to financial limitations.

Access to psychological and neuropsychological services is especially important for CMS beneficiaries when one considers the high rates of cognitive and mental health conditions in older and low-income populations (Goodman et al., 2017; https://www.medicaid.gov/medicaid/benefits/behavioral-health-services/index.html). Unfortunately, numerous factors have increased barriers to psychological and neuropsychological care for CMS beneficiaries and sparked opportunities for advocacy over the years. Two prominent platforms include (a) the fight for psychologists' inclusion in the CMS definition of "physician" and (b) championing fair rates of reimbursement for services.

Centers for Medicare & Medicaid Services Physician Designation

CMS guidelines state that a physician must oversee and supervise the clinical services and interventions provided by psychologists in certain settings, such as inpatient or partial hospitalization. Per the current CMS policy, a "physician" is defined as "any of the following types of professionals that are legally authorized by the state to practice," regardless of the CMS plan: Doctors of Medicine or Osteopathic Medicine, Doctors of Dental Medicine or Dental Surgery, Doctors of Podiatric Medicine, Doctors of Optometry, and Chiropractors (see https://cms.gov). As it stands by current law, psychologists are the only independently licensed doctoral-level provider that is not included in the CMS physician definition. This raises a significant issue regarding parity, in particular with respect to equivalence of status and pay. Exclusion of psychologists creates barriers to care for beneficiaries, limits access to provider incentive funds aimed at expanding services for underserved and/or rural populations, and prohibits access to CMS funds that promote training of postdoctoral residents. Because of these detrimental consequences to the public, national psychological and neuropsychological associations have engaged in advocacy efforts for many years to fight for the inclusion of psychologists in the CMS physician definition. One noteworthy recent advocacy effort was the development of a bipartisan bill, known as the Medicare Mental Health Access Act, the current iteration of which was initially introduced in the U.S. Senate and House of Representatives in 2019, with previous versions since at least 2010. If passed, this legislation would expand the current Medicare physician definition to include psychologists. This bill remains an active priority of the American Psychological Association (APA) and is still proceeding through legislative channels. Neuropsychological organizations have also provided steadfast support of this bill through letters, direct contact with members of Congress, and the development and distribution of fact sheets that provide evidence supporting the need for reducing barriers to mental health care. Advocacy on an individual level has also been, and will continue to be, important, given that more calls, letters, and evidence-based information can lead to broader congressional support.

Current Procedural Terminology Codes and Centers for Medicare & Medicaid Services Reimbursement Rates

Current Procedural Terminology (CPT) codes are used by insurance carriers nationwide and were developed to provide a universal system of medical service coding and billing. Because CMS funding is constrained by budgetary limitations, periodic audits of certain *CPT* codes are conducted to assess the need for revision of coverage or service fees—a process that can ultimately lead to a "proposed rule change" of reimbursement rates. Although these audits do not always yield a negative outcome, the results can lead to reduced payments and barriers to coverage for certain health care services.

The field of psychology, including the specialty of neuropsychology, has not been immune to *CPT* code audits. In fact, in 2016 there was the potential for CMS to enact deep cuts to the reimbursement rates assigned to psychological and neuropsychological testing *CPT* codes. The advocacy efforts made by the APA and its Practice Organization, along with supporting initiatives undertaken by other national, regional, and state psychological and neuropsychological organizations, helped ensure that cuts that would have devastated the profession and severely limited the public's access to clinical services were not enacted.

Master's Training in Psychological Practice

Since the 1949 Boulder Conference on Graduate Education in Clinical Psychology (Raimy, 1950), doctoral-level training has been recognized as the standard for practice as a psychologist. All versions of the APA Model Act for State Licensure of Psychologists, including the most recent 2010 version, affirm doctoral training as the standard for entry-level practice as a psychologist (APA, 2011). The Association for State and Provincial Psychology Boards' (ASPPB; 2018) Model Act for Licensure and Registration of Psychologists also establishes the doctoral degree as the standard for entry-level practice in the profession. Still, inconsistency exists across jurisdictions in the standards used to credential psychology practice, with 16 states currently granting licenses to people with master's degrees in psychology, despite recommendations by APA and ASPPB (APA Minority Fellowship Program, 2016; Buckman et al., 2018). In five of these jurisdictions a master's-level person may practice psychology independently without any distinction from doctoral-level licensed psychologists.

Why is this a problem? The lack of training standards has left state psychology licensing boards responsible for overseeing master's-level practitioners—but without clear criteria or metrics to evaluate first, who is competent to practice psychology and, second, what their scope of practice should be. The inconsistencies in licensing requirements across jurisdictions and allowance of master's-trained individuals to practice psychology have also contributed to the public's uncertainty of the definition of a "psychologist" and their associated expertise. This confusion is compounded by the fact that, with the exception of testing and evaluation services, in many states licensed professional counselors, marriage and family therapists, and licensed clinical social workers possess the same scope of practice as doctoral-level psychologists.

Furthermore, licensing of master's-level persons to practice psychology complicates psychologists' efforts to gain parity with physicians. Concern exists that equivalence between master's- and doctoral-trained persons dilutes the value of psychology within both the medical community and the eyes of the public. In contrast, an increase in the number of licensed master's-level trained clinicians would have the benefit of increasing access to mental health care services, in particular in underrepresented and marginalized communities.

Until recently, APA had not officially advocated for or against recognition of master's-level practitioners in the sequence of training for psychology. In December 2016, the APA Minority Fellowship Program held a summit on Master's Training in Psychological Practice to discuss whether APA should indeed recognize practitioners at the master's level and how such recognition might affect regulation of scope of practice and licensure, access to care, and potential accreditation of master's-level training programs. The consensus from the summit was that APA should continue to recognize the doctoral degree as requisite for entry-level practice of psychology and defining oneself a "psychologist" but that APA should also advocate for licensing and consistent titling of master's-trained people who themselves should be distinguished from other master's-level providers of behavioral health services (APA Minority Fellowship Program, 2016). In March 2018, APA's Council of Representatives voted to approve the process of developing formal accreditation guidelines for master's-level psychology training programs in an attempt to achieve increased accountability for training and practice standards while also addressing the increasing mental health workforce crisis. Continued advocacy in this area will surely prove necessary.

ADVOCATING FOR NEUROPSYCHOLOGY AS A SPECIALTY

Although the field of neuropsychology has an impressive history, it is still relatively young. Recognition of neuropsychology as a science and practice did not occur by chance. It was not until the mid-1960s that the International Neuropsychological Society was formed to share and proliferate new scientific knowledge. A decade later, the International Neuropsychological Society and the newly formed National Academy of Neuropsychology (NAN) began advocating for recognition of the specialty via creation of the new Division of Clinical Neuropsychology within APA. APA's Division 40, the Society for Clinical Neuropsychology (SCN), was established in 1980 and charged with advancing the specialty as a science and profession, as a means of enhancing human welfare. Creation of this division allowed for development of the initial education and training guidelines in neuropsychology, which were the foundation of the Houston Conference on Specialty Education and Training in Clinical Neuropsychology Policy Statement (Hannay et al., 1998). As neuropsychology advanced as a science and grew in numbers of trained practitioners, it became clear that recognition of the field as a specialty by APA was needed to identify the distinct knowledge and specialized skills requisite for competent practice and the advanced sequence of education and training needed in order to obtain those competencies. In 1996, professional neuropsychological organizations and their memberships were successful in their effort to have Clinical Neuropsychology approved by APA's Commission for the Recognition of Specialties and Proficiencies in Professional Psychology (now known as the Commission for the Recognition of Specialties and Subspecialties in Professional Psychology) as the first professional psychology specialty. This recognition has helped legitimize neuropsychology as a discipline and raise its presence and standing within psychology, across medical specialties, and in the eyes of the public.

Defining and Conducting Neuropsychological Assessment

The importance of understanding patients' cognitive capacities has grown among those in health care. Having objective and valid cognitive data leads to more accurate and early diagnoses and, subsequently, to the delivery of appropriate treatments (Donders, 2020). However, ambiguity and inconsistencies exist regarding the terminologies used for measuring cognition. Disagreement also exists as to who is qualified to conduct and interpret assessments of cognitive and neuropsychological functioning. Despite significant differences in formal education and training, numerous professions consider the assessment of cognitive functioning to fall within their scope of their practice. For example, neuropsychologists, psychologists without formal training in neuropsychology, physicians, speech-language pathologists, occupational therapists, nurse practitioners, social workers, and master's-level psychology clinicians all claim right to the ability to practice some level of cognitive assessment. Potential issues stemming from this situation include the increased probability of inadequate assessment, incorrect interpretation of clinical data, and provision of improper diagnoses when neuropsychological evaluations are conducted by clinicians who do not have the advanced, specialized training needed to develop basic competencies. In efforts to protect the public from such negative consequences, neuropsychologists have advocated for increased recognition of the competencies obtained solely through their advanced specialized training.

Neuropsychology professional organizations and individual practitioners have highlighted the specialized training and expertise needed to competently administer and interpret neuropsychological evaluations, thereby advocating for neuropsychological services to be performed solely by appropriately trained neuropsychologists and technicians under their supervision (Block et al., 2017; Roebuck-Spencer et al., 2017). Block and colleagues (2017) outlined the differences among cognitive screening, cognitive testing, and neuropsychological assessment. *Cognitive screenings* aim to determine one's likelihood of having cognitive impairment and/or need for a referral, through the use of brief measures that typically rely on cutoff scores. They can be administered by a range of providers with various levels of training and education. *Cognitive testing* aims to collect circumscribed cognitive data to, when normative corrections are applied, inform specific treatment goals and/or determine whether a referral for specialty assessment is warranted. It can be performed by licensed psychology providers with training in neuro-cognition and neuropsychological assessment. In contrast, *neuropsychological assessments* involve a comprehensive assessment of all cognitive domains along with the integration of neurological, medical, emotional, behavioral, demographic, and situational considerations. They are most commonly conducted to assist in differential diagnosis, inform medical and psychological treatment, provide an indicator of change, and/or provide insight into decision making capacity. They can be performed by neuropsychologists with training that conforms to the Houston Conference Guidelines (Hannay et al., 1998).

Across your own career, there will be opportunities to advocate for the appropriate use of neuropsychological measures. You can proactively work in your state and national psychological organizations, as well as in your institution and community, to educate others on the differences among measures, evaluation approaches, and the distinct expertise held by neuropsychologists.

Professional Organization Advocacy

Advocacy and leadership are closely linked (see Chapter 19, this volume), and professional organizations are at the front lines of advocacy initiatives in neuropsychology.

American Psychological Association

If asked, the majority of neuropsychologists would almost certainly identify their professional home as existing within at least one of the major national neuropsychological organizations. These organizations, namely, the International Neuropsychological Society, National Academy of Neuropsychology,

SCN, American Academy of Clinical Neuropsychology (AACN), American Board of Clinical Neuropsychology, Academy of the American Board of Professional Neuropsychology, American Board of Professional Neuropsychology, and American Academy of Pediatric Neuropsychology, certainly play important roles in advocating for diverse issues germane to the specialty; however, APA is arguably the most powerful and influential organization when it comes to advocating for psychologists, including neuropsychologists, and in igniting broad and significant change. In most areas of governance, such as on APA's Council of Representatives and Board of Directors, neuropsychology's presence and thus influence has been disproportionately low. Because APA's resources far exceed that of each professional neuropsychological organization, the interests of the specialty rest within its ability to identify, develop, and elect neuropsychologists into governance, thereby facilitating opportunities to direct policy and affect change from within.

Professional Neuropsychological Organizations

Most of the major professional neuropsychology organizations have committees designated to one or more forms of advocacy, including education of the public, promotion of professional development for members from underrepresented groups, and addressing diversity in patient populations. Some also have committees dedicated to practice- and policy-based advocacy. As examples, the SCN's Practice Advisory Committee, NAN's Professional Affairs and Information Committee, and AACN's Practice and Public Policy Committee are devoted to providing professional advocacy on behalf of the specialty and the public. Each committee distributes practice-related information to its membership; educates the public on the roles and value of neuropsychological services; and promotes the profession through advocacy work with medical professions, other allied health specialties, and local, state, and national health care organizations. In addition, the SCN Practice Advisory Committee, NAN's Legislative Action & Advocacy Committee, and the Practice and Public Policy Committee Legislative Subcommittee actively monitor and respond to issues, in particular, those pertinent to state and federal legislative and regulatory changes, which actively affect—or have the likelihood to affect—the professional practice of neuropsychology.

Although often unrecognized, the efforts and achievement of these committees and key neuropsychology leaders cannot be understated. Throughout the years, neuropsychologists have been faced with threats related to equitable reimbursement, scope of practice infringements, and attacks on psychologists' legal capacity to practice independently. These committees and their parent organizations have frequently led the charge on behalf of neuropsychologists in their advocacy work with key legislators and other stakeholders on these issues. They have also worked proactively to raise recognition of neuropsychology's value and secure, preserve, or expand the specialty's roles in multiple arenas, including the assessment of concussion and clinical use of functional magnetic resonance imaging. As neuropsychologists are increasingly tasked with providing evidence of effectiveness to support reimbursement for services, these professional organizations have undertaken important efforts to coalesce existing data, support further scientific inquiry, and broadly disseminate information demonstrating the benefit of neuropsychological services across patient health care and cost effectiveness outcomes.

Interorganizational Practice Committee

Differences in national, regional, and state health care regulations have hindered coordinated and effective advocacy efforts from APA; state, provincial and territorial psychological associations (SPTAs); and major professional neuropsychology organizations. The Inter Organizational Practice Committee (IOPC; https://iopc.online), which comprises the practice and advocacy chairs of the SCN, AACN, NAN, and American Board of Professional Neuropsychology and a representative from American Psychological Association Services, Inc., was formed in 2012 as one means of coordinating advocacy across each of these key organizations, to provide more influential and time sensitive responses. Creation of the Inter Organizational Practice Committee also helped reduce unnecessary reduplication of advocacy efforts and expanded the reach of grassroots advocacy for issues that have local and national implications through its 360 Degree Advocacy model (Postal et al., 2014).

Though formed only in 2012, the scope of issues undertaken by the Inter Organizational Practice Committee is broad. It has helped coordinate and champion advocacy efforts to expand the definition of physician to include psychologists, use technicians to administer and score neuropsychological measures under the supervision of the neuropsychologist, fight against the consolidation of psychology licensing boards with those overseeing other fields, promote and protect the qualifications of competencies of neuropsychologists, secure insurance coverage and fair reimbursement rates, and protect the integrity of tests in legal cases.

State and Regional Advocacy

The majority of the policies and regulations that directly affect psychological services are developed and implemented at the state, not national, level. To be specific, state legislatures determine the scope of practice of the profession, and licensing boards administer those regulations. Significant differences exist between states, as well as between states and national and regional health care regulations. The SPTAs play a critical role advocating for the needs of psychologists by responding to state-specific threats to the profession. Unfortunately, because SPTA membership includes people from all areas of psychology, issues most relevant to practicing neuropsychologists are often inadequately addressed.

To more specifically address the needs of its neuropsychologists, several states have developed neuropsychology societies. Some of these maintain a formal association with their SPTA and thus promote the option to leverage that relationship when conducting legislative advocacy work. In addition, there are some regional neuropsychological societies with professional affairs committees that devote significant effort to advocating on behalf of you and other neuropsychology constituents.

Through steadfast advocacy and collaboration with other stakeholders, neuropsychological societies and SPTAs have garnered important legislative wins. For years, New York prohibited the use of technicians in administering and scoring psychological and neuropsychological tests under supervision of the neuropsychologist. Not only did this prohibition have a detrimental impact on neuropsychologists' livelihood by limiting the use of lower cost assistants for test administration, but it unnecessarily reduced access to care, in particular, from persons in socioeconomically disadvantaged groups. The New York State Association of Neuropsychologists advocated for the use of technicians and, with the support from clinical psychologists across the country and other neuropsychological organizations, they ultimately secured this legal right in 2016. The North Carolina and Massachusetts Psychological Associations also saw successes in their ability to revise state laws to allow for neuropsychological assessments to be covered by insurance for a full range of medically necessary diagnoses and to force insurance companies to make medical necessity criteria sets transparent, respectively (Postal et al., 2014).

Institutional and Interprofessional Advocacy

Many medical and allied health professionals are unfamiliar with the specialty of neuropsychology. Even physicians who work more closely with neuropsychologists often possess a limited or inaccurate understanding of the roles, services, and benefits provided by neuropsychologists. The results of historically poor communication, and the subsequent poor awareness of the value associated with neuropsychological services, comes with a significant cost to patients, the public, and neuropsychologists. Such negative consequences include a dearth of referrals, inappropriate referrals, and a failure to adequately integrate neuropsychologists into multi- and interdisciplinary teams, all of which can in turn lead to missed or inappropriate diagnoses and poor health care outcomes (see Braun et al., 2011, for a review of the benefits of neuropsychological assessment). Although large-scale organizational efforts can serve to improve physicians' awareness of neuropsychological services, it is imperative that neuropsychologists take it upon themselves to advocate for the profession by proactively educating their colleagues about the benefits of neuropsychological services and the evidence base supporting appropriate utilization of said services.

Local and Community Advocacy

Efforts to increase public awareness of neuropsychology as a specialty are critically important. These may include community outreach to provide education about the nature, purposes, and benefits of neuropsychological services or research pertinent to the lives and well-being of specific populations or society as a whole. Providing lectures to patient and caregiver support groups; volunteering time with nonprofit health care organizations; and conducting interviews with local newspapers, radio stations, and television news organizations are effective ways to increase the visibility of neuropsychology. Engaging in community outreach increases awareness on various public health topics, such as education about concussion identification, proper management, and expected recovery timelines. For example, a recent video chronicling "a day in the life" of a neuropsychologist (Ochsner Health, 2020) received 457 views in 1 week, increasing the viewers' understanding of the types of services a neuropsychologist provides.

Social Justice Advocacy

As defined by Toporek and Liu (2001), "social justice advocacy" refers to actions that facilitate the removal of external barriers to opportunity and well-being. Social justice advocacy is consistent with APA's (2003) "Guidelines on Multicultural Education, Training, Research, Practice, and Organizational Change for Psychologists," which recommend that psychologists work to effect prosocial and social justice change. It is also consistent with APA's (2017) *Ethical Principles of Psychologists and Code of Conduct*, which require that psychologists remain aware of their responsibilities to society and recognize that all people are entitled to access and benefit from the contributions of psychology, as well as APA's newly developed strategic plan. The latter outlines guiding principles and specific objectives aimed at promoting human rights, fairness, diversity, and inclusion through the application of psychological science for society (APA & APA Services, Inc., 2019).

Psychologists' responsibility to actively combat individual and systemically supported oppression has become increasingly important over time, in particular, given psychologists' unique capability of addressing the complex influences of social, political, historical, and economic contexts on individuals' and groups' behavior (Melton, 2018). Psychologists can strive to promote the importance of treating patients of all identities with value and respect and provide culturally appropriate treatment goals and recommendations (Toporek & Williams, 2006). Psychologists can also work to reduce systemic barriers to accessing hospital- and/or community-based assessments, interventions, and other resources, by giving voice to oppressed patients and actively working to eliminate said barriers (Toporek & Williams, 2006). Often, this work includes promoting socially just acts and policies to legislative officials, regulators, and other stakeholders through the support of psychological research.

As awareness of the broad and detrimental effects of systemic oppression has grown, psychology training programs have been faced with increased demands to provide social justice advocacy training (Ali & Sichel, 2014; Mallinckrodt et al., 2014). APA has realigned their strategic plan to recognize social justice issues, new standards of accreditation have been adopted that include social justice considerations in training, and discussions have begun as to how to better integrate culture and diversity within training programs. You as a psychology student thus have a unique opportunity to contribute to institutional and prosocial change via advocacy within your training program and involvement in professional governance activities that address social justice issues.

ADVOCATES' ROLES AND RESPONSIBILITIES

As we have described, advocates and advocacy come in many forms, with roles and responsibilities varying depending on the specific circumstances and goals of each effort. People can often advocate for themselves, their work, profession, or specific causes without constraints. It might come across as unusual to formally declare that you are engaging in advocacy when talking with consumers about brain health or with colleagues about the specific role of neuropsychology with a particular patient population, for instance.

However, many employers have rules regarding employee behavior related to legislative advocacy or lobbying for a particular bill or legal outcome. It is therefore important to review guidelines to determine rules for identification and use of employer resources for legal or legislative advocacy.

Advocates have a responsibility to provide information accurately and that is based on the best research available at the time. Advocacy that is not tied to evidence may be effective in the moment but has the potential to negatively affect the profession's ability to advocate in the future, because targets of advocacy may perceive all arguments as opinion rather than fact based. People advocating on behalf of an organization often have specific responsibilities related to their role within that organization. A person representing an organization should identify themselves as such and define any conflicts of interest when presenting information. Psychologists often maintain memberships in multiple organizations at one time. For example, a person may be employed by an organization; maintain memberships in multiple local and national professional organizations; and be in a leadership position in organizations that have complementary, but at times competing, goals and missions. We encourage you to be explicit about whom you are representing when you engage in advocacy. For example, when identifying yourself in a grassroots letter-writing campaign about practice issues, you may specify that you are a psychologist and member of professional organizations, but you may have to include a statement clarifying that the opinions expressed do not represent those of you employer.

Tips on Becoming an Advocate for Neuropsychology

Becoming an advocate does not have to be scary; neither does it have to be done on a grand state or national level. Take every opportunity to educate your patients, their families, other professionals, and the community at large and consider these additional ideas to advocate.

Tip 1: Jump into advocacy. In short, start advocating! Any act of educating others regarding psychology, neuropsychology, patient issues, or other professional issues can be considered advocacy. That said, the word "advocacy" often raises anxiety (see Howe et al., 2010, for a detailed review). Howe et al. (2010) identified frequent barriers to engaging in advocacy, including attitudes such as "It's not in my backyard"; "Nothing is wrong, so we do not need to act"; "Others are taking care of it; there's no need for me to get involved"; "I can't make a difference, so why bother?"; "I don't have time; I don't know how to get involved, even if I wanted to"; and "Advocacy is uncomfortable because it is emotional, not scientific." Each individual should decide for themselves the degree to which they are comfortable engaging in advocacy and the manner in which they feel most competent and capable of providing information.

Tip 2: Educate yourself on the issues. The first step to becoming an effective advocate is to learn about issues that may require advocacy. This may involve learning the status of psychology in your workplace, developing an understanding of the needs of a particular patient group, or setting up legislative alerts for bills related to the practice of neuropsychology.

Tip 3: Lend financial support to professional organizations. Becoming involved in professional organizations as a dues-paying member is also an important form of advocacy because these organizations engage in promotion of the profession.

Tip 4: Express your opinion and exercise your rights. Voting in organizational, local, state, and national elections and donating to organizations or individual candidates are individualized and personal forms of advocacy.

Tip 5: Volunteer your time. On a more formal and public level, several organizations offer opportunities to become more visibly involved in advocacy through volunteer and leadership roles on committees or boards. Most professional organizations have a student/trainee committee that is actively involved in the organizational mission, including advocacy. In addition, many practice and advocacy committees have trainee positions. Formal leadership and advocacy training programs are also available in many local and national organizations (e.g., employer leadership programs, programs through national research funding agencies or governmental programs, formal leadership training through universities). APA offers training programs to volunteers in state and regional organizations, and those who meet particular criteria, such as women in leadership or individuals from diverse groups. They also have an Advocacy Coordinating Committee and a long-standing competitive congressional fellowship program to provide real-world training in public policy. Specific to neuropsychology, NAN offers the Leadership Ambassador Development Program (https://www.nanonline.org/nan/Professional_Resources/Ambassador_and_Leadership_Development_Program/NAN/_ProfessionalResources/Ambassador_and_Leadership_Development_Program.aspx?hkey=b2e7196c-eb3d-4f5a-906e-580491e5f9ee), which includes specific training in professional advocacy.

CONCLUSION AND FUTURE DIRECTIONS

Positive change, whether at the individual or systems level, is at the root of psychologists' work. Psychologists are ideally positioned for advocacy aimed at improving the welfare of patients, society, and the standing of the profession. All stewards of the profession, including neuropsychologists and neuropsychology students and trainees, have a responsibility to engage in advocacy (Howe et al., 2010). Failure to do so can lead to significant real-world consequences. Be it time spent educating colleagues about the value of neuropsychology or leading a legislative action committee, each moment engaged in advocacy is meaningful and necessary.

REFERENCES

Ali, A., & Sichel, C. E. (2014). Structural competency as a framework for training in counseling psychology. *The Counseling Psychologist, 42*(7), 901–918. https://doi.org/10.1177/0011000014550320

American Psychological Association. (2003). Guidelines on multicultural education, training, research, practice, and organizational change for psychologists. *American Psychologist, 58*(5), 377–402. https://doi.org/10.1037/0003-066X.58.5.377

American Psychological Association. (2011). Model Act for State Licensure of Psychologists. *American Psychologist, 66*(3), 214–226. https://doi.org/10.1037/a0022655

American Psychological Association. (2017). *Ethical principles of psychologists and code of conduct* (2002, Amended June 1, 2010, and January 1, 2017). https://www.apa.org/ethics/code/ethics-code-2017.pdf

American Psychological Association & American Psychological Association Services, Inc. (2019). *IMPACT APA: American Psychological Association strategic plan.* https://www.apa.org/about/apa/strategic-plan

American Psychological Association Minority Fellowship Program. (2016). *Proceedings of the Summit on Master's Training in Psychological Practice.* https://www.apa.org/pi/mfp/masters-summit/training-proceedings.pdf

Association of State and Provincial Psychology Boards. (2018). *ASPPB Model Act for Licensure and Registration of Psychologists.* https://cdn.ymaws.com/www.asppb.net/resource/resmgr/guidelines/model_act_for_licensure_and_.pdf

Block, C. K., Johnson-Greene, D., Pliskin, N., & Boake, C. (2017). Discriminating cognitive screening and cognitive testing from neuropsychological assessment: Implications for professional practice. *The Clinical Neuropsychologist, 31*(3), 487–500. https://doi.org/10.1080/13854046.2016.1267803

Braun, M., Tupper, D., Kaufmann, P., McCrea, M., Postal, K., Westerveld, M., Wills, K., & Deer, T. (2011). Neuropsychological assessment: A valuable tool in the diagnosis and management of neurological, neurodevelopmental, medical, and psychiatric disorders. *Cognitive and Behavioral Neurology, 24*(3), 107–114. https://doi.org/10.1097/WNN.0b013e3182351289

Buckman, L. R., Nordal, K. C., & DeMers, S. T. (2018). Regulatory and licensure issues derived from the Summit on Master's Training in Psychological Practice. *Professional Psychology: Research and Practice, 49*(5–6), 321–326. https://doi.org/10.1037/pro0000214

Donders, J. (2020). The incremental value of neuropsychological assessment: A critical review. *The Clinical Neuropsychologist, 34*(1), 36–87. https://doi.org/10.1080/13854046.2019.1575471

Garner, B. A., & Black, H. C. (2009). *Black's law dictionary* (9th ed.). West.

Goodman, R. A., Lochner, K. A., Thambisetty, M., Wingo, T. S., Posner, S. F., & Ling, S. M. (2017). Prevalence of dementia subtypes in United States Medicare fee-for-service beneficiaries, 2011–2013. *Alzheimer's & Dementia, 13*(1), 28–37. https://doi.org/10.1016/j.jalz.2016.04.002

Hannay, H. J., Bielaskus, L., Crosson, B. A., Hammeke, T. A., Hamsher, K., & Koffler, S. P. (1998). Proceedings of The Houston Conference on Specialty Education and Training in Clinical Neuropsychology. *Archives of Clinical Neuropsychology, 13,* 157–250. https://doi.org/10.1186/1472-6920-6-5

Howe, L. L. S., & Pliskin, N. (Eds.). (2010). Advocacy in neuropsychology [Special issue]. *The Clinical Neuropsychologist, 24*(3).

Howe, L. L. S., Sweet, J. J., & Bauer, R. M. (2010). Advocacy 101: A step beyond complaining. How the individual practitioner can become involved and make a difference. *The Clinical Neuropsychologist, 24*(3), 373–390. https://doi.org/10.1080/13854040903264154

Mallinckrodt, B., Miles, J. R., & Levy, J. J. (2014). The scientist–practitioner–advocate model: Addressing contemporary training needs for social justice advocacy. *Training and Education in Professional Psychology, 8*(4), 303–311. https://doi.org/10.1037/tep0000045

Melton, M. L. (2018). Ally, activist, advocate: Addressing role complexities for the multiculturally competent psychologist. *Professional Psychology: Research and Practice, 49*(1), 83–89. https://doi.org/10.1037/pro0000175

Ochsner Health. (2020, September 16). *A day in the life with neuropsychologist Robert John Sawyer II, PhD* [YouTube video]. https://youtu.be/sbTlzhkyJoQ

Postal, K. S., Wynkoop, T. F., Caillouet, B., Most, R., Roebuck-Spencer, T., Westerveld, M., Puente, A., & Pliskin, N. H. (2014). 360 Degree Advocacy: A model for high impact advocacy in a rapidly changing healthcare marketplace. *The Clinical Neuropsychologist, 28*(2), 167–180. https://doi.org/10.1080/13854046.2014.885087

Raimy, V. C. (1950). *Training in clinical psychology*. Prentice Hall.

Roebuck-Spencer, T. M., Glen, T., Puente, A. E., Denney, R. L., Ruff, R. M., Hostetter, G., & Bianchini, K. J. (2017). Cognitive screening tests versus comprehensive neuropsychological test batteries: A National Academy of Neuropsychology education paper. *Archives of Clinical Neuropsychology, 32*(4), 491–498. https://doi.org/10.1093/arclin/acx021

Toporek, R. L., & Liu, W. M. (2001). Advocacy in counseling: Addressing race, class, and gender oppression. In D. B. Pope-Davis & H. L. K. Coleman (Eds.), *The intersection of race, class, and gender in multicultural counseling* (pp. 285–413). Sage. https://doi.org/10.4135/9781452231846.n16

Toporek, R. L., & Williams, R. A. (2006). Ethics and professional issues related to the practice of social justice in counseling psychology. In R. L. Toporek, L. H. Gerstein, N. A. Fouad, G. Roysircar, & T. Israel (Eds.), *Handbook for social justice in counseling psychology: Leadership, vision, and action* (pp. 17–34). Sage. https://doi.org/10.4135/9781412976220.n2

Index

About the Editor

Cady Block, PhD, is an assistant professor and neuropsychologist in the Department of Neurology at Emory. Dr. Block's doctoral, internship, and fellowship training all included emphases in neuropsychology, comprising a PhD at the University of Alabama at Birmingham, an internship at the University of Oklahoma Health Sciences Center, and a postdoctoral fellowship at Baylor College of Medicine. She has published a number of peer-reviewed articles related to the training, education, and practice of neuropsychology in national journals. She has also served in a variety of leadership roles in national and international neuropsychological societies, including contributing to the development of the Taxonomy for Education and Training in Clinical Neuropsychology. In recognition of her work, she is a recipient of a number of awards, including the National Academy of Neuropsychology's Early Career Service Award, the Society for Clinical Neuropsychology's Presidential Citation Award, and the American Psychological Association's Early Career Champion Award.